Advances in Neurosurgery 7

Neurovascular Surgery

Specialized Neurosurgical Techniques

Edited by
F. Marguth M. Brock E. Kazner
M. Klinger P. Schmiedek

With 202 Figures in 249 Separate Illustrations
and 85 Tables

Springer-Verlag
Berlin Heidelberg New York 1979

Proceedings of the 29th Annual Meeting of the Deutsche Gesellschaft für Neurochirurgie and Joint Meeting with The American Academy of Neurological Surgery
Munich, October 22–25, 1978

ISBN-13: 978-3-642-67457-0 e-ISBN-13: 978-3-642-67455-6
DOI: 10.1007/978-3-642-67455-6

Library of Congress Cataloging in Publication Data. Deutsche Gesellschaft für Neurochirurgie. Neurovascular surgery. (Advances in neurosurgery; v. 7) "Proceedings of the 29th annual (joint) meeting of the Deutsche Gesellschaft für Neurochirurgie and the American Academy of Neurological Surgery, Munich, October 22–25, 1978." Bibliography: p. Includes index. 1. Nervous system – Blood-vessels – Surgery – Congresses. I. Marguth, Frank. II. American Academy of Neurological Surgery. III. Title. IV. Series. RD594.2.D48 1979 617'.48 79-26442

2127/3140-543210

Preface

This volume of **Advances in Neurosurgery 7** presents the papers held at the Joint Meeting of the American Academy of Neurological Surgery and the "Deutsche Gesellschaft für Neurochirurgie" in October 1978 in Munich.

This exchange of thoughts on scientific methods in neurosurgery on both sides of the globe, i.e., both in the United States and in Germany, covered a number of different topics in the field of neurosurgery, with special emphasis on the following subjects: Intracranial vascular surgery and specialized neurosurgical techniques used for different operative approaches to the skull, brain, pituitary gland, and peripheral nerves.

Contributions to the field of computer tomography, traumatology, functional and experimental neurosurgey, as well as chemotherapy rounded off the broad exchange of thoughts. In particular, the variety of the problems discussed, gives insight into the present state of our special field and shows progress and new points of departure.

Special gratitude is expressed to the Springer-Verlag for its help in editing the Advances in Neurosurgery, Volume 7.

München, September 1979 F. MARGUTH

Opening Oration

F. MARGUTH

I should like to welcome all of you wholeheartedly to the Joint Meeting of the American Academy of Neurological Surgery and the Deutsche Gesellschaft für Neurochirurgie. I welcome especially our collegues from the United States and the ladies.

This event is a historical one for the very special reason that, for the first time in the history of our field, an American and a German society are holding a joint congress. This does not mean that contacts between American and German colleagues are new. On the contrary, this congress is the result and expression of relationships that have existed for many years, through international and national meetings, as well as of exchanged visits.

The interaction between American and German developments in the field of medicine reaches back to the middle of the last century. First it was the German medical scene that had a strong influence on developments in America, until the turn of the century. Then this situation was reversed. Prior to, and especially after, the second World War strong American impulses and innovations were influential in the whole field of German medicine.

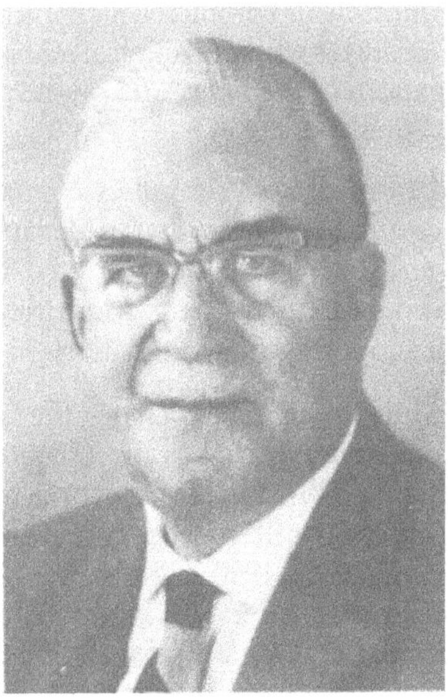

WILHELM TÖNNIS, 1898–1978

As concerns neurosurgery, HARVEY CUSHING and WALTER DANDY laid the foundation for a systematic and world-wide development. Their scientific findings are still of value today. This meeting also provides a special occasion to look back to the development of German neurosurgery.

On September 12, 1978 WILHELM TÖNNIS died, only a few months after having celebrated his 80th birthday. His name, the development of German neurosurgery and our society are closely interwoven. There is hardly any action that does not also carry his initials.

WILHELM TÖNNIS was born in Dortmund-Kley in Westphalia. He received his medical degree in 1922/1923 and presented his doctoral thesis in 1924. He became Dozent in 1929 in Würzburg. His surgical teacher supported his wish to devote himself to the field of neurosurgery. TÖNNIS was awarded a Rockefeller grant so that in 1932 he could start to specialize in neurosurgery with HERBERT OLIVECRONA at the Karolinska Institute in Stockholm. He then inaugurated the first neurosurgical department in Würzburg. In 1937 he was appointed to the first university chair of neurosurgery in Berlin, where he was able to start an ideal connection between clinical work and brain research. Thereafter he obtained the chairmanship of the Department of Brain Research and Experimental Pathology at the Kaiser-Wilhelm Institute, later to become the Max-Planck Institute. In 1936 TÖNNIS founded the "Zentralblatt für Neurochirurgie" edited by JOHANN AMBROSIUS BARTH in Leipzig, the first neurosurgical journal ever published. The organization of the treatment of brain and spinal cord injuries during the second World War by TÖNNIS is still basically valid and constitutes an excellent example, beginning with first aid and ending in rehabilitation. After the second World War, he started the rebuilding program at the Knappschaftskrankenhaus in Bochum-Langendreer, again as a general surgeon with a department of neurosurgery. In 1948 TÖNNIS obtained the first postwar chair of neurosurgery in Germany, founded by the Medical Faculty of the University of Cologne. In the following years he wrote many scientific papers, gathering his experience in the HANDBUCH FÜR NEUROCHIRURGIE (edited by him and OLIVECRONA). At the same time he completed his clinical and operative developments. Of paramount importance are his works on clinical management and diagnosis of brain tumors, vascular malformations of the brain, and on the pathophysiology of cerebral blood flow and intracranial pressure.

Neuroradiology also benefited from decisive impulses coming from WILHELM TÖNNIS. He is responsible for the creation of neurosurgical departments and chairs in 24 other German and foreign universities. In 1970 TÖNNIS created the foundation that bears his name and provides grants to young neurosurgeons to aid their training in foreign centers. His testament gives further support to this foundation.

His membership in 21 national and international societies, the fact that he was awarded a title of doctor honoris causa four times, as well as the OTFRID FOERSTER, the ERB, the HARVEY CUSHING, the PARACELSUS, and WALTER POPPELREUTER medals, and that he received the "Große Bundesverdienstkreuz mit Stern" show the great recognition of his work as a pioneer in German neurosurgey. In 1950 TÖNNIS proposed the creation of the FEDOR KRAUSE and of the OTFRID FOERSTER Lectures. Among other things, TÖNNIS wrote: "What has German neurosurgery done?" Certainly, for all of us, at the beginning stands the person and personality of HARVEY CUSHING, to whom we are grateful for having given us, through his systematic life-long work, fundamental knowledge about the operative treatment of brain tumors. The outstanding importance of HARVEY CUSHING is by no means minimized if we point out that prior to him, and at the same time, other pioneers were active in contributing essentials to our field, and to whom we all are also grateful. Therefore, the names of three German physicians should be remembered by every German neurosurgeon: ERNST VON BERGMANN, FEDOR KRAUSE, and OTFRID FOERSTER. The inivitation to such a lecture IN MEMORIAM represents the greatest honor our society has to offer a colleague.

In honoring others, it honors itself by remembering the words of HANS SACHS:

"Ehret Eure großen Meister,
dann bannt Ihr gute Geister".

Having said this, we should like to pay tribute to the memory of WILHELM TÖNNIS, who deserves great gratitude on the part of German neurosurgery.

He had a clear vision for the essential facts. He challenged and promoted his collegues and students. For his patients he was a physician as well as an aid in difficult times.

I should like to ask you now to honor WILHELM TÖNNIS, the great surgeon, with a standing ovation.

What a long way our field has gone since its beginnings! The rapid progress in basic sciences and technology was of decisive benefit. Let us review only the last 10 years: What great possibilities have been given to us by the operative microscope and by computer tomography. Neurosurgery of today, although recognized world-wide as an independent special field, is in danger of being fragmented. Certainly, activities and research programs concentrating on a limited field of activities have led again and again to new knowledge and talents, but they should remain under one roof and under one guiding chairmanship, integrating everything that goes together with the operative treatment of diseases of the central and peripheral nervous system, since the problems and the experiences of the different subspecialties overlap. They could lead to a fruitful and stimulating interaction. My concerned thoughts also include the fact that large operational needs for personnel and equipment do not make it recommendable to establish small departments, as experience seems to show.

We have arranged this meeting together with the American Academy (and hopefully are planning more meetings) to strengthen contacts. We are convinced that scientific discussions within a smaller framework as well as the exchange of personal points of view are very beneficial. Therefore, it is understandable that our program does not have a main subject but consists of a colorful presentation of different scientific and clinical problems.

Additionally to the exchange of scientific thoughts, we wish to show you a small part of our country. We should like you to get to know Munich and its countryside, and we gladly took efforts to arrange a program that will hopefully please you. Arriving in a foreign country, you are probably touched, and feel at home, by things and persons coming from your own homeland. This, too, we can offer you, namely two Americans. One from the past and one from the present. The name of the first is Mr. BENJAMIN THOMPSON. At the end of the eighteenth century he arrived at the royal courts of Munich and made a big career, there, under the reign of Kurfürst KARL THEODOR. In 1790 he abolished begging and provided occupation and food for the beggars. On his suggestion, a large park was built for the people: the English Garden of today, in the northern part of Munich. Sir Benjamin Thompson, Count of Rumford, also invented a special kind of potato soup. It carries his name: Rumford soup. Finally, he suggested the demolition of the walls and fences around the city.

The other American is sitting right among us. He stems from an old aristocratic Bohemian family, is an American citizen, and comes from the University of Notre Dame. He is Professor Dr. Nikolaus Lobkowicz, the president of the Ludwig-Maximilians University of Munich. In contrast to Mr. Thompson, he provided strong support for the walls protecting the University of Munich against attacks on the part of the government and permitting the University to defend itself against destructive political actions, for the preservation of the freedom of science and teaching.

Some Thoughts About the Future of Neurological Surgery

A. A. WARD, JR.

This joint meeting of the American Academy of Neurological Surgery and the Deutsche Gesellschaft für Neurochirurgie is a memorable occasion. For the benefit of our German hosts, I might make a few comments about the Academy. This is not a conventional professional organization. It has always had a limited membership and has always had more of the attributes of a large family than an organization. We would like to think that our membership encompasses the leadership of neurosurgery in North America. Perhaps more importantly, we are all good friends. We know each other well, and we know each other's families. We feel free to discuss matters among ourselves that we would not discuss in a more public forum. We feel free to make demands on each other that we would not make of other colleagues. It is an intellectual family. For these reasons you can understand why it is a particular honor to have the opportunity to serve this group. The honor is magnified this year since I have been given the opportunity to serve at a time when we meet jointly with one of the most renowned neurosurgical societies in the world. So, at the commencement of this joint meeting, I would like to express our thanks to our German hosts for the privilege of meeting with you.

It is useful, from time to time, for a profession to step back and view its current progress in a broad perspective. Neurosurgery is a new specialty that is barely 50 years old. It evolved with phenomenal success, and its initial growth was spectacular. Among surgical disciplines, we were considered the "Queen of the Arts". However, in recent years, there is a growing perception that the major excitement has left the field. We have been displaced by other areas of rapid progress such as open heart surgery, organ transplant, etc. We are becoming just another surgical speciality. Although the therapeutic horizons of our field continue to enlarge, it might be hard to document that there have been significant advances in our therapy of brain tumors, herniated disk, and trauma of the nervous system as compared to what the discipline provided 30 years ago.

A cynic might say that neurosurgery has developed into a mundane, routine field relegated to delivering standardized surgical treatment to the public, perhaps analogous to the current status of abdominal surgery. Certainly we need surgeons to carry out appendectomies and to remove gallbladders, and we will need neurosurgeons to remove brain tumors and subdural hematomas. If we are to be satisfied with such a role, a major opportunity will have been lost.

At this point in time when the momentum of progress in neurosurgery is faltering, it is ironic that the broad field of neuroscience is now just coming into full flower. There is, at this time, more intellectual excitement and potential in neuroscience than any field of biologic research. Some 2 years ago, the President of the United States appointed a Presidential Biomedical Research Panel, and I would like to quote one of their key recommendations:

> Perhaps the ultimate challenge to biomedical research, representing the very pinnacle of our understanding of the human organism, lies in neurobiology: how the brain and nervous system develop, how they function in health and disease, how thought occurs, how memory is stored, how we reason, how we are motivated, and how we interact with our physical and social environment... The study of brain and mind deserves greatly increased attention not only in the programs of the Federal Government, but also from the many different disciplines of biomedical and behavioral sciences... This Panel commends neurobiology as a compelling long-range interest worthy of national attention.

This is high praise and it comes from a group of scientists, clinicians, and experts from all fields. This potential is well-recognized by our young people. Neuroscience is attracting the bright young brains who have interests in biomedical research, but how can neurosurgery be a part of this new adventure? It will not occur without involvement by our discipline and not without some changes. We cannot place all the responsibility for progress on our colleagues who are Ph. D. scientists. Clinicians must be involved in the process. The future answers will be slow to evolve without access to the experiments of nature as they occur in human disease. The field of neurosurgery must play an active role in this process.

What needs to be done? We need the right people and the right environment. An old German recipe on how to make hasenpfeffer begins "First you must catch the right rabbit". We must attract the young people into our discipline with the right motivations and goals, and we must then provide the unusually talented individuals with an environment where they can be productive. They must have an opportunity to interact with a spectrum of research scientists. They must be shielded from nonproductive activities. We must make it possible for them to obtain support for their research. If they are clinicians, they must be protected from an overwhelming clinical load that saps their time and innovative energies. Academic centers in the United States have been making progress in the past in recruiting some such individuals and providing them with the necessary environment where research is possible. I am sorry to say that this effort is currently declining. In Germany, it has not been the custom for neurosurgical centers to develop along these lines. In contrast to America, I am happy to see that you are building greater momentum in the direction of providing research training and opportunities for young people. However, as you can judge better than I, some fundamental changes in the structure and function of neurosurgical centers will be necessary before major progress along these lines is possible. Such an effort is expensive. It requires more manpower and more facilities. The health care system as well as the profession must support such changes. We need research that is ultimately relevant to man. This is essential if the future viability of neurosurgery is to be assured.

The history of significant advances in other fields clearly shows that a broad base of knowledge is necessary upon which to build clinical advances. Open heart surgery is such an example. It is hardly accidental that GIBBON began his long research program on a heart-lung machine in 1934 – the very year that heparin became commercially available. Furthermore, it is important to remember that GIBBON spent 13 years trying to perfect the heart-lung machine, not for open heart surgery, but to allow time for a surgeon to remove an embolus blocking the pulmonary artery. It was only in 1947 that, on the urging of ALFRED BLALOCK (of blue baby fame), he switched his goal to providing an instrument that would permit the repair of cardiac defects. We in neurosurgery are also dependent on a broad base of innovative research, and we must have clinicians involved in the research process to guide and extend the research effort into areas relevant to human problems. Most importantly, we must have active clinicians interfacing with the research efforts so that, like BLOLOCK, we can identify the clinical potential of new knowledge. Otherwise it will not occur.

Once a body of knowledge has accumulated that leads to a potential new therapeutic approach, we must devise better methods for clinical trial. In the past, this process has been haphazard, inefficient and, at times, dangerous to the public.

The development of portocaval shunts is a lesson that we can hopefully avoid. The first experimental portocaval shunts were carried out in animals in 1877, but attempts to apply the procedure in patients resulted in no long-term survivors and the procedure fell into disuse. It was reintroduced for the treatment of esophageal varices in patients suffering from cirrhosis of the liver by WHIPPLE in 1945. Soon after, the apparent success of the operation was such that it was many years before the value of the procedure came into serious question. It was not until 1954 that it was recognized that portal systemic shunt in man is often followed by a severe intermittent encephalopathy – now recognized to be related to alterations of amine metabolism in brain. For these reasons, undertaking the operation for prophylactic reasons was discredited, and by now, the value of therapeutic shunts in patients who had already bled from varices is being questioned. From this brief history, it is obvious that at least 30 years were wasted by the failure to introduce standardized or randomized clinical trials from the beginning.

We have had similar experiences in neurosurgery. Aneurysm surgery was well-established before an effort was made to objectively determine the therapeutic effectiveness of the operation as compared to the natural history of this condition. A similar situation is developing with respect to the extracranial-intracranial bypass graft operation for occlusive disease of intracranial vessels. The National Institute of Health in the United States has sponsored a controlled study to determine the efficacy of this procedure, but already the operation is becoming so popular that it may be too late to undertake an appropriate study of this kind. We may be in the same position as the field of cardiac surgery and the coronary bypass operation that they have developed. The surgeons are enthusiastic about their clinical results, and the operation is popular with the public, but there is still no firm evidence that this cardiac operation prolongs life.

I think the time is past when new therapeutic approaches can be developed and utilized in the haphazard way that has been the custom in the past. Appropriate techniques are available for safely developing new procedures and instituting controlled clinical trials. We know what to do. Furthermore, the public is also aware that operations can be developed with appropriate safety and that they should be carefully evaluated by clinical trials before they are generally adopted. If the neurosurgical profession does not undertake this task, I suspect that society will do so. This will, however, involve the known inefficiencies and burdens of governmental involvement. It is our obligation to the public to improve our capability to help the sick and suffering and to do so in a safe, responsible, and accountable way.

Thus, I would propose that the field of neurological surgery has an exciting future as a part of the rapidly expanding field of neuroscience, but we must make some effort to plan our destiny.

Contents

Neurovascular Surgery

Specialized Neurosurgical Techniques

Free Topics

List of Editors and Senior Authors

BONGARTZ, E. B.: Neurochrirurgische Klinik, Universitätsklinikum Essen, Hufelandstrasse 55, D-4300 Essen 1 (FRG)

BRANDT, F.: Neurochirurgische Klinik, Universitätsklinikum Essen, Hufelandstrasse 55, D-4300 Essen 1 (FRG)

BROCK, M.: Universitätsklinikum Steglitz, Neurochirurgische Klinik und Poliklinik, Freie Universität Berlin, Hindenburgdamm 30, D-1000 Berlin 45 (FRG)

BRODKEY, J. S.: University Hospitals, Case Western Reserve University, School of Medicine, 2065 Adelbert Road, Cleveland, OH 44106 (USA)

BUSHE, K.-A.: Neurochirurgische Klinik und Poliklinik der Universität Würzburg, Josef-Schneider-Strasse 11, D-8700 Würzburg (FRG)

CÁRDENAS, J.: Department of Neurosurgery, The American British Cowdray Hospital, Mexico City (Mexico)

CORRELL, J. W.: Departments of Neurological Surgery and Neuroradiology, Neurological Institute of New York, Columbia Presbyterian, Medical Center New York, 710 West 168th Street, New York, NY 10032 (USA)

DIECKMANN, G.: Neurochirurgische Universitätsklinik, D-6650 Homburg/Saar (FRG)

DISTELMAIER, P.: Neuroradiologische Abteilung der Neurochirurgischen Universitätsklinik, D-5300 Bonn-Venusberg (FRG)

FAHLBUSCH, R.: Neurochirurgische Klinik, Klinikum Grosshadern, Ludwig-Maximilians-Universität München, Marchioninistrasse 15, D-8000 München 70 (FRG)

FOLTZ, E. L.: University of California Irvine, California College of Medicine, 101 City Drive, South Orange, CA 92668 (USA)

GARNER, J. T.: University of Southern California, 744 Fairmount Avenue, Pasadena, CA 91105 (USA)

Grote, W.: Neurochirurgische Universitätsklinik, Klinikstrasse 55, D-6300 Giessen (FRG)

Harper, R. L.: Baylor University Medical School, 6410 Fannin Street, Houston, TX 77025 (USA)

Hoffmann, H. J.: Department of Surgery, Division of Neurosurgery, Hospital for Sick Children, 555 University Avenue, Toronto, (Canada M 5G, IX 8)

Holbach, K.-H.: Neurochirurgische Universitätsklinik, Annaberger Weg, D-5300 Bonn-Venusberg (FRG)

Hunt, W. E.: Division of Neurologic Surgery, Department of Surgery, The Ohio State University, College of Medicine, 410 West 10th Avenue, N 907, Columbus, OH 43210 (USA)

Kazner, E.: Neurochirurgische Klinik im Klinikum Charlottenburg der Freien Universität Berlin, Spandauer Damm 130, D-1000 Berlin 19 (FRG)

Klinger, M.: Neurochirurgische Klinik der Universität Erlangen-Nürnberg, Schwabachanlage 6 (Kopfklinikum), D-8520 Erlangen (FRG)

Llewellyn, R. C.: Department of Neurological Surgery, Tulane University School of Medicine, 1430 Tulane Avenue, New Orleans, LA 70012 (USA)

Lucas, J. T.: University of Maryland Hospital, 22 S. Greene Street, Baltimore, MD 21201 (USA)

Marguth, F.: Neurochirurgische Klinik, Klinikum Grosshadern, Ludwig-Maximilians-Universität München, Marchioninistrasse 15, D-8000 München 70 (FRG)

Menzel, J.: Neurochirurgische Abteilung des Chirurgischen Zentrums der Universität Heidelberg, Im Neuenheimer Feld 110, D-6900 Heidelberg 1 (FRG)

Miltner, F. O.: Neurochirurgische Klinik der Universität Würzburg, Josef-Schneider-Strasse 11, D-8700 Würzburg (FRG)

Müke, R.: Neurochirurgische Abteilung, Universitätsklinik Hamburg-Eppendorf, Martinistrasse 52, D-2000 Hamburg 20 (FRG)

Nashold, B. S.: Duke University, Medicine Center, Durham, NC 27706 (USA)

Ojemann, G. A.: Department of Neurological Surgery, RR 744 HSB, RI – 20, University of Washington School of Medicine, Seattle, WA 98195 (USA)

Onofrio, B. M.: Mayo Clinic, Section of Neurosurgery, 200 1st Street, Rochester, MN 55901 (USA)

Pia, H. W.: Neurochirurgische Universitätsklinik, Klinikstrasse 29, D-6300 Giessen (FRG)

Pudenz, R. H.: University of Southern California, 744 Fairmont Avenue, Pasadena, CA 91105 (USA)

Richard, K. E.: Neurochirurgische Universitätsklinik Köln, Joseph-Stelzmann-Strasse 9, D-5000 Köln 41 (FRG)

Samii, M.: Neurochirurgische Klinik, Krankenhaus Nordstadt, Haltenhoffstrasse 41, D-3000 Hannover 1 (FRG)

Sano, K.: Department of Neurosurgery, University of Tokyo School of Medicine, 7-3-1 Hongo, Bunkyo-Ku, Tokyo 113 (Japan)

Schäfer, M.: Abteilung für Allgemeine Neurochirurgie, Klinikum der Johann Wolfgang Goethe-Universität, Schleusenweg 2–16, D-6000 Frankfurt 71 (FRG)

Schmiedek, P.: Neurochirurgische Klinik, Klinikum Grosshadern, Ludwig-Maximilians-Universität München, Marchioninistrasse 15, D-8000 München 70 (FRG)

Schubert, R.: Neurochirurgische Universitätsklinik, Langenbeckstrasse 1, D-6500 Mainz (FRG)

Schürmann, K.: Neurochirurgische Universitätsklinik, Langenbeckstr. 1, D-6500 Mainz (FRG)

Senter, H. J.: Department of Surgery, Section of Neurosurgery, Yale University, School of Medicine, 333 Cedar Street, New Haven, CT 06510 (USA)

Shelden, C. H.: University of Southern California, School of Medicine, 734 Fairmount Avenue, Pasadena, CA 91105 (USA)

Sprung, Ch.: Neurochirurgische Abteilung im Klinikum Charlottenburg, Spandauer Damm 130, D-1000 Berlin 19 (FRG)

Steudel, W. I.: Abteilung für Allgemeine Neurochirurgie, Klinikum der Johann Wolfgang Goethe-Universität, Schleusenweg 2–16, D-6000 Frankfurt 71 (FRG)

Stochdorph, O.: Institut für Neuropathologie der Universität München, Thalkirchner Strasse 36, D-8000 München 2 (FRG)

Story, J. L.: Division of Neurosurgery, University of Texas Health Science Center, 7703 Floyd Curl Drive, San Antonio, TX 78229 (USA)

STRUPPLER, A.: Neurologische Klinik der Technischen Universität München, Möhlstrasse 28, D-8000 München 80 (FRG)

SUNDT, T. M.: Mayo Clinic, Section of Neurological Surgery, 200 1st Street, Rochester, MN 55901 (USA)

SWEET, W. H.: Harvard Medical School, Massachusetts General Hospital, Neurological Surgery, One Longfellow Place, Boston, MA 02114 (USA)

WALLENFANG, T.: Neurochirurgische Universitätsklinik, Langenbeckstr. 1, D-6500 Mainz (FRG)

WAPPENSCHMIDT, J.: Neuroradiologische Abteilung der Neurochirurgischen Universitätsklinik, D-5300 Bonn-Venusberg (FRG)

WARD, A. A., JR.: Department of Neurological Surgery, University of Washington, School of Medicine, Seattle, WA 98195 (USA)

WINKELMÜLLER, W.: Neurochirurgische Klinik der Medizinischen Hochschule Hannover, Karl-Wiechert-Allee 9, D-3000 Hannover 61 (FRG)

YAMAMOTO, L. Y.: The Cone Laboratory for Neurosurgical Research, Montreal Neurological Institute, McGill University, 3801 University Street, Montreal, Quebec (Canada)

Neurovascular Surgery

Positron Emission Tomography: a New Method for Examination of the Circulation and Metabolism of the Brain in Man

Y. L. YAMAMOTO, C. J. THOMPSON, E. MEYER, J. LITTLE, and W. FEINDEL

Historical Note

The physical advantages of positron-emitting tracers for localizing brain tumors were advocated by WRENN and his associates in 1951 (11). The positive electron, or positron, was identified by CARL ANDERSON in 1932 from cloud chamber tracks produced by the action of cosmic rays. In 1965 SWEET and BROWNELL described the application of positron emitters for brain tumor detection using ^{74}Ar (9).

Positrons have the property of undergoing annihilation radiation with a pair of photons being emitted in exactly opposite directions at 511 KeV. Coupled with coincidence counting, this serves as a basis for precise localization in the brain. However, the introduction of iodine, mercury and technetium compounds for brain scanning proved more practical than the positron emitters available 20 years ago.

KUHL and his associates in 1964 introduced horizontal tomographic scanning using gamma emitters (4). This gave a more useful anatomic survey of the brain than detectors placed at a right angle to the head, which gave foreshortening or external detectors that looked at the head from a static position and showed only a core of tissue of heterogeneous make up. At about the same time, the development of a gallium generator and a better positron camera stimulated the return to positron scanning.

Then in 1966 YAMAMOTO and ROBERTSON at Brookhaven reported on the feasibility of a circular detector array (8,12). Using ^{79}Kr, they were able to obtain cross sectional images of regional cerebral blood flow, which was the first physiologic application of positron emission. In 1968 BROWNELL and BURNHAM and associates introduced the multicrystal positron camera and in 1975 TER-POGOSSIAN, PHELPS and HOFFMAN developed the hexagonal array of crystals with interposed gaps in the circle (7).

The Brookhaven device transferred to Montreal in 1975 became operational for cerebral blood flow results in patients shortly after that. Some 300 patients were examined using ^{68}Ga for steady-state scanning and ^{77}Kr from the McGill Synchrocyclotron for focal cerebral blood flow studies (13). Enhancement of some 15 times over sodium iodide crystals was obtained by THOMPSON, YAMAMOTO and MEYER when they used for the first time bismuth germanate crystals in a positron camera (10). This unit, using 64 crystals in a circular array, provides a colour code of horizontal cross sections of the brain (Fig. 1). The enhancement of data can be translated either into increased speed of scanning or a finer resolution of brain compartments defined on the cross sectional image (10,13,15).

The use of ^{11}C labeled glucose by the Washington University group, as reported in 1975, opened up an avenue to metabolic studies of brain activity by positron techniques. The modification of this, using ^{18}F deoxyglucose, introduced by SOKOLOFF and his associates, now provides a firm experimental base from which patient studies can be investigated as technologic improvement is developed (6,7).

Ten or more centers are now energetically developing the application of positron tomography to neurological disorders. Some of these are concentrating on complete or partial circular array of detectors, while others are exploiting multiwire proportional chamber cameras.

Application and Results

The advantages of measuring cerebral blood flow by this avenue are substantial. The method is noninvasive; it provides an anatomic map on a horizontal plane. This gives exact localization of both superficial and deep areas and ready comparison with CT scanning (Fig. 2a and b). Ischemia restricted to the cortical territory of the middle cerebral artery can be readily defined (Fig. 3). The injection of major arteries supplying the brain, which is associated with some risk, particularly in patients suffering from occlusive vascular disease while at the same time being unpleasant to the patient, is not necessary with the inhalation method using positron emitters. A global view on the horizontal section of blood flow is also demonstrated in contrast to the restricted view using, for example, the xenon techniques and arterial injection where only the territory on the injected artery is displaced with no data being provided on some two-thirds of three-quarters of the remainder of the cerebral hemispheres.

Because of the low risk and absence of discomfort to the patient and the fact that the isotopes used have a short physical half-life that reduces the radiation dose, the physiologic positron scans can be repeated judiciously to provide important information in the natural course of neurological disorders and particularly to evaluate the longterm results of various therapies.

An example of the unique role that positron blood flow measurement can play in the evaluation of new techniques is the series that have been reported at the Montreal Neurological Institute where patients have been subjected to vascular bypass from a scalp artery to a cerebral artery for cerebrovascular occlusive disease (5). Pre- and postoperative positron blood flow studies, supported by fluorescein angiography and xenon miniregional blood flow measurements at the time of surgery, have provided firm quantitative data on the changes in cerebral blood flow with this procedure that had not before been available (15). Areas of focal ischemia are temporarily reduced with inhalation of 5% carbon dioxide and are made considerably less after surgical bypass from the scalp to the intracerebral arterial system (Fig. 4).

Furthermore, in a series of angiomas examined during the past few years by the positron method, we have obtained maps of abnormal flow and distribution that indicate the presence of cerebral steal (Fig. 5) (1,2,3).

However, by far the most exciting aspect of positron emission tomography is the extraordinary potential for chemical studies by positron tracer techniques of major neurological problems, such as stroke, epilepsy, brain tumors, dementia and the many mysterious metabolic affections of the cerebrum. The reviews of the development of brain imaging by OLDENDORF and of emission computer tomography by PHELPS catalogue in more detail the technical and experimental background for this new field (6,7).

Conclusion

Positron tomography at present is almost cyclotron dependent and will necessarily be limited to a relatively small number of medical centers in the first instance. The history of radionuclide scanning itself and more recently of computer tomography indicates eventual wider acceptance of this promising clinical tool.

As we have stated elsewhere (14), CT scanning has given us splendid still-life-pictures of the brain. Despite its remarkable contribution to neurological diagnosis, however, it has not so far led to any significant new therapeutic in-roads on neurological disease. The great attraction of positron imaging is that it can show us not only how the brain looks but how it works. We can reasonably expect that this technique will yield information to develop new methods of treatment for some of the many unsolved neurological disorders that affect the human brain and mind.

Positron-emitting tracers can be mapped on horizontal cross sections of the human brain in vivo using a circular array of detectors designed with bismuth germanate crystals and an improved logic circuit and computer program. ^{68}Ga and ^{77}Kr have been used to provide steady-state scans and dynamic blood flow measurements, respectively. The value of this brain-imaging technique as a supplementary to CT scanning and as a marked improvement over xenon CBF measurement after intravascular injection is illustrated here. Two series of examples, surgical bypass procedure to the brain and the circulatory investigation of cerebral angiomas, demonstrate the value of the method. Future applications of short physical half-life tracers and labeled metabolites offer a promising potential for the investigation of many brain disorders.

References

1. FEINDEL, W., PEROT, P.: Red cerebral veins: A report on arteriovenous shunts in tumors and cerebral scars. J. Neurosurg. 22, 315-325 (1965)
2. FEINDEL, W., YAMAMOTO, Y.L., HODGE, C.P.: Red cerebral veins and the cerebral steal syndrome. Evidence from fluorescein angiography and microregional blood flow by radio-isotopes during excision of an angioma. J. Neurosurg. 35, 167-179 (1971)
3. FEINDEL, W., YAMAMOTO, Y.L., HODGE, C.P., BRANAN, R., MEYER, E.: Reversal of cerebral steal during surgery of arteriovenous malformations: Evidence from fluorescein angiography and focal cortical blood flow measurement. Meeting of American Association of Neurological Surgeons. Toronto, April 1977
4. KUHL, D.E., EDWARDS, R.Q.: Cylindrical and section radioisotope scanning of the liver and brain. Radiology 83, 926-936 (1964)
5. LITTLE, J., YAMAMOTO, Y.L., FEINDEL, W., MEYER, E., HODGE, C.P.: Superficial temporal artery anastomosis. Intraoperative evaluation by fluorescein angiography and Xenon-133 clearance. J. Neurosurg. 50, 560-569 (1979)

6. OLDENDORF, W.H.: The quest for an imaged brain: A brief historical and technical review of brain imaging techniques. Neurology (Minneap.) 28, 517-577 (1978)

7. PHELPS, M.E.: Emission computer tomography. Semin. Nucl. Med. 7, 337-365 (1977)

8. ROBERTSON, J.S., MARR, R.B., ROSENBLUM, M., RADEKA, V., YAMAMOTO, Y.L.: 32-crystal positron transverse section detector. In: Tomographic imaging in nuclear medicine. FREEDMAN, G.S. (ed.), pp. 142-153. New York: Society of Nuclear Medicine 1973

9. SWEET, W.H., BROWNELL, G.L.: Localization of intracranial lesions by scanning with positron-emitting arsenic. J.A.M.A. 157, 1183 (1955)

10. THOMPSON, C.J., YAMAMOTO, Y.L., MEYER, E.: A positron-imaging system for measurement of regional cerebral blood flow. Proc. Soc. Photo-Optical Inst. Eng. 96, 263-268 (1976)

11. WRENN, F.R., Jr., GOOD, M.L., HANDLER, P.: The use of positron-emitting radio-isotopes for the localization of brain tumors. Science 113, 525 (1951)

12. YAMAMOTO, Y.L., ROBERTSON, J.S.: Study of quantitative assessment of section micro-regional cerebral blood flow in man by multipole positron detecting system using Krypton-79. BNL Med. Dept. Circ. No. 28 (1966)

13. YAMAMOTO, Y.L., THOMPSON, C., MEYER, E., ROBERTSON, J.S., FEINDEL, W.: Dynamic positron emission tomography for study of cerebral hemodynamics in a cross-section of the head using positron emitting Gallium-68 EDTA and Krypton-77. J. Comput. Assist. Tomogr. 1, 43-56 (1977)

14. See also papers from the First International Symposium on Positron Emission Tomography. J. Comput. Assist. Tomogr. 2, 637-638, 650-651, 662-663 (1978)

15. YAMAMOTO, Y.L., LITTLE, J.R., MEYER, E., THOMPSON, C., FEINDEL, W.: Topographical regional cerebral blood flow by positron emission tomography with Krypton-77 before and after vascular bypass to the brain. J. Neurosurgery (in press)

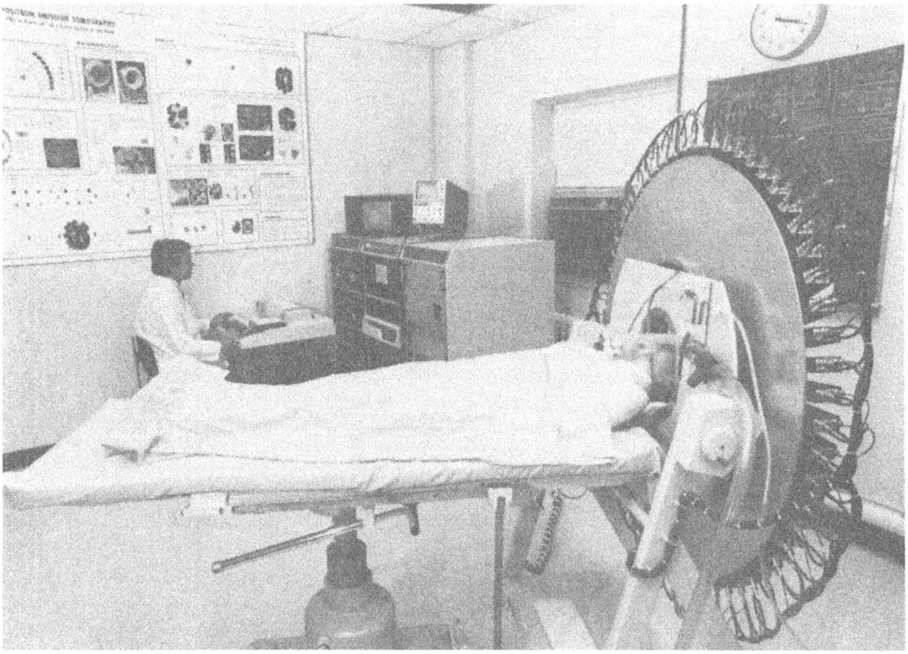

Fig. 1. Positome II using 64 detectors of bismuth germanate crystals. The patient is breathing ^{77}Kr for measurement of focal regional cerebral blood flow imaged on a horizontal cross section of the head

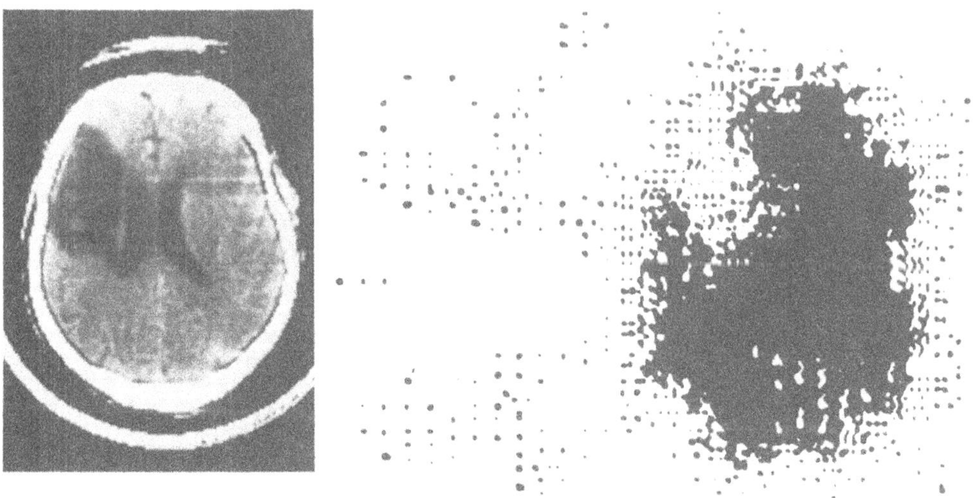

a b

Fig. 2 a,b. CT scan and positron scan of patient showing a large infarct in the left frontal region, to demonstrate correspondence of the two images

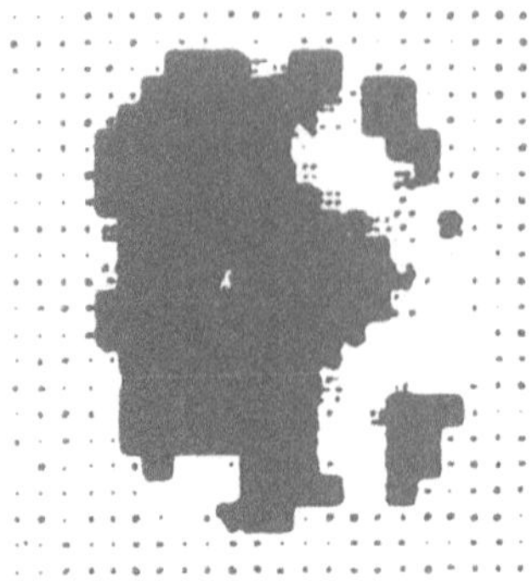

Fig. 3. ^{68}Ga study in a patient with middle cerebral artery occlusion. The white area denotes ischemia. The subcortical circulation of the abnormal hemisphere remains intact. Image obtained from the 32-detector camera, now obsolete

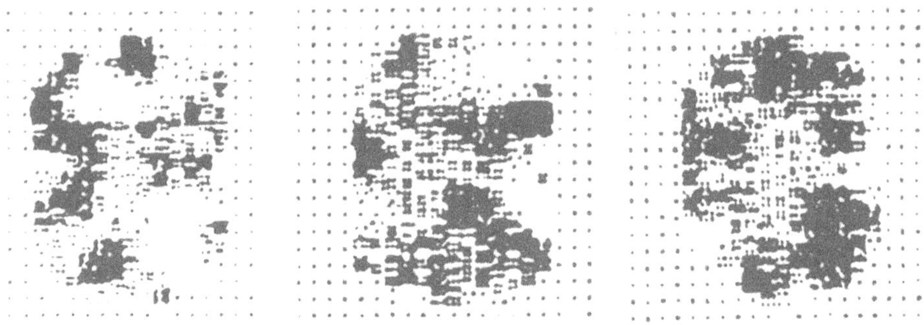

Fig. 4. Positron scan of a patient with multiple areas of focal ischemia, before *(left)* and after *(right)* surgical anastomosis of the superficial temporal artery to the middle cerebral arterial cortical branch. Note improvement in circulation indicated by *darkening* of the image. Temporary improvement was shown after inhalation of 5% CO_2 *(center)*

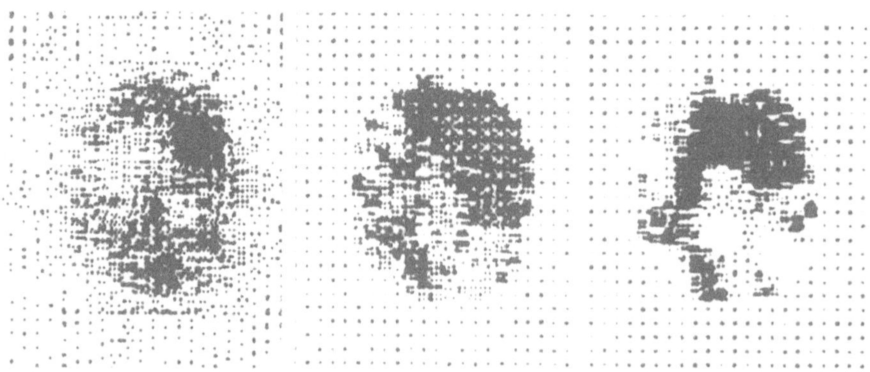

Fig. 5. ^{68}Ga scans in patient with a right frontal angioma. Note increased flow indicated by the *dark area* and decreased flow by the *light area*. Areas of cerebral steal *(right)* is shown in the parieto-occipital region. Orientation of scans is similar to the horizontal planes of CT scans

Lateralized Changes in Cognitive Function Following Carotid Endarterectomy

J. T. GARNER, J. ROSENSTOCK, T. D. FIELD, R. M. TAGER, and D. B. JACQUES

The neurosurgical procedure of carotid endarterectomy is commonly undertaken to prevent stroke in patients with carotid artery occlusion (22,27,28). Recent studies disclose that this procedure can lead to restoration of cognitive function in some cases (6,11,12,14), thus providing a better quality of life for those individuals. Our preliminary findings suggest that the type of cognitive improvement associated with this procedure is a function of the side of the brain receiving the increased blood flow.

Several reports indicate that increased blood flow to the brain can lead to improved cognitive function. DRAKE and colleagues (6) report significant improvement in mentation in their private hospital patients following carotid endarterectomy. Six patients of GOLDSTEIN and co-workers (11) who exhibited symptoms of transient ischemic attacks preoperatively were assessed for alteration in mentation following surgery. Although IQ scores remained relatively stable, improvement was noted on certain tasks requiring concept formation, auditory pattern discrimination, and motor speed. HORNE and ROYLE (14) report improvement in visuospatial performance subsequent to carotid endarterectomy. Significant changes in IQ, particularly regarding visuospatial perceptual and motor abilities, were noted by HAYNES and colleagues (12) following this neurosurgical procedure. JACQUES and GARNER (15) were able to improve speech function by augmenting cerebral blood flow. These reports confirm the proposal that increasing blood flow to the brain can serve a restorative as well as a prophylactic function.

The above-mentioned studies have investigated changes in cognitive function following cerebrovascular augmentation procedures in a generalized manner. Because the two hemispheres of the brain appear to be specialized for different functions, it might be expected that improved mentation following unilateral increase in blood flow should bear some relationship to the side of the brain affected. For the majority of the population, the left hemisphere is thought to be generally superior to the right in processing verbal information, whereas the right hemisphere is considered relatively more efficient in analyzing nonverbal information (8,16,18). Therefore, one would expect to see a greater improvement in cognitive processes underlying verbal function following a left-sided vascular augmentation procedure, while nonverbal function should be relatively more affected by a right-sided procedure. Although this investigation is still in the preliminary stages, our initial findings support the concept of lateralized differences in cognitive changes following enriched perfusion. Two representative cases of our series are presented that illustrate this pattern.

In this investigation cognitive function was assessed both pre- and postoperatively for all patients by the Wechsler Adult Intelligence Scale (WAIS). The various subtests that comprise this test battery are classified as belonging to either a Verbal Scale or a Performance Scale. Performance on the former generally reflects the examinee's verbal abilities, including vocabulary, judgment and reasoning abilities, abstract thought processes, and long-term memory. In contrast, the Performance Scale of the WAIS assesses visuospatial perceptual and motor abilities, in that it requires the examinee to copy block designs, assemble pictures in puzzle form, and identify missing parts of pictures. Studies of factor analysis basically support the functional distinction WECHSLER assigns to the two groups of subtests (20). Information, Comprehension, Similarities, and Vocabulary share a common "verbal" factor, whereas Block Design, Object Assembly, Picture Completion, and Picture Arrangement are reported to load on a separate "visuospatial" factor. In addition to the WAIS, the Ray Auditory Verbal Learning Task, Closure Flexibility (Concealed Figures), and Closure Speed Test (Gestalt Completion) are administered in cases where the patient's preoperative cognitive status is high enough to warrant the use of more subtle assessment procedures.

In the first of our two representative cases, patient R.S. showed preoperative IQ scores as measured by the WAIS of 96 Verbal, 89 Performance, and 93 Total (Fig. 1). Following a left-sided carotid endarterectomy, IQ scores increased to 122 Verbal, 107 Performance, and 117 Total. As expected, there was a relatively larger score increment on the Verbal Scale of the WAIS than on the Performance Scale. This pattern of change would be consistent with a relatively greater improvement of left hemisphere verbal capacities, as compared with the nonverbal skills of the right hemisphere.

In our second case, preoperative IQ scores for patient E.O. as measured by the WAIS were 105 Verbal, 104 Performance, and 105 Total (Fig. 2). Following right-sided carotid endarterectomy, IQ scores for this patient were 108 Verbal, 114 Performance, and 111 Total on the WAIS. The relatively greater improvement on the Performance Scale, which relies so heavily on nonverbal ability, suggests improved cognitive function of the right hemisphere of the brain following right-sided carotid endarterectomy.

Our preliminary findings of recovery of function following increased blood flow to the brain are of interest not only as a clinical achievement, but also as an experimental model for lateralized representation of function. Previous studies have investigated lateralization of function in one of three ways: (1) analysis of deterioration or impairment of function resulting from stroke, brain tumor, or other forms of brain damage; (2) examination of function associated with each hemisphere in vacuo in the commissurotomized patient; and (3) study of normal subjects. We suggest that a fourth method be taken into consideration as a model in the investigation of brain function. Against the background of a structurally intact (albeit functionally depressed) brain, we have sought to investigate function by attempting to reconstitute its normality.

Regardless of the technique used, the results of previous studies generally support the concept of the existence of a functional dichotomy with regard to the two hemispheres of the brain (see MILNER 1971, for review). The dominant (usually left) hemisphere is more highly developed for verbal skills, whereas the nondominant (usually right) hemisphere is superior in visuospatial perception and other nonverbal processes. Since the earliest observations of BROCA (2), it has been noted that aphasia is common following left hemisphere lesion in right-handed people, whereas it rarely coincides with damage to the right hemisphere. Damage to the right hemisphere, on the other hand, leads to visuospatial perceptual disorders that are more frequent and more severe than those following left hemisphere damage (13,24). In addition, facial recognition (5) and discrimination of position and slope of a line (29) are particularly impaired following right hemisphere injury. Reports on commissurotomized patients are consistent with findings from the brain-damaged population. Following commissurotomy, it is the left hemisphere that can express itself through propositional speech and writing (10). Commissurotomized patients are more adept at copying geometric designs (1) and visualizing spatial relations (9) with the left hand. In line with the clinical findings, the left brain of normal right-handed subjects also appears to excel in language function by processing verbal material more efficiently than the right. In dichotic listening tasks, there is a distinct right ear advantage for recognition of digits, words, and consonants (4,17, 26), in contrast to a left ear advantage for recognition of nonverbal environmental sounds (3,19), melodies (17), two-click thresholds (23), and simple pitch patterns (4). In the visual sphere, tachistoscopic studies indicate a right visual field advantage for perception of alphabetic material (16) whereas there is a left visual field superiority for facial recognition (25) and discrimination of the slope of lines (7). Our findings, though tentative, are impressive in that they suggest an alternative approach to investigation of lateralization of brain function that produces results consistent with studies using traditional techniques. The current study demonstrates a restoration of function that is in accord with a "verbal dominant hemisphere" and a "visuospatial" nondominant hemisphere.

The findings in the two cases presented above are consistent with the proposal that change in cognitive function following cerebrovascular augmentation procedures should reflect the area of the brain receiving the increased blood flow. Performance of patient R.S. on the Verbal Scale of the WAIS improved dramatically following a left-sided procedure. In our second case, a similar improvement was noted in performance on tasks with a strong nonverbal component subsequent to right-sided operation. We conclude that our initial results look encouraging in regard to a model of lateralized differences in cognitive changes following increased cerebral blood flow and that these procedures offer to a select group of patients hope for enhanced cortical function and improved quality of life.

References

1. BOGEN, J.E.: The other side of the brain. 3. The corpus callosum and creativity. Bull. Los Angeles Neurol. Soc. 34, 191-220 (1969)
2. BROCA, R.: Remarques sur le siege de al faculte du language articule. Bull. Soc. Antrhop. 6, 337-93 (1865)
3. CURRY, F.K.W.: A comparison of left-handed and right-handed subjects on verbal and non-verbal dichotic listening tasks. Cortex 3, 343-352 (1967)
4. DARWIN, D.J.: Dichotic backward masking of complex sounds. Q. J. Exp. Psychol. 23, 386-392 (1971)
5. DE RENZI, E., FAGLIONI, P., SPINNLER, H.: The performance of patients with unilateral brain damage on face recognition. Cortex 4, 17-34 (1968)

6. DRAKE, W.E., Jr., BAKER, M., BLUMENKRANTZ, J.: The quality and duration of survival in bilateral carotid occlusive disease: a preliminary survey of the effects of thromboendarterectomy. TOOLE, J.F., SIEKERT, R., WHISNANT, J. (eds.). 6th Princeton Conference. New York: Grune & Stratton 1968

7. DURNFORD, M., KIMURA, D.: Right hemisphere specialization for depth perception reflected in visual field differences. Nature 231, 394-395 (1971)

8. GAZZANIGA, M.S.: One brain - two minds. Am. Sci. 60, 311-317, (1972)

9. GAZZANIGA, M.S., BOGEN, J.E., SPERRY, R.W.: Observations on visual perception after disconnection of the cerebral hemispheres in man. Brain 88, 221-236 (1965)

10. GAZZANIGA, M.S., SPERRY, R.W.: Language after section of cerebral commissures. Brain 90, 131-148 (1967)

11. GOLDSTEIN, S.G., KLEINKNECHT, R.A., GALLO, Jr., A.E.: Neuropsychological changes associated with carotid endarterectomy. Cortex 6, 308-322 (1970)

12. HAYNES, C.D., GIDEON, D.A., KING, G.D., DEMPSEY, R.L.: The improvement of cognition and personality after carotid endarterectomy. Surgery 80, 399-407 (1976)

13. HECAEN, H., PENFIELD, W., BERTRAND, C., MALMO, R.: The syndrome of apractognosia due to lesion of the minor cerebral hemisphere. A.M.A. Arch. Neurol. Psychiatry 75, 400-434 (1956)

14. HORNE, D.J., ROYLE, J.P.: Cognitive changes after carotid endarterectomy. Med. J. Aust. 1, 316-318 (1974)

15. JACQUES, S., GARNER, J.T.: Reversal of aphasia with superficial temporal artery to middle cerebral artery anastomosis. Surg. Neurol. 5, 143-145 (1976)

16. KIMURA, D.: Dual functional asymmetry of the brain in visual perception. Neuropsychologia 4, 275-285 (1966)

17. KIMURA, D.: Functional asymmetry of the brain in dichotic listening. Cortex 3, 163-178 (1967)

18. KIMURA, D.: The asymmetry of the human brain. Sci. Am. 228, 70-78 (1973)

19. KNOX, C., KIMURA, D.: Cerebral processing of nonverbal sounds in boys and girls. Neuropsychologia 8, 227-237 (1970)

20. LEZAK, M.D.: Neurophychological assessment. New York: Oxford University Press 1976

21. MILNER, B.: Interhemispheric differences in the localization of psychological processes in man. Br. Med. Bull. 27, 227-272 (1971)

22. MURPHEY, F., MACCUBIN, D.A.: Carotid endarterectomy. A long-term follow up study. J. Neurosurg. 23, 156-168 (1965)

23. MURPHY, E.H., VENABLES, P.H.: Ear asymmetry in the threshold of fusion of two clicks: A signal detection analysis. Q. J. Exp. Psychol. 22, 288-300 (1970)

24. PATTERSON, A., ZANGWILL, O.L.: Disorders of visual space perception associated with lesions of the right cerebral hemisphere. Brain 67, 331-358 (1944)

25. RIZZOLATTI, G., UMILTA, C., BERLUCCHI, G.: Opposite superiorities of the right and left cerebral hemispheres in discriminatiive reaction time to physiognomical and alphabetical material. Brain 94, 431-442 (1971)

26. SHANKWEILER, D., STUDDERT-KENNEDY, M.: Identification of consonants and vowels presented to left and right ears. Q. J. Exp. Psychol. 19, 59-63 (1967)

27. SUNDT, Jr., T.M.: Surgical therapy of occlusive vascular diseases of the brain. Surg. Annu. 6, 393-411 (1974)

28. THOMPSON, J.E.: Surgery for cerebrovascular insufficiency (stroke) with special emphasis on carotid endarterectomy. Springfield/Ill.: Thomas 1968

29. WARRINGTON, E.K., RABIN, P.: Perceptual matching in patients with cerebral lesions. Neuropsychologia 8, 475-487 (1970)

TABLE OF SCALED SCORE EQUIVALENTS*

Scaled Score	RAW SCORE											Scaled Score
	Information	Comprehension	Arithmetic	Similarities	Digit Span	Vocabulary	Digit Symbol	Picture Completion	Block Design	Picture Arrangement	Object Assembly	
19	29	27-28		26	17	78-80	87-90					19
18	28	26		25		76-77	83-86	21		36	44	18
17	27	25	18	24		74-75	79-82		48	35	43	17
16	26	24	17	23	16	71-73	76-78	20	47	34	42	16
15	25	23	16	22	15	67-70	72-75		46	33	41	15
14	23-24	22	15	21	14	63-66	69-71	19	44-45	32	40	14
13	21-22	21	14	19-20		59-62	66-68	18	42-43	30-31	38-39	13
12	19-20	20	13	17-18	13	54-58	62-65	17	39-41	28-29	36-37	12
11	17-18	19	12	15-16	12	[illegible]	58-61	15-16	35-38	26-27	34-35	11
10	[illegible]	[illegible]	11	13-14	11	40-46	52-57	14	31-34	23-25	31-33	10
9	13-14	15-16	10	11-12	10	32-39	47-51	[illegible]	28-30	20-22	28-30	9
8	11-12	14	[illegible]	9-10		26-31	41-46	10-11	25-27	18-19	25-27	8
7	9-10	12-13	7-8	7-8	9	22-25	35-40	8-9	21-24	15-17	22-24	7
6	7-8	10-11	6	5-6	[illegible]	18-21	29-34	6-7	17-20	[illegible]	19-21	6
5	5-6	8-9	5	[illegible]		14-17	23-28	5	13-16	9-11	15-18	5
4	4	6-7	4	3	7	11-13	18-22	4	10-12	8	11-14	4
3	3	5	3	2		10	15-17	3	[illegible]	7	[illegible]	3
2	2	4	2	1	6	9	13-14	2	3-5	6	5-7	2
1	1	3	1		4-5	8	12	1	2	5	3-4	1
0	0	0-2	0	0	0-3	0-7	[illegible]	0	0-1	0-4	0-2	0

Preoperative		Postoperative	
WAIS		WAIS	
Verbal IQ	96	Verbal IQ	122
Performance IQ	89	Performance IQ	107
Total IQ	93	Total IQ	117

Fig. 1. Illustrating test reporting form and scores for patient 1 (left carotid endarterectomy)

TABLE OF SCALED SCORE EQUIVALENTS*												
	RAW SCORE											
Scaled Score	Information	Comprehension	Arithmetic	Similarities	Digit Span	Vocabulary	Digit Symbol	Picture Completion	Block Design	Picture Arrangement	Object Assembly	Scaled Score
19	29	27-28		26	17	78-80	87-90					19
18	28	26		25		76-77	83-86	21		36	44	18
17	27	25	18	24		74-75	79-82		48	35	43	17
16	26	24	17	23	16	71-73	76-78	20	47	34	42	16
15	25	23	16	22	15	67-70	72-75		46	33	41	15
14	23-24	22	15	21	[illegible]	63-66	69-71	19	44-45	32	40	14
13	21-22	21	14	19-20		59-62	66-68	18	[illegible]	30-31	38-39	13
12	19-20	20	13	17-18	13	54-58	62-65	17	39-41	28-29	36-37	12
11	[illegible]	19	[illegible]	[illegible]	12	47-53	[illegible]	[illegible]	35-38	[illegible]	34-35	11
10	15-16	[illegible]	11	13-14	11	[illegible]	52-57	14	31-34	23-25	31-33	10
9	13-14	15-16	10	11-12	10	32-39	47-51	12-13	28-30	20-22	28-30	9
8	11-12	14	9	9-10		26-31	41-46	10-11	25-27	18-19	[illegible]	8
7	9-10	12-13	7-8	7-8	9	22-25	35-40	8-9	21-24	15-17	22-24	7
6	7-8	10-11	6	5-6	8	18-21	29-34	6-7	17-20	12-14	19-21	6
5	5-6	8-9	5	4		14-17	23-28	5	13-16	9-11	15-18	5
4	4	6-7	4	3	7	11-13	18-22	4	10-12	8	11-14	4
3	3	5	3	2		10	15-17	3	6-9	7	8-10	3
2	2	4	2	1	6	9	13-14	2	3-5	6	5-7	2
1	1	3	1		4-5	8	12	1	2	5	3-4	1
0	0	0-2	0	0	0-3	0-7	0-11	0	0-1	0-4	0-2	0

Preoperative		Postoperative	
WAIS		WAIS	
Verbal IQ	105	Verbal IQ	108
Performance IQ	104	Performance IQ	114
Total IQ	105	Total IQ	111

Fig. 2. Illustrating test reporting form and scores for patient 2 (right carotid endarterectomy)

Cerebral Revascularization: Cervical Carotid Artery-Intracranial Arterial Long Graft Bypass

J. L. STORY, W. E. BROWN, JR., E. EIDELBERG, K. V. AROM, J. R. STEWART, and B. D. SMITH [1]

Introduction

The superficial temporal-middle cerebral artery (STA-MCA) bypass procedure as introduced by DONAGHY and YASARGIL (5,25) has been demonstrated to the satisfaction of many neurosurgeons to increase cerebral blood flow (1,21) and appears to protect against transient cerebral ischemia and completed stroke (10,18,26). It is the mainstay of cerebral revascularization. Occasionally, however, the STA-MCA bypass procedure is not practical for a variety of reasons (22).

We have been interested in methods by which immediate high volume blood flow may be accomplished. To this end a long graft from the cervical carotid to intracranial vessels has been employed. The site of distal anastomosis in one bypass procedure was to the supraclinoid carotid artery and in two others the distal middle cerebral artery.

The purpose of this report is to present our follow-up of these procedures. The grafts were 18-22 cm in length and 4-5 mm in internal diameter. The three grafts are all functioning well at 12 months, 13 months, and 18 months, respectively.

Case Presentations

Patient 1, C.R., a 45-year-old male with dementia related to bilateral internal carotid artery occlusion. In March 1977, he underwent a common carotid to intracranial internal carotid artery bypass procedure utilizing a saphenous vein graft as described by WORINGER and KUNLIN (24) and by LOUGHEED (15).

Follow-up at 18 months reveals that the vein graft remains large in caliber. The proximal and distal anastomotic sites continue to be widely patent. The angiogram also demonstrates that the disease in the supraclinoid internal carotid artery has not progressed and generous bilateral hemispheral perfusion persists (Figs. 1 and 2).

This procedure does have limitations, however (22). Hoping to avoid some of these, we turned to cervical carotid-distal middle cerebral artery bypass (22,23). The technical feasibility of this bypass pro-

1 The authors acknowledge the generous contributions of the Science Unlimited Research Foundation and Mr. Milton B. Clapp in their support of the University of Texas Health Science Center Neurosurgical Research Laboratories, in which this surgical procedure was developed.

cedure was demonstrated in laboratory animals by KHODADAD in 1972 and by MAROON and DONAGHY in 1973 (16). The following two patient presentations are examples of this procedure.

Patient 2, G.S., a 65-year-old male, experienced a right internal carotid artery occlusion and subsequently multiple episodes of transient left hemiparesis. Occlusion of the cervical internal carotid artery on the right was found at angiography. The right middle cerebral circulation filled only from the left vertebral circulation and ophthalmic collaterals. Furthermore, a severe stenosis of the right posterior communicating artery made circulation to the right cerebral hemisphere extremely tenuous.

In August 1977, a common carotid to middle cerebral artery bypass was performed employing a saphenous vein graft. The details of the procedure have been described previously (22). The proximal anastomotic site at 13 months postoperative is widely patent (Fig. 3). The vein graft, distal anastomosis and middle cerebral vessels at 13 months postoperative are filling well as demonstrated angiographically (Figs. 4 and 5).

Patient 3, X.D., a 57-year-old diabetic male, experienced several episodes of transient left hemiparesis due to middle cerebral artery stenosis near the trifurcation (Fig. 6). In September 1977, a proximal external carotid to middle cerebral artery bypass utilizing an expanded polytetrafluoroethylene tube graft (Gore-tex, W.L. Gore and Associates, Flagstaff, Arizona) was performed (23).

Twelve months postoperative the graft is functioning well. The origin of the graft from the external carotid artery is widely patent (Fig. 7). Selective external carotid angiography demonstrates excellent filling of the graft and excellent middle cerebral circulation at 12 months postoperative (Figs. 8 and 9).

Discussion

The first patient has not significantly improved by the procedure. The second and third patients, however, have been asymptomatic and neurologically normal since bypass procedures were performed. Failure of improvement in the first patient did not result from failure of the graft. However, it does emphasize the current difficulty with the dementia-hypoperfusion complex.

With respect to patients 2 and 3, we elected to use the distal middle cerebral artery because of the convenience of performing an anastomosis on the surface of the brain. It is striking that a 2-mm cortical artery can receive such an apparent large blood volume and provide sufficient run-off to prevent occlusion of such a sizeable conduit. We chose to use the expanded polytetrafluoroethlyene tube graft in our third patient because vascular disease in his lower extremities made the acquisition of a saphenous vein unattractive.

Several clinical and experimental animal studies have shown favorable results with the use of polytetrafluoroethlyene (2-4,7,9,17) and other synthetic (19) grafts for small arterial replacement. Additionally, long-term successful function of a small diameter prosthesis for aortocoronary bypass has been reported (20).

How long the grafts in our patients will remain patent is not known. The somewhat analagus aorto coronary bypass experience with saphenous veins at 5 year follow-up reveals the patency rate approximating 80% with less than 5% graft failure after the 1st year (6,8,11,13,14). Whether or not we can approach this patency rate with carotid to middle cerebral artery bypass remains to be seen. We are indeed encouraged by the appearance of the grafts in all three of our patients at 12-18 months postoperative.

Conclusion

Three patients with cerebral ischemia have undergone cervical carotid-intracranial arterial bypass procedures. All three grafts, two saphenous veins and a synthetic tube, are functioning well at 12 months, 13 months, and 18 months as demonstrated by angiography.

Two of the patients, cervical carotid to middle cerebral artery bypass, are asymptomatic at 13 months and 14 months postoperative. Failure of improvement in patient 1 reflects our limitations in patient selection, particularly in the difficult hypoperfusion dementia categories.

References

1. AUSTIN, G., LAFFIN, D., HAYWARD, W.: Microcerebral anastomosis for the prevention of stroke. In: Microneurosurgery. HANDA, H. (ed.), pp. 47-67. Maryland: Baltimore University Park Press 1975
2. CAMPBELL, C.D., BROOKS, D.H., WEBSTER, M.W., BAHNSON, H.T.: The use of expanded microporous polytetrafluoroethlyene for limb salvage: A preliminary report. Surgery 79, 485-491 (1976)
3. CAMPBELL, C.D., BROOKS, D.H., WEBSTER, M.W., BONDI, R.P., LLOYD, J.C., HYNES, M.F., BAHNSON, H.T.: Addendum: Aneurysm formation in expanded polytetrafluoroethlyene prosthesis. Surgery 79, 491-493 1976
4. CAMPBELL, C.D., GOLDFARB, D., ROE, R.: A small arterial substitute: Expanded microporous polytetrafluoroethlyene. Patency versus porosity. Ann. Surg. 182, 138-143 (1975)
5. DONAGHY, R.M.P., YASARGIL, M.G.: Extra-Intracranial blood flow diversion. 36th Annual Meeting of the American Association of Neurological Surgeons. Chicago, April 11 1968.
6. FLEMMA, R.J., JOHNSON, W.D., LEPLEY, D., Jr., TECTOR, A.J., WALKER, J., GALE, H., BEDDINGFIELD, G., MANLEY, J.E.: Late results of saphenous vein bypass grafting for myocardial revascularization. Ann. Thorac. Surg. 14, 232-242 (1972)
7. FLORIAN, A., COHN, L.H., DAMMIN, G.J., COLLINS, J.J., Jr.: Small vessel replacement with Gore-Tex (expanded polytetrafluoroethlyene). Arch. Surg. 111, 267-270 (1976)
8. GARRETT, H.E., DENNIS, E.W., DEBAKEY, M.E.: Aortocoronary bypass with saphenous vein graft: Seven-year follow-up. J.A.M.A. 223, 792-794 (1973)
9. GAZZANIGA, A.B., LAMBERTI, J.J., SIEWERS, R.D., SPERLING, D.R., DIETRICK, W.R., ARCILLA, R.A., REPLOGLE, R.L.: Arterial prosthesis of microporous expanded polytetrafluoroethlyene for construction of aorta-pulmonary shunts. J. Thorac. Cardiovasc. Surg. 72, 357-363 (1976)
10. GRATZL, O., SCHMIEDEK, P., OLTEANU-NERBE, V.: Long-term clinical results following extra-intracranial arterial bypass surgery. In: Microsurgery for stroke. SCHMIEDEK, P. (ed.), pp. 271-275. Berlin, Heidelberg, New York: Springer 1977

11. GRONDIN, C.M., LESPERANCE, J., BOURASSA, M.G., PASTERNAC, A., CAMPEAU, L., GRONDIN, P.: Serial angiographic evaluation in 60 consecutive patients with aorto-coronary artery vein grafts 2 weeks, 1 year, and 3 years after operation. J. Thorac. Cardiovasc. Surg. 67, 1-6 (1974)

12. KHODADAD, G.: Extracranial-intracranial bypass grafts. J. Neurol. Neurosurg. Psychiatry 35, 522-526 (1972)

13. LAWRIE, G.M., LIE, J.T., MORRIS, G.C., Jr., BEAZLEY, H.L.: Vein graft patency and intimal proliferation after aortocoronary bypass; early and long-term angiopathologic correlations. Am. J. Cardiol. 38, 856-862 (1976)

14. LAWRIE, G.M., MORRIS, G.C., Jr., CHAPMAN, D.W., WINTERS, W.L., LIE, J.T.: Patterns of patency of 596 vein grafts up to seven years after aorta-coronary bypass. J. Thorac. Cardiovasc. Surg. 73, 443-448 (1977)

15. LOUGHEED, W.M., MARSHALL, B.M., HUNTER, M., MICHEL, E.R., SANDWITH-SMYTH, H.: Common carotid to intracranial internal carotid bypass venous graft. J. Neurosurg. 34, 114-118 (1971)

16. MAROON, J.C., DONAGHY, R.M.P.: Experimental cerebral revascularization with autogenous grafts. J. Neurosurg. 38, 172-179 (1973)

17. MATSUMOTO, H., HASEGAWA, T., FUSE, K., YAMAMOTO, M., SAIGUSA, M.: A new vascular prosthesis for a small caliber artery. Surg. 74, 519-523 (1973)

18. POPP, A.J., CHATER, N.: Extracranial-to-intracranial vascular anastomosis for occlusive cerebrovascular disease: Experience in 110 patients. Surg. 82, 648-654 (1977)

19. SAUVAGE, L.R., BERGER, K.E., MANSFIELD, P.B., WOOD, S.J., SMITH, J.C., OVERTON, J.B.: Future directions in the development of arterial prostheses for small and medium caliber arteries. Surg. Clin. North Am. 54, 213-228 (1974)

20. SAUVAGE, L.R., SCHLOEMER, R., WOOD, S.J., LOGAN, G.: Successful interposition synthetic graft between aorta and right coronary artery: Angiographic follow-up to sixteen months. J. Thorac. Cardiovasc. Surg. 72, 418-421 (1976)

21. SCHMIEDEK, P., GRATZL, O., STEINHOFF, H., OLTEANU-NERBE, V., MARGUTH, F.: Blood flow and cerebral revascularization. Clinic. Neurosurg. 23, 270-286 (1976)

22. STORY, J.L., BROWN, W.E., Jr., EIDELBERG, E., AROM, K.V., STEWART, J.R.: Cerebral revascularization: Common carotid to distal middle cerebral artery bypass. Neurosurg. 2, 131-134 (1978)

23. STORY, J.L., BROWN, W.E., Jr., EIDELBERG, E., AROM, K.V., STEWART, J.R.: Cerebral revascularization: Proximal external carotid to distal middle cerebral artery bypass with a synthetic tube graft. Neurosurg. 3, 61-65 (1978)

24. WORINGER, E., KUNLIN, J.: Anastomose entre la carotide primitive et la carotide intra-cranienne ou la sylvienne par greffon selon la technique de la suture suspendue. Neurochirurgie 9, 181-188 (1963)

25. YASARGIL, M.G.: Microsurgery Applied to Neurosurgery. Stuttgart: Thieme 1969

26. YASARGIL, M.G., YONEKAWA, Y.: Results of microsurgical extra-intracranial arterial bypass in the treatment of cerebral ischemia. Neurosurg. 1, 22-24 (1977)

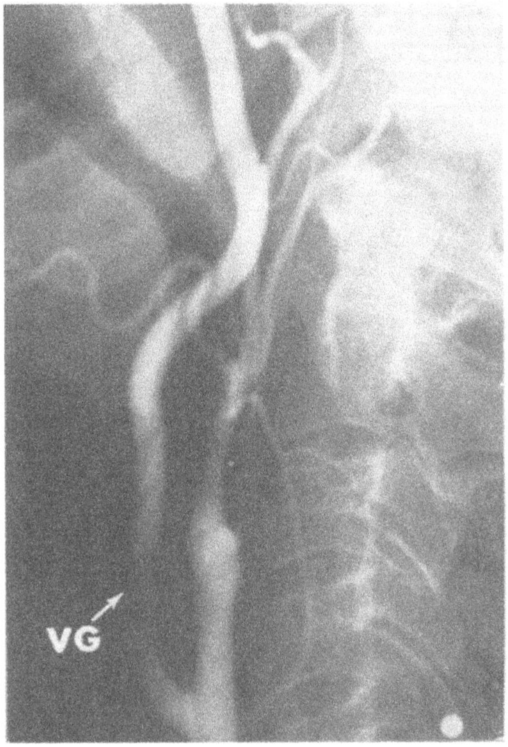

Fig. 1. Lateral angiogram 18 months postoperative demonstrating the origin of the saphenous vein graft *(VG)* from the common carotid artery

Fig. 2. Anteroposterior view of the common carotid angiogram demonstrating the vein graft, distal anastomosis with the supraclinoid carotid artery, and bilateral hemispheral perfusion at 18 months postoperative

▽

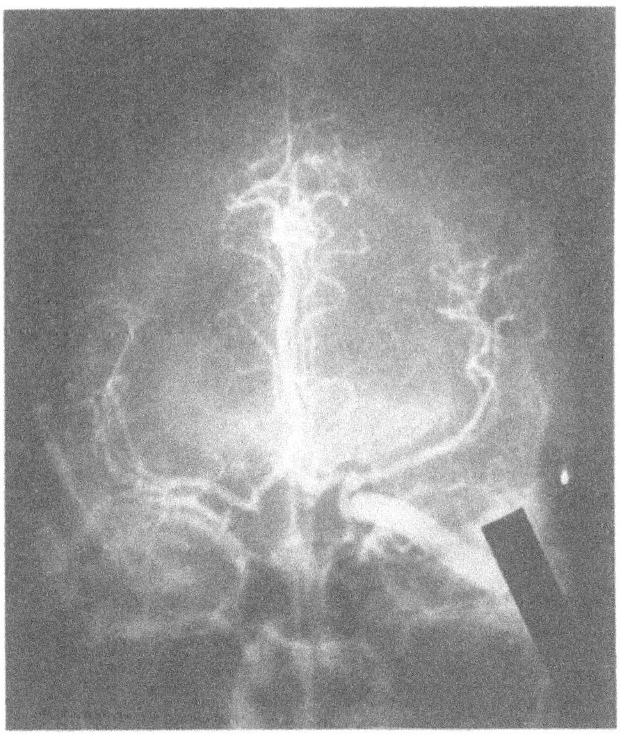

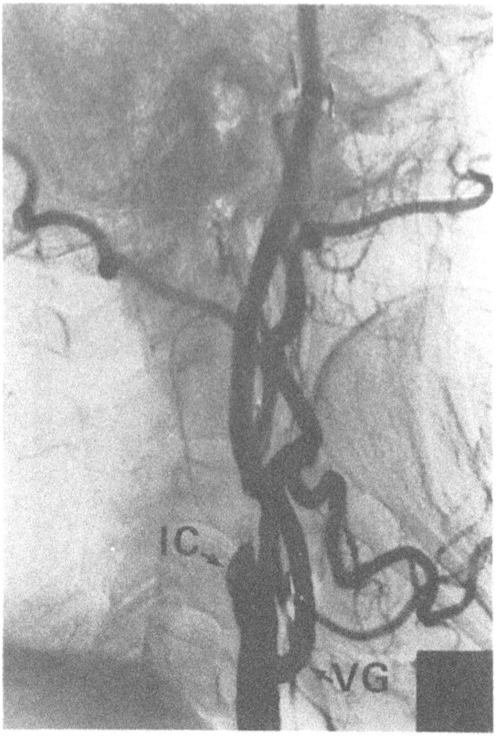

Fig. 3. Lateral angiogram at 13 months postoperative demonstrating the occluded internal carotid artery *(IC)* and the origin on the vein graft *(VG)* from the common carotid artery

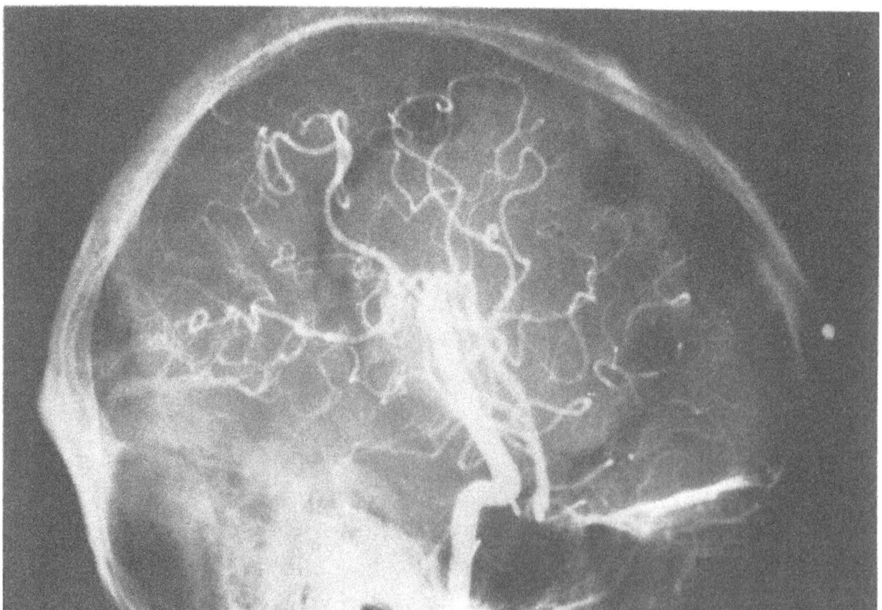

Fig. 4. Lateral angiogram 13 months postoperative demonstrating the vein graft, distal anastomosis, and the middle cerebral circulation

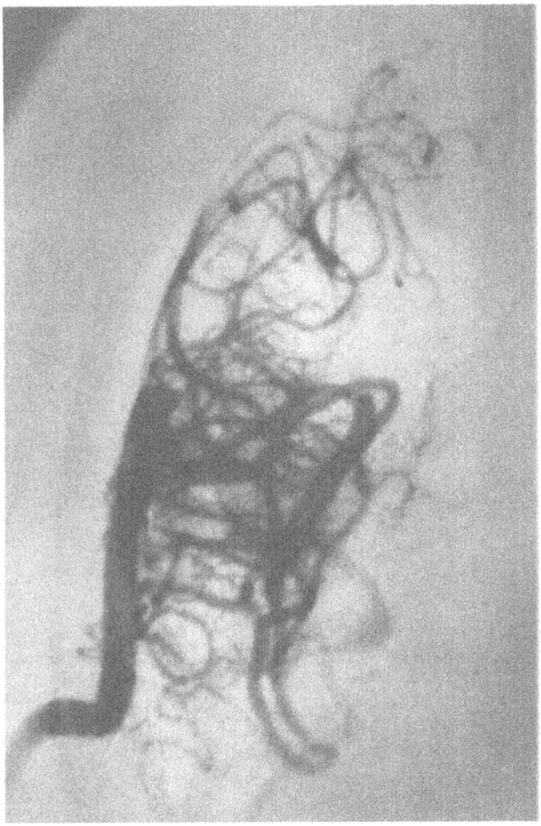

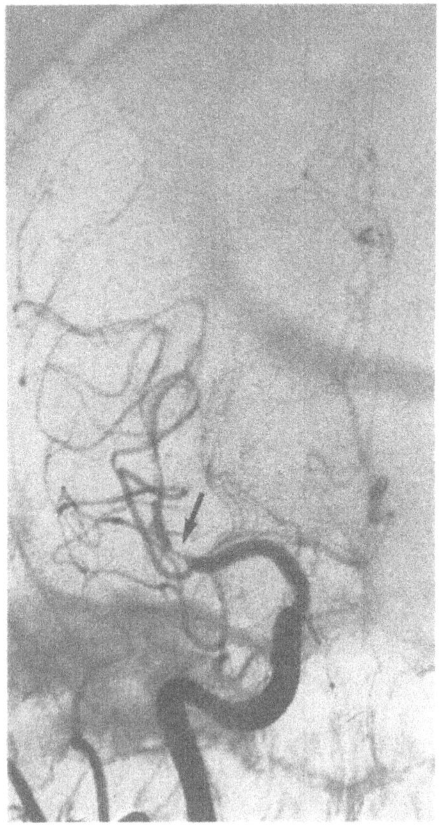

Fig. 5 Fig. 6

Fig. 5. Anteroposterior angiogram 13 months postoperative demonstrating the vein graft of the middle cerebral

Fig. 6. Anteroposterior view of the right common carotid angiogram demonstrating stenosis of the middle cerebral artery *(arrow)*

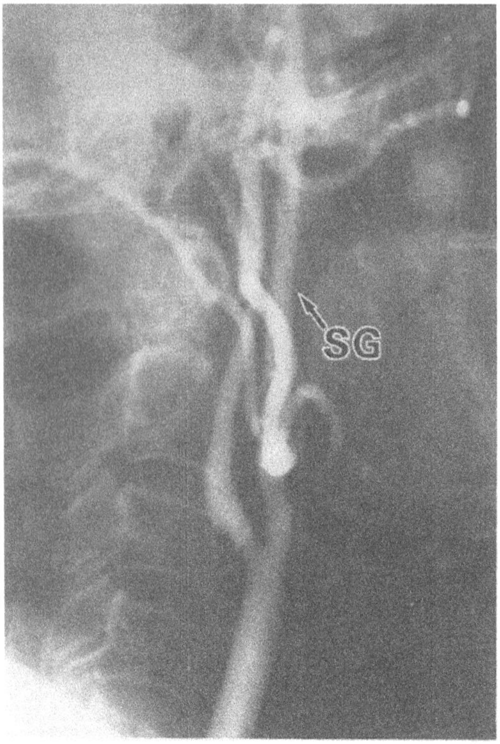

Fig. 7. Twelve months postoperative lateral angiogram demonstrating the origin of the synthetic graft *(SG)* from the external carotid artery

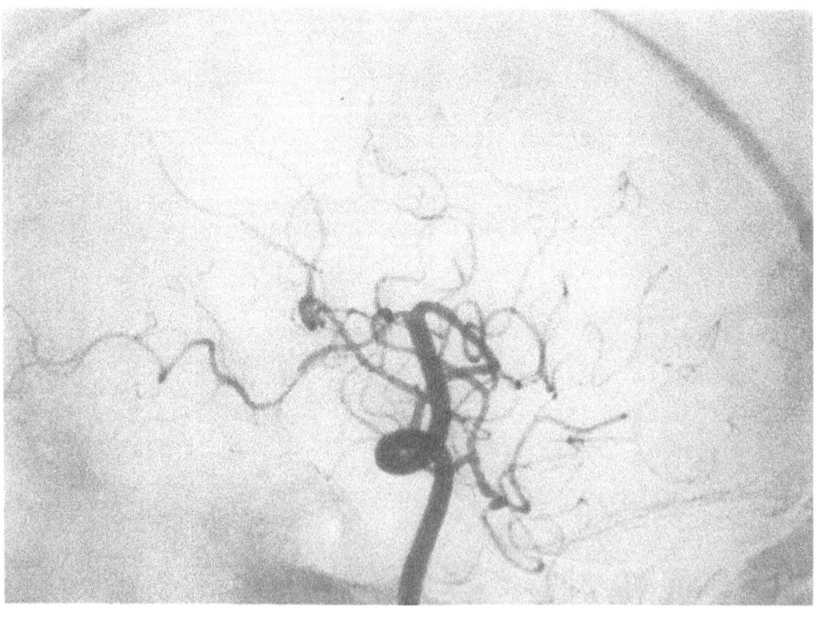

Fig. 8. Lateral view of the 12-month postoperative angiogram demonstrating the synthetic graft and antegrade and retrograde filling of the middle cerebral vessels

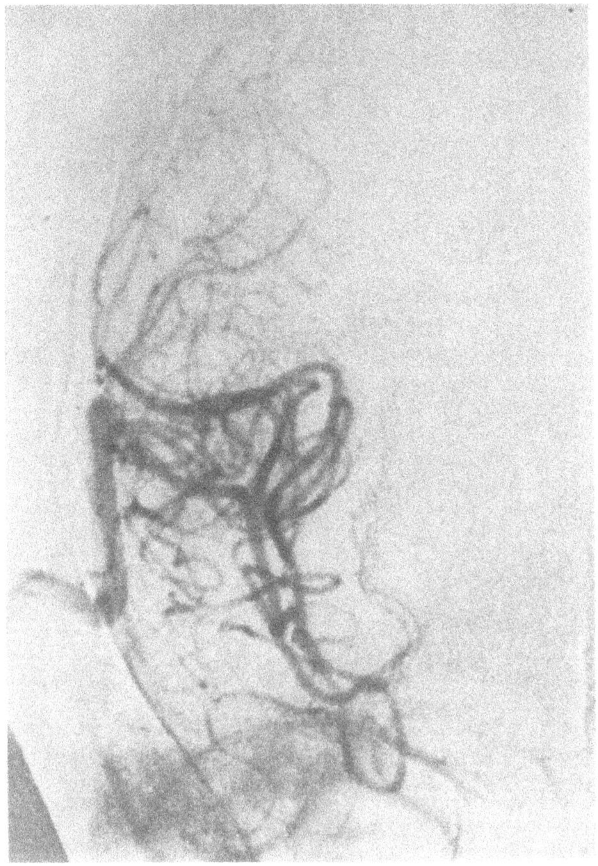

Fig. 9. Anteroposterior view of the 12-month postoperative angiogram demonstrating the synthetic graft and filling of the middle cerebral vessels via the graft

Microneurosurgery and Hyperbaric Oxygenation in Chronic Stroke

K.-H. HOLBACH and H. WASSMANN

A completed stroke (CS) is most frequently due to an occlusive vascular lesion resulting in cerebral hypoxia, ischemia, or a combination of these (2). Whether in such post-stroke states the neurological disorder is due to reversible or irreversible neuronal alterations cannot be predicted. If the neurons have lost their function but are still alive, it appears reasonable to assume that improving the oxygenation of the brain tissue by increasing either arterial oxygen concentration or cerebral blood supply may result in an improvement of the neurological deficit.

Material and Methods

We studied 112 patients (90 males, 22 females, mean age 50.3 years) with CS. They had persisting neurological deficits due to internal carotid occlusion in 99 cases and due to middle cerebral artery occlusion in 13 patients. They were considered suitable for extra-intracranial arterial bypass (EIAB) surgery if necessary. Among these patients there were 26 with mild neurological deficit who had EIAB surgery and 86 with severe neurological deficit who were randomily assigned to a surgical or a medical treatment group. Each of the 112 patients underwent hyperbaric (HO) treatment prior to either surgical or medical treatment. The average time elapsed between the CS and a series of 15 single daily HO sessions. These were performed under spontaneous respiration of oxygen at a pressure of 1.5 atm and an exposure time of 40 min.

Neurological examinations were carried and EEG analysis out on each patient before, during, and at the conclusion of the HO treatment. To assess the immediate effect of breathing oxygen at 1.5 atm on cerebral functions, EEGs were also recorded and analyzed from the hyperbaric chamber prior to pressurization under spontaneous respiration of air, during the respiration of air, and after respiration of oxygen at 1.5 atm, and 15 min after the change from oxygen to air respiration at normal ambient pressure (1.0 atm). Long-term follow-up neurological assessment and EEG analysis were done in all patients during a period ranging from 1/2 to 3 1/2 years. The EEG interval amplitude analysis system previously described (1) enabled us to obtain values for the local electric brain activity in the form of electric power equivalent (EPE) values for each classical EEG range.

We tried to quantify the motor deficits by applying seven grades of severity (6; normal physical strength; 5; slight paresis; 4; active movement of extremities against moderate resistance; 3; active movement of extremities against gravity; 2; active movement of extremity upon exclusion of gravity; 1; visible contraction without any effect on mobility; 0; paralysis). These were separately assessed for the arm, hand, and leg. Aphasic disturbances were graded by applying five grades of severity (4; undisturbed speech; 3; slight dysphasia; 2; moderate dysphasia; 1; severe dysphasia; 0; total aphasia). The classification of the motoric and aphasic disorders was made by a neurologist particularly interested in dysphasia.

Results

A typical case is presented here to demonstrate the procedure of this study. A 54-year-old man suddenly developed aphasia and right-sided hemiparesis in December 1974. Before admission to our clinic in March 1975, he was under intensive medical management. At this time we found that he had a spastic right hemiparesis and motor dysphasia. Angiography revealed an occlusion of the left internal carotid artery with moderate retrograde filling of the ophthalmic artery feeding some suprasylvian arteries as well as a stenosis of the right internal carotid artery. HO therapy was begun subsequent to angiography, i.e., after the neurological deficit had already persisted for 3 1/2 months.

The EEG analyses, performed immediately before and during the first HO session, showed a lower α- and β-wave activity over the affected left hemisphere than over the contralateral side (Fig. 1). Thirty minutes after the change from breathing air to oxygen at 1.5 atm there was a bilateral increase of α-wave activity, in particular over the left side of the brain, and also a minor increase of β-wave activity. At the conclusion of this HO session, i.e., after the change from breathing oxygen to air at 1.0 atm (normal ambient pressure), the improvement of the EEG receded almost completely. After the conclusion of the HO therapy consisting of a series of 15 single sessions, there was mainly a considerable increase of the α-wave activity over the left affected hemisphere (Fig. 2). At this time the neurological examination revealed an increase of motor function in the right hand and an improvement of the speech disorder.

Subsequently EIAB surgery was carried out on the left side. Two days after the operation, angiography revealed a patent anastomosis irrigating most of the middle cerebral territory.

EEG analyses performed 6 weeks and 6 months following surgery showed a distinct increase of the α-wave activity over the affected left side as well as over the contralateral side of the brain. Also the β- and frequent θ-wave activity showed slight increases. At the same time, the neurological examination revealed further recovery of the right hemiparesis.

After this satisfactory clinical course, we suggested the disobstruction of the right internal carotid artery. The patient, however, did not agree with this surgical procedure. The postoperative neurological condition persisted until December 1975. At this time the patient abruptly developed a left-sided hemiplegia and a renewed speech disorder. One month later he was admitted to our clinic with only little change in the severe left-sided neurological deficit.

Angiography revealed an occlusion of the right internal carotid artery. Follow-up EEG analyses indicated a distinct bilateral reduction of the α- and β-wave activity. This was more pronounced over the right - at this time the mainly affected hemisphere - than over the contralateral side, which was perfused by the EIAB. Again, HO therapy was given. At the conclusion of this treatment, i.e., after 15 sessions, we found an improvement of the left neurological deficit and a bilateral increase of the α- and β-wave activity. Subsequently, a right EIAB was carried out. Following surgery the speech disorder, the impaired motor functions, and the reduced mental activity improved. Finally, the patient became able to walk on his own and to take care of himself. The postoperative follow-up EEG analyses showed further improvement, which has been maintained so far. At this time we studied the effect of a 2-min digital compression of the enlarged right superficial temporal artery on EEG (Fig. 2). This short interruption of blood flow through the right EIAB resulted in a considerable temporary reduction in electric brain activity over both cerebral hemispheres.

The last postoperative repeat angiography, done 3 1/2 years after the left and 2 1/2 years after the right EIAB surgery, revealed that the left EIAB was filling the territory of the left middle cerebral artery and that the right EIAB was irrigating the complete right hemisphere and also the territory of the left anterior cerebral artery, i.e., both cerebral hemispheres of this patient were completely perfused by the extra-intracranial anastomoses (Fig. 3a and b).

The following results were obtained in 111 patients with completed stroke (Table 1). During the first HO session, under respiration of oxygen at 1.5 atm, an improvement of the EEG was defined as at least a 15% increase in the sum of the EPE values of the α and β range. Generally, these improvements receded partly or completely after changing from oxygen to air at ambient pressure following the first HO session. After conclusion of the HO therapy, i.e., after a series of 15 single sessions, the EEG was considered to be improved where we had, at least, a persistent 25% increase in the sum of the EPE values of the α and β range in relation to the initial values.

Table 1. Effects of hyperbaric oxygenation and EIAB on EEG and neurological status (NS) in completed stroke (CS) patients with mild and severe neurological deficits (ND)

		Under O_2 respiration at 1.5 ATA	After conclusion of HO-therapy		Follow-up results after 1/2 - 3 1/2 years	
		EEG	EEG	NS	EEG	NS
CS	Improved	84%	67%	67%	83%	87%
Mild ND	Unchanged	16%	33%	33%	13%	9%
(N=26 pat.)	Worsened	-	-	-	4%	4%
	Died	-	-	-	-	-
CS	Improved	55%	58%	56%	61%	59%
Severe ND	Unchanged	45%	42%	44%	33%	35%
With EIAB	Worsened	-	-	-	4%	4%
(N=46 pat.)	Died	-	-	-	2%	2%
CS	Improved	47%	59%	55%	30%	30%
Severe ND	Unchanged	53%	41%	45%	30%	28%
Without surgery	Worsened	-	-	-	23%	25%
(N=40 pat.)	Died	-	-	-	17%	17%

We considered patients neurologically improved when impaired motor function had improved either at least two grades in one extremity or one grade in both members of the affected side, or when the speech disorder had improved at least one grade. During the long-term follow-up examinations, made 1/2 to 3 1/2 years following either conclusion of the HO therapy (in patients assigned to the medically treated group) or EIAB surgery subsequent to HO treatment, EEG was considered to be improved when an increase of at least 25% in the sum of the EPE values of the α and β range was observed beyond the level found at the conclusion of the HO therapy. The neurological condition was considered to be improved whenever some further recovery of the impaired neurological functions found at the conclusion of the HO therapy had occurred, or when at this time the motor function had improved at least two grades, or the speech disorder had improved one grade in relation to the initial neurological deficit. While the percent of improved patients with severe neurological deficits was significantly higher in the surgically treated group, the percent of worsened and dead patients was significantly higher in the conservatively group treated. During the long-term post-operative follow-up, we found that the percent of improved patients with mild neurological deficits was significantly higher than the percentage of improved patients with severe neurological deficits. Furthermore, we assessed the relationship between the effects of HO and EIAB surgery on impaired neurological functions and found that patients with a favorable electroenecephalographic and/or neurological response to HO showed a positive response to EIAB surgery, while patients in whom HO treatment was considered to be ineffective showed no or little change in the impaired neuronal functions subsequent to EIAB surgery. This correlation was found in over 90% of these patients.

These findings in patients with completed stroke indicate that

a) HO treatment can improve hypoxic-ischemic alterations of the brain.

b) Subsequent EIAB surgery can additionally improve neurological deficit and maintain the level of improved neurological function.

c) The evaluation of the effect of HO treatment on hypoxic-ischemic alterations of the brain, particularly by EEG interval amplitude analysis, can be helpful in differentiating reversible and irreversible post-stroke changes.

   Consequently, the response to HO treatment may be used as a criterium to determine the prognosis of a cerebrovascular lesion and also for the selection of patients for EIAB surgery.

References

1. HOLBACH, K.-H., WASSMANN, H., HOHELÜCHTER, K.L.: Reversibility of the chronic post-stroke state. Stroke 7, 296-300 (1976)

2. INGVAR, D.H.: The pathophysiology of stroke related to findings in EEG and to measurements of regional cerebral blood flow. In: Stroke, Thule Internat. Symposia. ENGEL, A., LARSSON, T. (eds.). Stockholm: Nordiska 1967

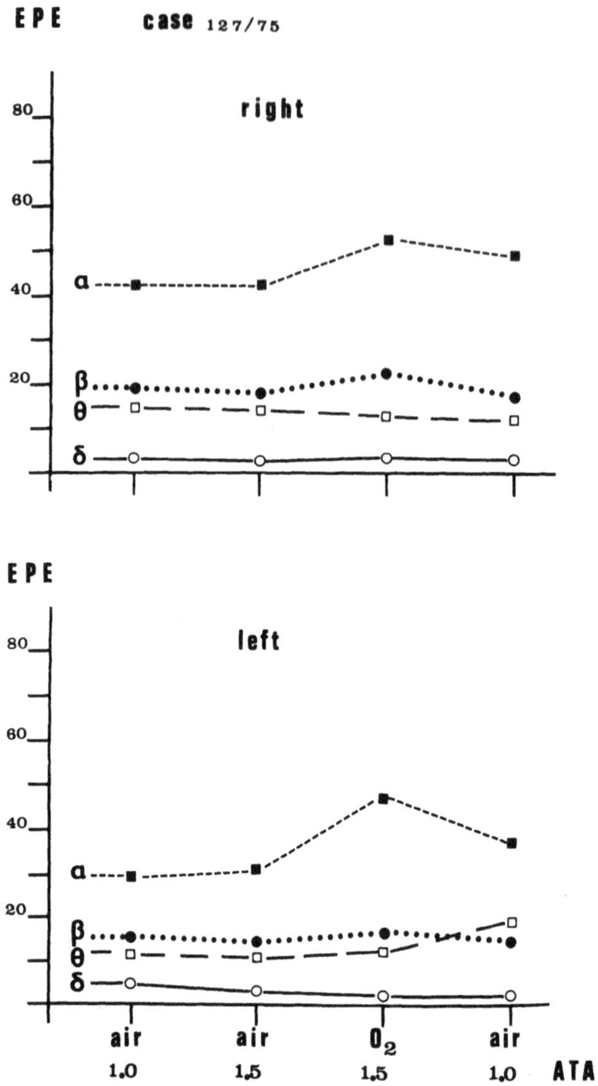

Fig. 1. EEG analyses before and during a hyperbaric oxygenation session. *EPE*, electric power equivalent value; *ATA*, atmospheres absolute

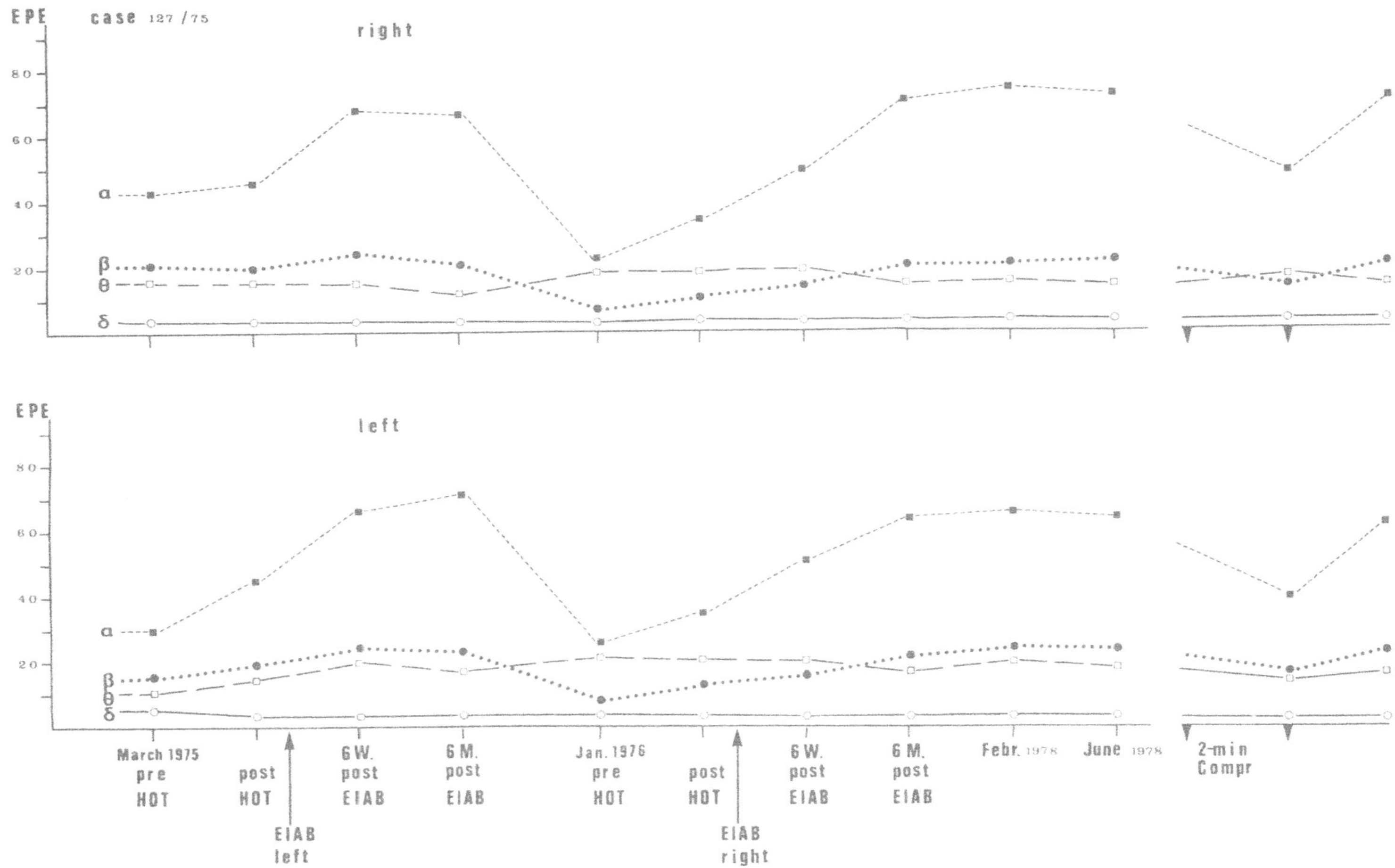

Fig. 2. Follow-up EEG analyses and their changes during a 2-min digital compression *(Compr)* of the right superficial temporal artery. *EPE*, electric power equivalent values

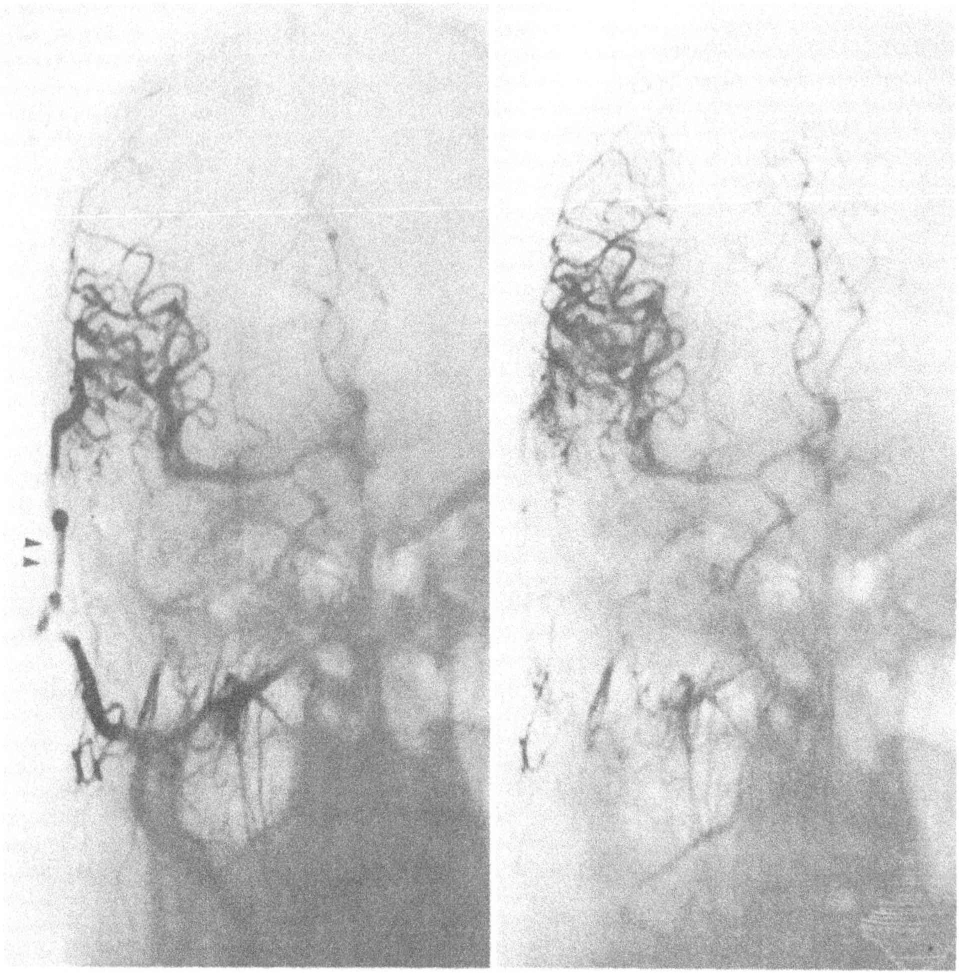

Fig. 3. a Postoperative right carotid angiography

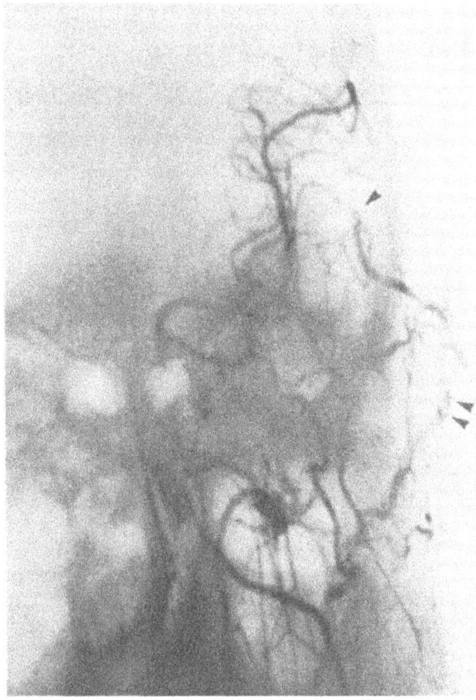

Fig. 3. b Postoperative left carotid angiography

Nine Years of Experience with Extra-Intracranial Bypass Surgery for Cerebral Ischemia

P. SCHMIEDEK, O. GRATZL, V. OLTEANU-NERBE, U. STEUDE, and F. MARGUTH

Extra-intracranial bypass surgery has become increasingly popular, particularly during the last few years (4,5,6,7,11). However, it cannot be considered an established treatment modality for cerebral ischemia. This is mainly due to the uncertainty in the evaluation of the effectiveness of this treatment in view of the complex, interrelated hemodynamic factors and the unpredictable natural history of individual patients with cerebrovascular disease. Secondly, the selection of patients thought to be good candidates for cerebromicrovascular management still remains controversial. Cerebral revascularization was started at our institution in 1970, only 3 years after the original description of the technique by DONAGHY and YASARGIL (2,13). Hence, the favorable and probably to an even greater extent the unfavorable experiences with this procedure since then have led us to finally arrive at some more definite conclusions that will be summarized in the present report.

Clinical Material

Our series includes 260 patients in whom a total number of 272 revascularization procedures have been carried out. The first 250 consecutive cases have been analyzed for this study. The age and sex distribution of our surgically treated cases was as follows. There were 196 men with a mean age of 50.9 years and 54 women with a mean age of 45.2 years (Fig. 1). Except for one recent case with an occipital artery to posterior inferior cerebellar artery (PICA) anastomosis for posterior circulation insufficiency, all patients had an end-to-side anastomosis between the superficial temporal artery (STA) or the occipital artery and a branch of the middle cerebral artery (MCA). The surgical technique has been the subject of minor modifications over the years. Instead of turning a scalp flap as originally proposed by YASARGIL (14), we are now using a linear skin incision over the donor artery and a small craniectomy over the recipient vessel. Postoperative morbidity was encountered in 34 patients (Table 1). This total rate of Almost 14% appears to be relatively high; however, when subdividing it according to the severity of symptoms, a more acceptable figure of about 5% with major complications remains. Ten patients died postoperatively (Table 2). Again, the individual case analysis reveals that the death was coincident with but definitely not related to surgery in three cases, whereas of the remaining seven cases five would no longer have been candidates for the operation with our present criteria for surgery. The documented graft patency, using either postoperative angiography or the Doppler technique was found to be 91%.

Table 1. Postoperative morbidity in 250 surgically treated cases

	No.	%
Scalp flap necrosis	12	4.8
Epidural hematoma	1	0.4
Subdural hematoma	3	1.2
Intracerebral hematoma	1	0.4
Temporary worsening of neurological status	12	4.8
Permanent worsening of neurological status	5	2.0
Total	34	13.6

Table 2. Postoperative mortality in 250 surgically treated cases

Case No.	Age	Sex	Neurological symptoms[a]	Cause of death	Interval between surgery and death
70/1	61	M	Acute CS	Brain swelling, cardiac failure	6 days
70/2	46	M	Acute CS	Brain swelling	1 day
70/7	57	M	CS	Contralateral glioma	5 mo
70/9	45	M	Acute CS	Brain swelling	4 days
71/18	49	F	SIE	No autopsy	23 days
71/19	62	M	SIE	Renal failure	5 days
75/78	53	M	CS	Septicemia	14 days
75/89	28	M	PRIND	Acute basilar thrombosis	2 mo
75/95	50	M	PRIND	Myocardial infarction	1 day
76/106	30	F	CS	Epidural hematoma	7 days

a CS, completed stroke; SIE, stroke in evolution; PRIND, prolonged reversible neurological deficit.

Criteria for Selection of Suitable Candidates for Surgery

In an attempt to simplify a complicated matter, the following conceptual decision tree has been developed, showing the criteria that we presently use to decide whether or not to operate on a patient (Fig. 2). The first and doubtlessly most decisive single parameter is represented by the *patient's history and clinical examination.* The rationale for surgery is based on two assumptions. The first is that revascularization influences the incidence of further strokes, and the second is that in some patients the neurological symptoms can be improved by an increase in collateral blood supply. Therefore, indications generally agreed on include patients with transient ischemic attacks (TIAs) and those with prolonged reversible ischemic neurological deficits (PRINDs) (Table 3). The indication for surgery

Table 3. Clinical classification of cerebrovascular disease

I.	Transient cerebral ischemic attack (TIA) Focal ischemic cerebral dysfunction followed by complete recovery within 24 h
II.	Prolonged reversible ischemic neurological deficit (PRIND) Focal ischemic cerebral dysfunction persisting longer than 24 h showing a subsequent tendency to clear
III.	Completed stroke (CS) Focal ischemic cerebral dysfunction with permanent and fixed neurological deficit
IV.	Stroke in evolution (SIE)
V.	Progressive stroke (PS)

is less clearly defined for patients with a completed stroke and usually will depend on the results of additional diagnostic studies. From our early experience, acute cerebral ischemia has to be considered a definite contraindication for bypass surgery (3).

The practical application of this experience is demonstrated in Fig. 3, which shows the change over the time of the relative percent of the different neurological subgroups in our surgically treated patients with a steadily increasing rate of those with either TIAs or PRINDs.

The following actual diagnostic work-up of potential candidates for bypass surgery usually starts with *computer tomographic (CT)* scanning of the brain to demonstrate the extent of any morphologic alterations secondary to cerebral ischemia. The interpretation of CT results in terms of selecting suitable surgical candidates is largely based on empiric evidence but is further established by a comparative analysis of CT findings and the results of regional cerebral blood flow (rCBF) measurements (9). Accordingly, patients with massive cerebral infarction, which is mostly associated with severe stroke, are easily excluded (Fig. 4a). The rationale for not operating on patients with so-called strategic infarction (Fig. 4b) is derived from anatomic considerations because these infarcts are primarily caused by deep seated ischemic events that cannot be expected to be influenced by any measures to increase the cortical brain blood flow. Finally, CT scanning enables us to detect the occasional patient whose ischemic symptoms are possibly caused by a brain tumor.

It should be emphasized that the diagnostic work-up of patients must also include a careful search for any potential *risk factors* that are generally considered contraindications to surgery, such as cardiac arrhythmias, severe hypertension, or uncontrolled diabetes.

Cerebral angiography then provides definite information for planning the further management of the patient. For practical reasons it has proved to be very useful to differentiate between accessible and inaccessible lesions within the craniocerebral vasculature (12). In the presence of an accessible lesion that is located proximally to the mandibular-mastoid conncetion line, it has become our policy to refer the patient for standard vascular surgery. The most common anatomic lesions, on the other hand, suitable for extra-intracranial arterial anastomosis are complete occlusion of the internal carotid artery, internal carotid artery siphon stenosis, and lesions within the middle cerebral artery territory. Angiographic findings in our series are listed in Table 4.

Table 4. Preoperative angiographic findings in 250 surgically treated cases

	No.	%
Internal carotid artery occlusion	110	44.0
Internal carotid artery stenosis	32	12.8
Middle cerebral artery occlusion	20	8.0
Middle cerebral artery stenosis	16	6.4
Multiple vessel disease	28	11.0
Small vessel disease	16	6.4
Within normal limits	13	5.4

At this point, it might be appropriate to briefly comment on the significance of *regional cerebral blood flow studies*. In the past, we made intensive use of this method, which then allowed us to differentiate between six different groups of cerebral blood flow patterns that can be commonly found in patients with cerebrovascular disease. Of these, only two were found to be suitable for bypass surgery, namely, the focal and the relative focal ischemic CBF pattern (8). Although rCBF studies still represent a very delicate and extremely useful adjunct in combination with the other diagnostic procedures, the frequency of preoperative rCBF studies has considerably decreased in our more recent patient material. This, however, is simply due to the fact that we are now making practical use of what we learned from our previous rCBF studies. Measurement of rCBF is now performed in only selected cases and for the evaluation of special problems related to bypass surgery. There are, however, two situations during the preoperative investigation of patients where the rCBF study continues to be of decisive importance. One is the borderline case in which some of the quantitative data provided by rCBF studies is helpful in deciding whether or not to operate on a patient, e.g., a patient with severe general reduction of his CBF. The other is the patient with a normal angiogram in spite of a history of or even obvious symptoms of cerebral ischemia. We think that it is justified to do a bypass operation in this patient, provided he has a focal or relatively focal reduction of his CBF (10). This is illustrated by the postoperative angiogram of a patient with a normal angiogram who had been operated on because of an abnormal rCBF study 2 1/2 years earlier (Fig. 5).

Comment

In summary, we think that following these guidelines for patient selection will eventually result in a more rational approach to revascularization microneurosurgery for cerebral ischemia. The ultimate effectiveness of these operations, however, will hopefully be established through a multicenter cooperative randomized clinical trial, which is presently being carried out in institutions in North America and Western Europe (1).

References

1. Cooperative study of extracranial/intracranial arterial anastomosis (EC/IC Bypass Study) Research Protocol

2. DONAGHY, R.M.P.: What's new in surgery? Neurological surgery. Surg. Gynecol. Obstet. 134, 269-271 (1972)

3. GRATZL, O., SCHMIEDEK, P., SPETZLER, R., STEINHOFF, H., MARGUTH, F.: Clinical experience with extra-intracranial arterial anastomosis in 65 cases. J. Neurosurg. 44, 313-324 (1976)

4. GRATZL, O., SCHMIEDEK, P., SPETZLER, R.: Extracranial-intracranial arterial bypass for cerebral ischemia. Prog. Neurol. Surg. (in press)

5. Microneurological anastomoses for cerebral ischemia. AUSTIN, G.M. (ed.). Springfield, Ill.: Thomas 1976

6. Microvascular anastomoses for cerebral ischemia. FEIN, J.M., REICHMANN, O.H. (eds.). Berlin, Heidelberg, New York: Springer 1978

7. Microsurgery for stroke. SCHMIEDEK, P., GRATZL, O., SPETZLER, R. (eds.). Berlin, Heidelberg, New York: Springer 1977

8. SCHMIEDEK, P., GRATZL, O., SPETZLER, R., STEINHOFF, H., ENZENBACH, R., BRENDEL, W., MARGUTH, F.: Selection of patients for extra-intracranial arterial bypass surgery based on rCBF measurements. J. Neurosurg. 44, 303-312 (1976)

9. SCHMIEDEK, P., LANKSCH, W., OLTEANU-NERBE, V., KAZNER, E., GRATZL, O., MARGUTH, F.: Combined use of regional cerebral blood flow measurement and computerized tomography for the diagnosis of cerebral ischemia. In: Microsurgery for stroke. SCHMIEDEK, P., GRATZL, O., SPETZLER, R. (eds.). Berlin, Heidelberg, New York: Springer 1977

10. SCHMIEDEK, P., OLTEANU-NERBE, V., GRATZL, O., MARGUTH, F.: Extra-intracranial arterial bypass surgery for cerebral ischemia in patients with normal angiograms (in press)

11. SPETZLER, R.: Extracranial-intracranial arterial anastomosis for cerebrovascular disease (in press)

12. TEW, J.M.: Reconstructive intracranial vascular surgery for prevention of stroke. Clin. Neurosurg. 22, 264-280 (1975)

13. YASARGIL, M.G.: Microsurgery applied to neurosurgery, pp. 105-155. New York: Academic Press 1969

14. YASARGIL, M.G., KARYENBÜHL, H.A., JACOBSON, J.H.: Microneurosurgical arterial reconstruction. Surgery 67, 221-233 (1970)

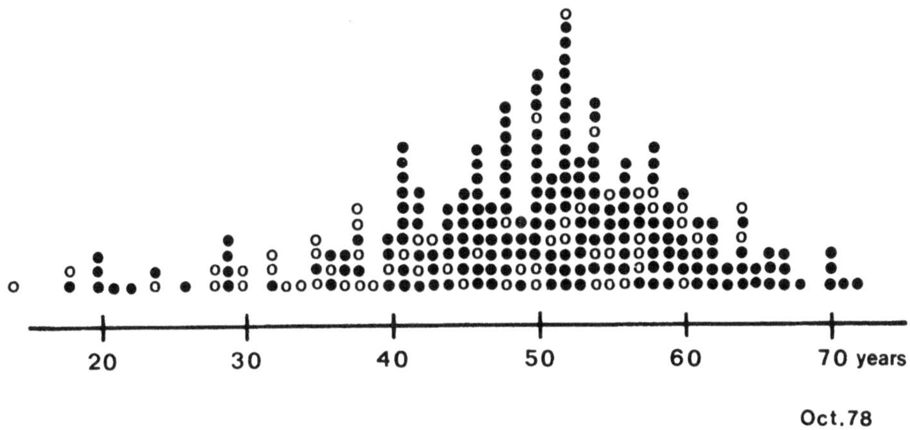

Fig. 1. Age and sex distribution of 250 surgically treated cases
●, M No. 196 (50.9); o, F No. 54 (45.2)

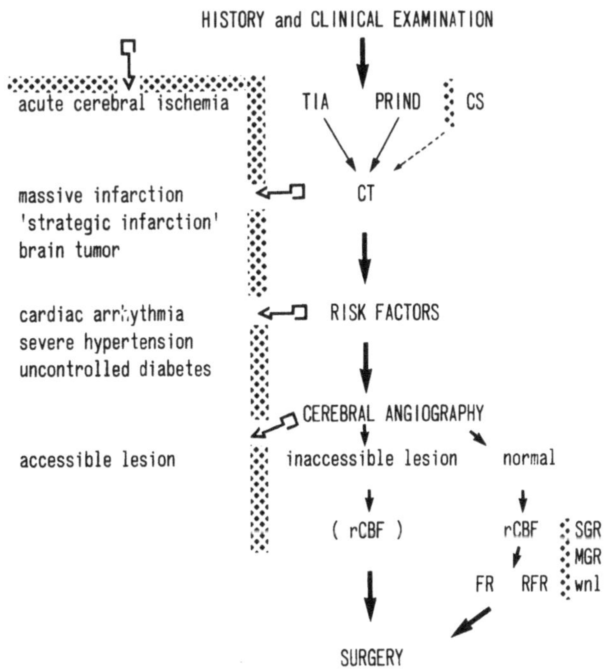

Fig. 2. Criteria for the selection of patients for extra-intracranial bypass surgery. *TIA*, transient cerebral ischemic attack; *PRIND*, prolonged reversible ischemic neurological deficit; *CS*, completed stroke; *CT*, computer tomography; *rCBF*, regional cerebral blood flow; *SGR*, severe generalized reduction; *MGR*, moderate generalized reduction; *FR*, focal reduction; *RFR*, relative focal reduction; *WNL*, within normal limits

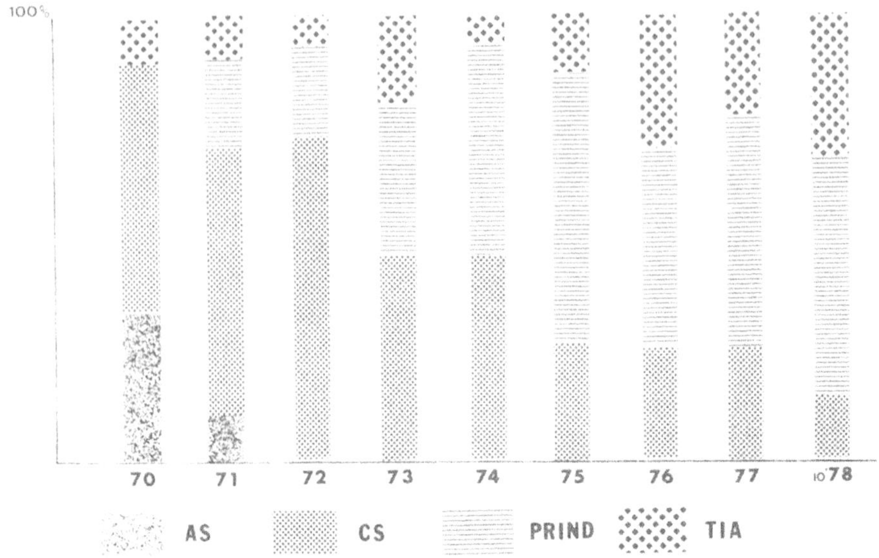

Fig. 3. Distribution and relative percent of different neurological subgroups in our surgically treated series from 1970 until October 1978. *AS*, acute stroke; *CS*, completed stroke; *PRIND*, prolonged reversible ischemic neurological deficit; *TIA*, transient ischemic attack

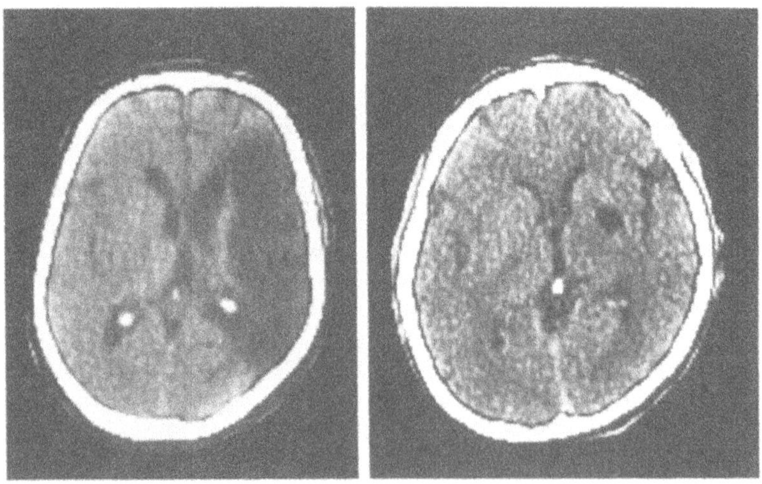

Fig. 4. CT finding in a patient with a massive infarction *(left)* and *(right)* with a strategic infarction

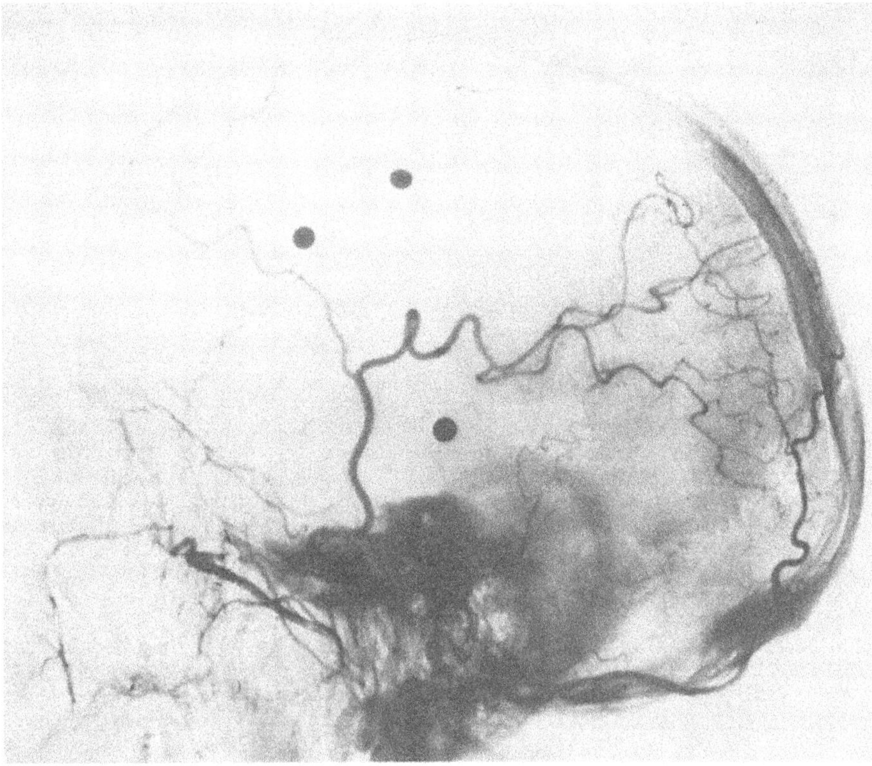

Fig. 5. Postoperative angiogram in a patient with normal preoperative angiography

Vertebrobasilar Insufficiency Relieved by Carotid Surgery

J. W. CORRELL, J. STERN, J. ZYROFF, and M. WHELAN

Introduction

Vertebrobasilar insufficiency (VBI) is one of the most common diagnoses in neurological practice (1). Transient ischemic attacks (TIAs) in the territory of the vertebrobasilar (VB) complex produce symptoms referable to the brain stem, cerebellum, or occipital cortex. These symptoms are usually characterized by one or a combination of the following: diplopia, dysarthria, ataxia; unilateral, bilateral, or alternating limb weakness; paresthesias with focal sensory loss; vertigo, unilateral or bilateral visual field disturbances; drop attacks; and single or multiple cranial nerve palsies.

One-third of patients with carotid symptomatology also demonstrate VBI (6), but exact figures are not available on the number of patients with VBI also having TIAs referable to the anterior circulation. The variations in the clinical picture demonstrated from one patient to another may be explained by the anatomic variations in the circle of Willis, the effectiveness of collateral pathways, the variability in location of occlusive or stenosing lesions, and the coexistence of two or more areas of occlusive disease. Occlusive disease within the circle of Willis or a congenitally small or absent communicating vessel may preclude collateral flow from one system to the other.

A small number of reports have been published on the role of carotid endarterectomy for the relief of TIAs in the posterior circulation (2,3,4,5). Because of the conflicting nature of these reports, the present study was undertaken. Special attention has been paid to the angiographic findings in an attempt to discriminate between those patients in whom carotid surgery was of benefit and those patients who derived no relief of their symptoms.

Materials and Methods

The records of 1000 patients with TIAs who had undergone either unilateral or bilateral carotid endarterectomy performed by the senior author (JWC) were reviewed. Criteria for entry into the present study were: (1) TIAs referable to the VB and carotid circulation, (2) attacks referable only to the VB circulation, (3) availability of angiograms demonstrating both extra- and intracranial vessels, and (4) adequate follow-up.

A TIA was defined as a focal neurological defect of sudden onset that resolved completely within 24 h. Patients with completed strokes or prolonged ischemic neurological deficit at the time of surgery were excluded from the study. No attempt was made to assess the frequency of TIAs prior to surgery. The frequency of attacks and the development of a permanent neurological deficit during the follow-up period was recorded.

Angiograms of all patients including both an arch study and intracranial vessel studies were reviewed. The radiologists were not informed about the patient's clinical findings. The arteriograms were evaluated for the following: (1) degree of stenosis and evidence of ulceration at the origin of both carotid and both vertebral arteries, (2) the presence and size of both posterior communicating arteries (PCAs), (3) the presence or absence of intracranial vascular disease.

Follow-up data was obtained by contacting the patients or their personal physicians. In most instances, the patients had also been seen at least once, and frequently more often, during the 1st postoperative year by the senior author.

Results

There were 44 men and 22 women entered into the study. The average age at the time of surgery was 60 years, with a range of 42-77. The average duration of follow-up was 24 months, with approximately 80% having been followed for 18 months.

Patients with TIAs were classified into two major groups: (1) 26 patients with nonhemispheric symptoms and (2) 40 patients with both hemispheric and nonhemispheric attacks.

Group I

Of the 26 patients with pure VB symptoms, 14 underwent bilateral carotid endarterectomy. Of these, there were eight patients whose disease was confined to the anterior circulation with angiographically normal, nonstenotic vertebrals. Six patients in this group had complete relief of their symptoms. These patients all had either large or normal PCAs. One patient who had persistent but fewer TIAs had bilaterally small PCAs. Another patient who had normal caliber PCAs developed total relief of symptoms for 1 year after which the symptoms reappeared. A repeat angiogram showed bilateral recurrent carotid disease. She underwent a second bilateral carotid endarterectomy and is again asymptomatic.

The other nine patients who underwent bilateral carotid endarterectomy had varying degrees of vertebral disease but all had normal or large caliber PCAs. Four of these patients had relief of symptoms despite the fact that each had one occluded vertebral. Two patients had fewer TIAs, both having bilateral high-grade vertebral disease. One patient who continued to have symptoms had an ulcerative plaque in one vertebral, and another patient who developed a brain stem stroke had bilateral vertebral ulcers. The last patient in this group had occlusion of the right vertebral and 50% stenosis of the left vertebral. This patient also developed a brain stem stroke.

In group I there were nine patients who underwent unilateral carotid endarterectomy. Five on the left and four on the right. Criteria for deciding the side upon which to operate were (a) the angiographically "worse" lesion, usually that lesion demonstrating ulceration, (b) if both lesions looked equally "bad", the operation was performed on the dominant hemisphere, or (c) if one carotid was totally occluded, the other carotid was chosen for operation.

Six patients had total relief. These patients, in general, were those who had no vertebral lesions, normal or large caliber PCAs, and had evidence of an ulcerated lesion in only the operated carotid. Two patients had fewer TIAs; the first also had an ulcer in the left vertebral, the other patient had angiographically normal vertebrals and PCAs. One patient who had a brain stem stroke had bilateral carotid ulcers, occlusion of one vertebral with 50% stenosis of the other, and bilaterally small PCAs.

Group II

Twelve patients with combined hemispheric and nonhemispheric TIAs underwent bilateral carotid endarterectomy. Seven of these patients had both normal vertebral and PCAs. Six had total relief of symptoms. One patient had relief of the hemispheric symptoms but had persistent although fewer TIAs in the VB distribution. The other five patients who underwent bilateral endarterectomy had vertebral disease. None of these patients had total relief of symptoms. Four have persistent and one has fewer symptoms.

Twenty-eight patients underwent unilateral endarterectomy; 12 on the right and 16 on the left. The carotid appropriate for the hemispheric symptoms was chosen for operation. Seventeen unilateral endarterectomies were performed on patients with normal vertebral arteries. Twelve patients became asymptomatic despite the fact that nine had ulcerative lesions in both their carotids. Three patients with persistent symptoms had small or absent PCAs. One patient with bilateral carotid ulcers and bilaterally small PCAs had resolution of his hemispheric symptoms with persistent VBI. Another patient in this subgroup had removal of his ulcerative lesion; the other carotid was occluded and he had bilaterally normal caliber PCAs; however, this patient also continued TIAs in a nonhemispheric distribution.

Eleven unilateral endarterectomies were performed in patients with diseased vertebral arteries. Seven of these patients became asymptomatic. Three of these patients had evidence of an ulcerative lesion in the vertebral. Six had significant lesions in the unoperative carotid. Two patients had persistent symptoms; both had vertebral lesions, one with small PCAs. Two patients in this subgroup had brain stem strokes. Both had bilateral carotid ulcers, bilateral vertebral ulcers, and bilaterally small PCAs.

Discussion

We have previously demonstrated (7) that carotid endarterectomy may relieve posterior fossa TIAs in patients with persistent hypoglossal or trigeminal arteries and ulcerative lesions in the carotid. It seems apparent that if blood flow to the basilar artery is derived largely or entirely from the internal carotid artery that lesions in the internal carotid artery could easily result in symptoms of vertebrobasilar insufficiency.

Conflicting reports from the literature (3,4,5) have prompted us to review this series of patients who had either pure VB symptoms or combined VB and carotid symptoms and who underwent either unilateral or bilateral endarterectomy. Patients with pure nonhemispheric symptoms and normal vertebral arteries who underwent bilateral endarterectomy all benefited from surgery. Only one patient in this group did not have total relief. The source of this patient's symptoms may be based on

(1) a vertebral or basilar lesion not appreciated on angiography or (2) decreased blood flow that could only be partially compensated for in the face of his bilaterally small PCAs.

All patients with combined symptoms and normal vertebral arteries who underwent bilateral endarterectomy also benefited from surgery. One patient with normal caliber PCAs continued to have VBI but no hemispheric TIAs. It seems probable that a lesion in the vertebral or basilar artery escaped detection.

Patients who underwent bilateral endarterectomy for either VBI alone or combined symptoms and also had vertebral disease did poorly. Despite normally sized PCAs, the persistence of symptoms or development of a VB stroke is probably related to the occlusive lesion in the vertebral or basilar artery.

In those patients whose symptoms were limited to VBI, relief of the symptoms consistently occurred after unilateral carotid endarterectomy only when evidence of vertebral disease was absent and the PCAs were normal or large. In these cases, operations on the carotid demonstrating ulceration proved most effective. If symptoms are not relieved, operating on the opposite side should be considered. The unoperated carotid may harbor an ulcerative lesion not readily visible on angiogram and responsible for the patient's symptoms.

When deciding which carotid to operate upon in patients with combined symptoms, it is best to start with that vessel responsible for the hemispheric TIAs. Here too, if symptoms persist in the face of apparently normal vertebral and basilar arteries, thought should be given to operating on the contralateral carotid.

Conclusion

The ability of a carotid lesion to produce vertebrobasilar symptoms and for carotid surgery to be of benefit is directly related to the freedom of communication between the carotid and basilar arteries.

References

1. BRADSHAW, P.: The syndrome of vertebro-basilar insufficiency. Q.J. Med. 32, 279 (1963)
2. CORRELL, J.W., STERN, J.: Carotid artery lesions causing vertebral-basilar insufficiency. Stroke 9, 107 (1978)
3. FORD, J. J., BAKER, W.H., EHERNHAFT, J.L.: Carotid endarterectomy for nonhemispheric transient ischemic attacks. Arch. Surg. 110, 1314 (1975)
4. HUMPHRIES, A.W., YOUNG, J.R., BEVEN, E.G., LEFEVRE, F.A., DEWOLFE, V.G.: Relief of vertebrobasilar symptoms by carotid endarterectomy, Surgery 57, 48 (1952)
5. McNAMARA, J.O., HEYMAN, A., SILVER, D., MANDEL, M.E.: The value of carotid endarterectomy in treating transient cerebral ischemia of the posterior circulation. Neurology (Minneap.) 27, 682 (1977)
6. NATALI, J., MARAVAL, M., KIEFFER, E.: Surgical treatment of stenosis and occlusion of the internal carotid and vertebral arteries. J. Cardiovasc. Surg. (Torino) 13, 14 (1972)
7. STERN, J., CORRELL, J.W., BRYAN, N.: Persistent hypoglossal artery and persistent trigeminal artery presenting with posterior fossa transient ischemic attacks. J. Neurosurg. 49, 614 (1978)

Bypass Surgery for Vertebral Artery Occlusive Disease: Technique and Complications[1]

T. M. Sundt, Jr., and D. G. Piepgras

We have previously reported our experience with bypass surgery for occlusive disease involving the posterior circulation and correlated our work with pathologic studies (2,3,4,5,6,8,12,15) focusing on vascular disease involving the vertebrobasilar system. We have considered the rationale, indications, and results of this operation (14) and compared this procedure to that for carotid system disease (1,7,9,10,11,13,14,15,16). It is our purpose here to focus attention only on the technical aspects and complications of the operation.

Case Material

This operation has been performed in 24 patients for a variety of ischemic symptomatology attributable to occlusive disease of the posterior circulation. These symptoms included progressing stroke, transient ischemic attacks (TIAs), minor brain stem infarcts, and orthostatic cerebral ischemia. Each patient suffered from more than one symptom complex. The grouping of the cases and typical case reports have been reported previously (1,2).

Surgical Technique

The operation is performed with the patient in the sitting position. The head is flexed anteriorly and secured into position with a pinion headholder. A hockey-stick incision is made (Fig. 1a) and the midline avascular plane identified. The musculature is swept unilaterally from the arch of C1 and the occiput. The cutting current is not used for the scalp incision but is useful to reflect the deep neck muscles from the occiput as far laterally as the mastoid process (Fig. 1b). The occipital artery is identified in its muscular plane and is best located by palpation in the mastoid groove just posterior and medial to the mastoid process (Fig. 1c). This vessel is then dissected free from the surrounding tissue using small blunt scissors. Small branching vessels are coagulated with the bipolar coagulator before their division. This is perhaps the most difficult part of the operation as the vessel is intimately adherent to the surrounding tissue and is much more difficult to isolate than is the superficial temporal artery (Figs. 1d and e). It is surrounded by a venous plexus and distally joins a facial sheath shared by the occipital nerve. The vessel is followed to its point of entrance into this muscular bed at the mastoid

1 Supported by grants from the McKnight Foundation, Minneapolis, Minnesota; Vernon and Earline Dale Foundation, LaCrosse, Wisconsin; and the National Institutes of Health, U.S. Public Health Service NS 6663.

groove. In its transplanted course it lies at the base of the occiput and follows a straight path from the mastoid groove to the point of anastomosis. It is important to mobilize this vessel as far proximally as possible to obtain adequate length for the graft. Proximal dissection often permits the resection of the distal 1-2 cm of the vessel. This mobilization of the occipital artery can be facilitated by the resection of the superior oblique muscle, which lies deep to the occipital artery as this vessel sweeps posteriorly from the mastoid groove. The digastric muscle, the splenious capitis, and the longissimus capitis all lie superficial to this vessel. The semispinalis capitis forms the primary bed for the artery.

A small unilateral suboccipital craniectomy is effected along with a unilateral resection in the arch of C1 (Fig. 1f). The dura is opened in the linear fashion and the margins sutured to adjacent tissue (Fig. 1g). The medullary loop of the posterior inferior cerebellar artery (PICA) is identified as this vessel passes around the brain stem on its course to the vermis (Fig. 1h). A small rubber dam is temporarily placed deep to this artery and the vessel elevated by suturing the superior end of the dam to the margin of the bone and the inferior end to the muscle or reflected dura (Fig. 1i). Miniature Mayfield clips are placed on either side of the area selected for arteriotomy. A small linear incision is made in the PICA with a broken razor blade on an appropriate holder. The arteriotomy is extended in both directions with small microscissors. The donor vessel (previously prepared for the anastomosis by resection of excess lenght, removing excessive soft tissue, and fish-mouthing the end) is sewn to the apex of the arteriotomy with a double-armed 9-0 monofilament nylon suture (Fig. 1j and k). This initial suture is an important one and is placed in both vessels from the inside to the outside. The remaining portion of the vessel is then anastomosed in a routine fashion by techniques described previously (Fig. 1l and m). Interrupted sutures are used throughout the closure; 9-0 monofilament nylon suture is preferred to 10-0 monofilament nylon as the wall of the occipital artery is thicker than the temporal artery and tends to bend the smaller needles provided for 10-0 monofilament suture. We are currently using a short double-armed suture with BV-5 needles.

Flow is restored by removing the clips on the recipient artery initially and the clip on the donor vessel last. Small bleeding points, if they occur, usually cease within a few minutes from light pressure applied using Gelfoam. However, on occasion it is necessary to place an additional suture if the bleeding does not terminate with light pressure. The temporary rubber dam is removed, and a dural graft is then sewn into place. Dural closure is facilitated by a separate incision in the lateral of the dura for entrance of the artery into the subarachnoid space (Fig. 1c). Nevertheless, a completely watertight closure is not possible because of the necessity of allowing adequate room for the occipital artery as it passes through the dural opening. Accordingly, a very tight muscle closure is necessary, and this in turn is made possible by retaining a muscular cuff in the transverse portion of the muscle incision and taking the patient out of the "flexed position" prior to closure. Sutures are left in place for 2 weeks. The transplanted occipital artery lies deep in the wound and follows a directly transverse course to the point of anastomosis (Fig. 1n). However, it is still possible to palpate an occipital pulse posterior to the mastoid process and the absence of a pulse in this area suggests an occlusion of the vessel.

Complications

Neurological

Two patients developed neurological deficits not present prior to operation (unilateral hearing loss, one patient; homonymous hemianopsia, one patient). The cause for the unilateral hearing loss was not determined. The cause of the homonymous hemianopsia was related to a lateral sinus occlusion and a secondary venous infarction (see below). Two patients had a transient increase in ataxia following surgery but had returned to preoperative function by the time of hospital discharge.

Subdural Hematomas

One patient developed bilateral subdural air collections that required burr holes for release 36 h after the operation. Another patient developed a unilateral subdural hematoma over one cerebral convexity that became symptomatic 6 weeks after the operation. These patients in general have a significant degree of cortical atrophy and, therefore, represent a higher risk for subdural air or fluid collection than patients operated in a sitting position for brain tumors. Nevertheless, the advantages of the sitting position for this operative procedure outweigh these possible complications, and it is our feeling that these complications must be accepted as possible risks of the operation. Neither of these two patients developed a permanent neurological deficit related to the subdural fluid or air accumulation.

Epidural Hematoma

One patient developed a postoperative epidural hematoma that was the result of a small bleeding point on the donor graft. This complication has been described in some detail in a previous communication (2). The bleeding point was repaired with a clip graft.

Pulmonary Complications

Three patients developed minor pulmonary complications and one major pulmonary complication. In each patient these complications were related to lower cranial nerve palsies present prior to surgery, and the complications responded to appropriate standard measures of respiratory therapy. However, in patients with a considerable degree of dysphagia prior to surgery, it is wise to consider a nasotracheal airway for 2 or 3 days following the operation. This has been our recent practice.

Graft Occlusion

Two patients occluded the bypass graft postoperatively. The cause of occlusion in each case was probably the absence of a perfusion gradient across the site of anastomosis. The PICA remained patent in each case.

Lateral Sinus Thrombosis

In one patient occlusion of the lateral sinus occurred from bone wax placed in a large mastoid emissary vein that was opened as the deep neck muscles were reflected from the occiput. This patient developed a sinus thrombosis 7 days following the operative procedure, and the sinus thrombosis resulted in a venous infarction in the hemisphere opposite the side of the sinus occlusion. This individual had only one patent sinus prior to the operation. Fortunately, collateral drainage did develop in this patient, and she did not lose vision in the opposite field nor did she develop symptomatology of increasing intracranial pressure. The complaints for which she was originally operated, viz., frequent transient ischemia attacks, orthostatic cerebral ischemia, and a slowly progressing ataxia, resolved following the operation.

Analysis of Complications

Our primary problems in connection with this operative procedure have been related to the marginal neurological status of these patients prior to surgery. Respiratory complications have been frequent and usually have resulted from previous impairment in the cranial nerve function as indicated above.

Surgery with the patient in a sitting position presents risks related to emboli, hypotension, and convexity subdural collections of fluid or air. However, it is our judgment that these risks are far outweighed by the exposure achieved from this position. All patients should receive adequate blood volume replacement on a unit for unit basis, which helps to prevent air amboli by maintaining a high venous pressure and also helps to avoid hypotension. These patients have areas in the brain in which autoregulation is no longer preserved, and they are extraordinarily vulnerable to fluctuations in perfusion pressure and cardiac output. Accordingly, it is imperative to maintain an adequate perfusion pressure throughout the operation.

To maintain a patent graft, it is necessary that a perfusion gradient be present across the site of anastomosis. Also, it is imperative that there be a patent PICA to serve as recipient artery. A typical postoperative angiogram is illustrated in Fig. 2. Angiograms of other grafts, some with higher flows, have been published previously.

Summary

Twenty-four operations in which the occipital artery was anastomosed to the posterior inferior cerebellar artery were performed for occlusions or inaccessible stenotic lesions of the vertebral arteries proximal to the site of the origin of the posterior inferior cerebellar artery. Patients were divided into two groups: those with no major focal neurological deficits but considered to be a high risk for posterior circulation infarct (group I, ten patients) and those patients severely or moderately disabled before the operation from ischemic related deficits in the posterior circulation (group II, 14 patients). Postoperative angiography revealed that 22 of the 24 grafts were patent. Technical aspects of the procedure, complications, and indications will be reviewed. A 4-min movie taken through the operating microscope will illustrate technical aspects of the anastomosis. The results and possible role of this operation will be considered.

References

1. AUSMAN, J.I., LEE, M.C., KLASSEN, A.C.: Stroke: What's new? Cerebral revascularization. Minn. Med. 59, 223-227 (1976)
2. CAPLAN, L.R., ROSENBAUM, A.E.: Role of cerebral angiography in vertebrobasilar occlusive disease. J. Neurol. Neurosurg. Psychiatry 38, 601-612 (1975)
3. CASTAIGNE, P., LHERMITTE, F., GAUTIER, J.C.: Arterial occlusions in the vertebro-basilar system. A study of 44 patients with post-mortem data. Brain 96, 133-154 (1973)
4. FISHER, C.M., CAPLAN, L.R.: Basilar artery branch occlusion: a cause of pontine infarction. Neurology (Minneap.) 21, 900-905 (1971)
5. FISHER, C.M., KARNES, W.E., KUBIK, C.S.: Lateral medullary infarction - the pattern of vascular occlusion. J. Neuropathol. Exp. Neurol. 20, 323-379 (1961)
6. FISHER, C.M., GORE, I., OKABE, N.: Atherosclerosis of the carotid and vertebral arteries - extracranial and intracranial. J. Neuropathol. Exp. Neurol. 24, 455-476 (1965)
7. KHODADAD, G., SINGH, R.S., OLINGER, C.P.: Possible prevention of brain stem stroke by microvascular anastomosis in the vertebrobasilar system. Stroke 8, 316-321 (1977)
8. LHERMITTE, F., GAUTIER, J.C., DEROUESNE, C.: Nature of occlusions of the middle cerebral artery. Neurology (Minneap.) 20, 82-88 (1970)
9. REICHMAN, O.H.: Extracranial-intracranial arterial anastomosis. In: SANDOK, B.A., WHISNANT, J.P. (eds.). Cerebral vascular diseases: ninth conference, pp. 175-185. New York: Grune & Stratton 1975
10. SCHMIEDEK, P., GRATZL, O., SPETZLER, R.: Selection of patients for extra-intracranial artery bypass surgery based on rCBF measurements. J. Neurosurg. 44, 303-312 (1976)
11. SPETZLER, R., CHATER, N.: Microvascular bypass surgery. Part 2: Physiological studies. J. Neurosurg. 45, 508-513 (1976)
12. STEIN, B.M., McCORMICK, W., RODRIQUEZ, J.N.: Incidence and significance of occlusive vascular disease of the extracranial arteries as demonstrated by post-mortem angiography. Trans. Am. Neurol. Assoc. 86, 60-66 (1961)
13. SUNDT, T.M., Jr., SIEKERT, R.G., PIEPGRAS, D.G.: Bypass surgery for vascular disease of the carotid system. Mayo Clin. Proc. 51, 677-692 (1976)
14. SUNDT, T.M., Jr., WHISNANT, J.P., PIEPGRAS, D.G.: Intracranial bypass grafts for vertebral-basilar ischemia. Mayo Clin. Proc. 53, 12-18 (1978)
15. TEW, J.M., Jr.: Reconstructive intracranial vascular surgery for prevention of stroke. Clin. Neurosurg. 22, 264-280 (1975)
16. YASARGIL, M.G., KRAYENBUHL, H.A., JACOBSON, J.H.: Microneurosurgical arterial reconstruction. Surgery 67, 221-233 (1970)

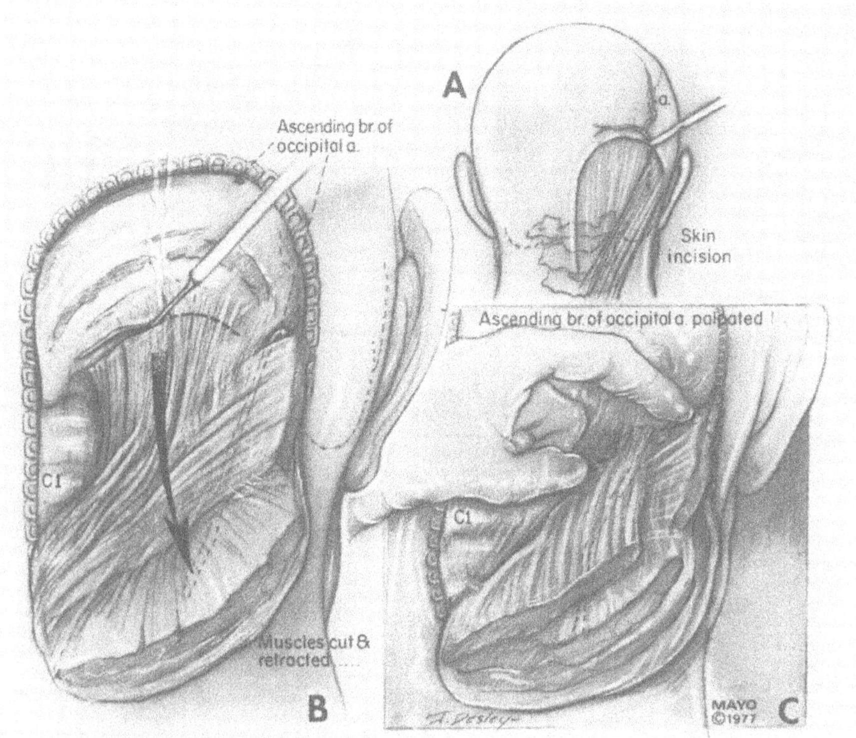

Fig. 1 A-N. Sketch of surgical procedure
A Hockey stick incision extending above level of superior nuchal line.
B Deep neck muscles cut from their insertion leaving a cuff of tissue for closure. C Occipital artery identified in mastoid groove posterior and superior to mastoid process

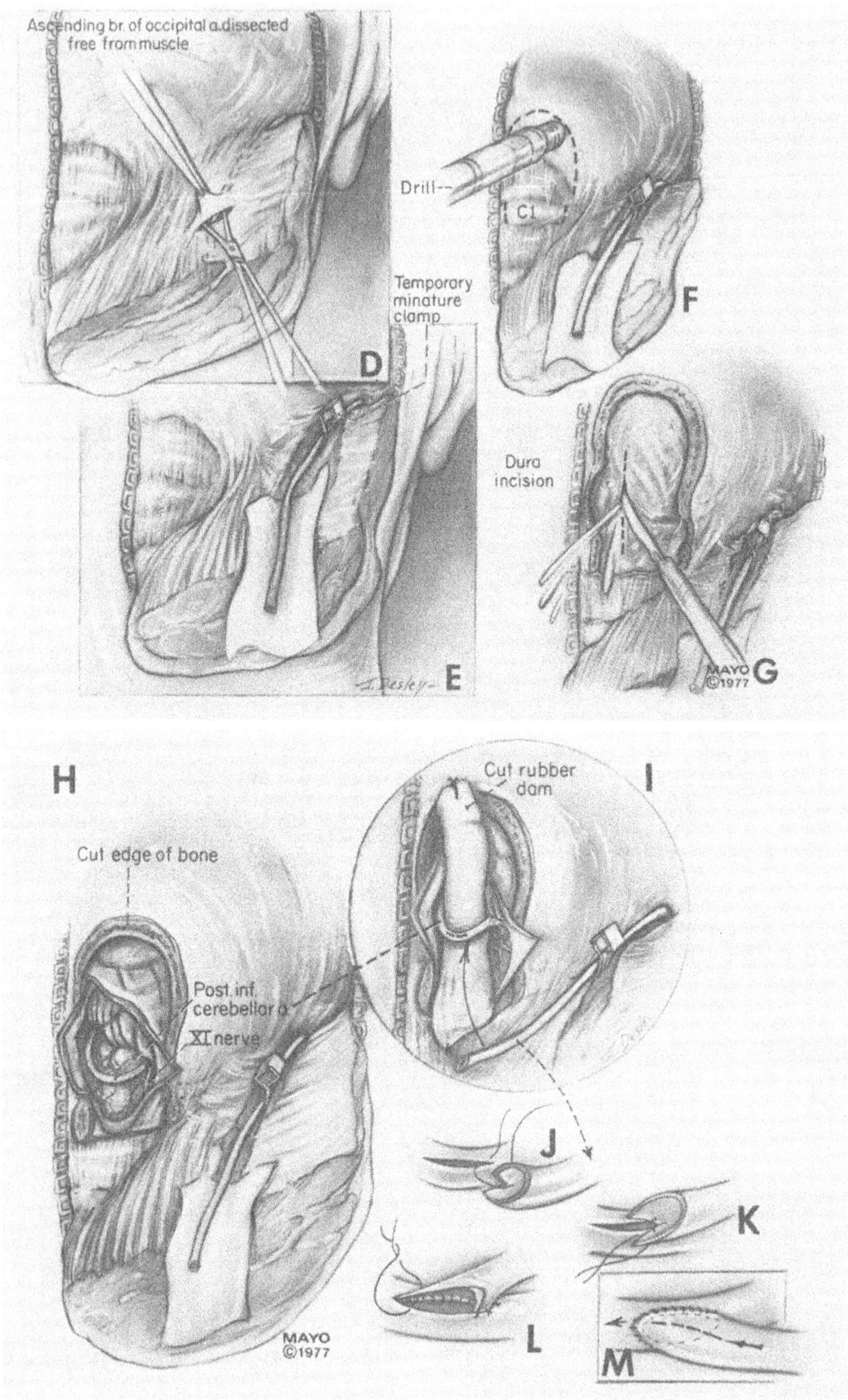
Ascending br. of occipital a. dissected free from muscle
D
Temporary minature clamp
E
Drill
C1
F
Dura incision
MAYO ©1977
G
H
Cut edge of bone
Post. inf. cerebellar a.
XI nerve
MAYO ©1977
Cut rubber dam
I
J
K
L
M

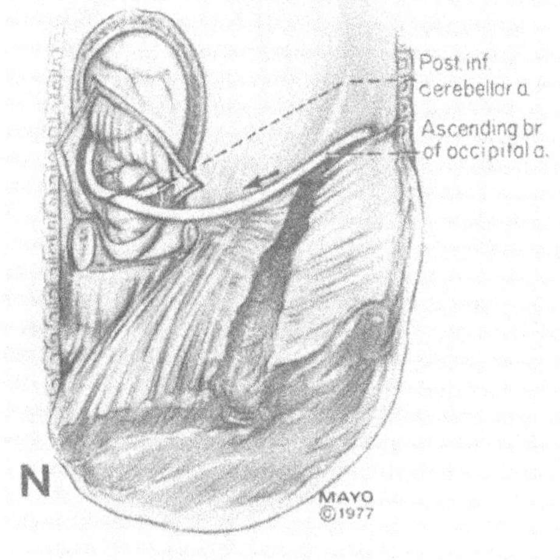

Fig. 1 A-N. Sketch of surgical procedure
D Occipital artery dissected free from adjacent tissue, this vessel lies deep to splenius capitis and longissimus capitis, the dissection is simplified by maintaining this tissue plane. E Occipital artery lying free in muscle bed from which it was dissected. F Small unilateral suboccipital craniectomy along with unilateral resection of arch of C_1. G Dura opened with straight incision. H Dura sutured to margins of craniectomy, medullary loop of PICA identified. I PICA elevated by means of a temporary rubber dam. J PICA opened with linear incision, occipital artery fish-mouthed. K and L Anastomosis performed with interrupted 9-0 monofilament nylon sutures. M Completed anastomosis.
N Transplanted course of occipital artery

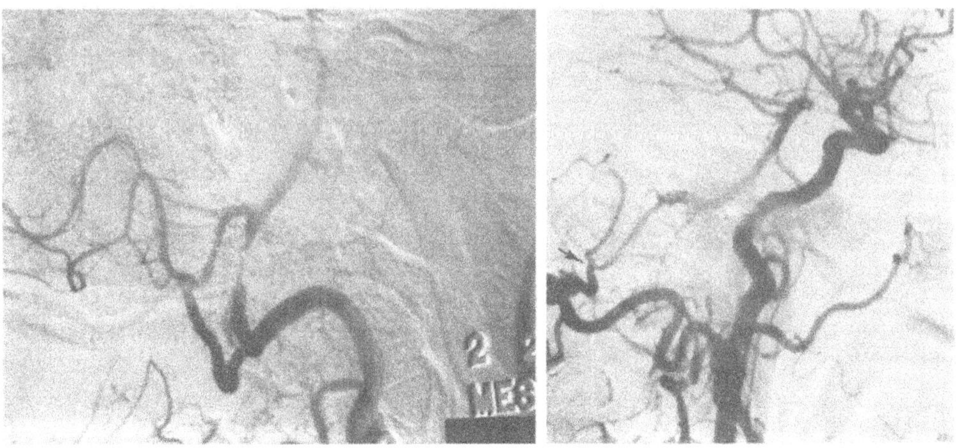

Fig. 2. Typical postoperative angiograms on patients following bypass surgery for intracranial occlusive disease of the vertebral artery proximal to the origin of the posterior inferior cerebellar arteries

Informational Value and Therapeutic Applications of Selective Angiography

J. WAPPENSCHMIDT and E. LINS

Selective arteriography has been frequently used in previous years. Our experience with this method is based on 207 superselective angiographies of the external and internal carotid and 74 superselective investigations of the spinal segmental arteries.

We would like to present some examples that demonstrate the informative value of this method. Among the brain tumors, the meningioma is the ideal lesion for studying the vascular pathology. In meningiomas we distinguish between:

1) Physiologic feeding arteries
2) Intratumoral distributive arteries
3) Capillary vessels

The first case (Fig. 1) shows the superselective arteriography of a fronto-lateral convexity meningioma. The tip of the catheter was placed at the origin of the middle meningeal artery. The large and tortuous branch of the middle meningeal artery is the feeding vessel, running along the lateral side of the tumor to its hilus. Within the tumor it ramifies in a radial fashion. The capillary nutrient vessels appear later - known as the "tumor cloud". It is important to note that the draining veins do not go to the sinus but run along the dura and bone the base of the skull where they join a basal plexus. This means that the part of the tumor fed by the meningeal branches may be drained by the veins of the dura and bone. Another important point is that the homogeneous appearence of the posterior side of the tumor is not well demarcated.

Selective angiography of the internal carotid artery, however, clearly shows that the tumor is also fed by branches of the middle cerebral artery (Fig. 2). It shows the posterior segment of the tumor with its limits clearly demarcated (Fig. 2). This means, that the whole tumor is divided into two segments, one supplied by branches of the internal carotid artery and the other supplied by branches of the external carotid artery.

In another case, internal carotid angiography clearly showed the side of the frontolateral convexity meningioma facing the brain, while the opposite side of the tumor is not clearly demarcated. Selective external carotid arteriography shows the part of the tumor close to the skull to be fed by the frontal branches of the middle meningeal artery and also by the frontal branches of the superficial temporal artery. Special attention must be paid to the vessels of scalp supplying the tumor since the tumor has usually infiltrated the skull.

Regarding subsequent embolization, the multipedicular supply is of a great importance. The tumors best suited for embolization are the meningiomas fed only by the external carotid artery. In such cases the selective arteriography of the external carotid artery shows the entire tumor as a complete circumscribed mass fed only by the middle meningeal artery. Meningosarcomas and hemangiopericytomas are very vascularized tumors with multipedicular feeding, that are also suited for embolization. The feeding arteries of the meningosarcomas are the superficial temporal artery and the occipital arteries. Hemangiopericytomas are fed by branches of the internal and external carotid arteries. Figure 3 demonstrates a metastasis of the right nostril. The catheter is placed in the facial artery. The physiologic feeding artery is a single branch of it.

Glomus tumors are also very vascularized. We observed a case of glomus jugulare metastasis located in the frontal region of the skull. The feeding vessels were branches of the superficial temporal artery and meningeal arteries. The tumor had a homogeneous structure.

Embolization can be best performed in angiomas of the galea, but they are particularly difficult to study angiographically.

Arteriovenous angiomas of the brain show a multipedicular feeding in most cases. Figure 4 shows an angioma located in the parietal region. Selective angiography shows that the main blood supply comes from the parietal branch of the superficial temporal artery and from the retro-auricular artery. The occipital artery also supplies the tumor through numerous lateral branches.

The value of selective angiography consists in:

1) The exact demonstration of the feeding arteries
2) The exact demonstration of the whole tumor and the differentiation between meningeal and cerebral arteries feeding the lesion
3) Sharply circumscribed appearance in cases of poorly opacified tumors

Furthermore, superselective angiography is a definite prequisite for embolization. Before discussing the results of embolization, there are some technical points that should be stressed. The aim is to introduce the embolizing material into the tumor vessels or into the physiologic feeding arteries near the tumor. If the occlusion of the physiologic feeding artery is distant from the tumor, collateral supply may revascularize the lesion. This means that at the beginning of the embolization very small emboli must be used, and larger emboli can only be used later.

Figure 5 shows a typical example: in a case of a parasagittal meningioma there were two feeding vessels from the middle meningeal artery. They were occluded near the tumor. The tumor opacification disappeared (Fig.6). As shown in a previous report (2), neuropathologic examination of an embolized hemangioendothelioma revealed numerous Gelfoam particles and a necrosis within the tumor. In the case of an external carotid cavernous fistula, we were able to occlude the feeding vessel and exophthalmus disappeared (1).

We have performed embolization in 67 patients. We prefer to use materials that are easily absorbed such as Gelfoam, lyophilized dura, and Tabotamp. Embolization was performed in 43 cases of malignant tumor of the skull and the face, the epipharynx, and the glomus jugulare. In cases where surgery was indicated, embolization was used as a preoperative method to reduce the intraoperative bleeding. In cases where surgery could not be performed, embolization was used to interfere with the tumoral metabolism. The main indication for embolization is an angioma. Good results were obtained in fistulas and low-flow angiomas. In angiomas with blood supply from the external carotid artery or multipedicular feeding from different vessels, we can obtain a remarkable temporary reduction of the blood supply. The advantage in using embolization is the reduction of the blood supply, permitting surgical removal of angiomas originally too large for surgery. In cases of meningioma, the indication for embolization is controversial. The optimal tumor is one supplied only by the external carotid artery. In cases of an additional supply from the internal carotid artery, a tumor steal syndrome can appear after occlusion of the branches of the external carotid artery. In these cases, embolization can only be used as a preoperative measure to reduce the blood supply, and surgery must be done shortly thereafter.

References

1. LINS, E., WAPPENSCHMIDT, J.: Transfemorale Embolisation einer Carotis-externa-Sinus-cavernosus-Fistel. Roentgenblaetter 30, 621-625 (1977)
2. WAPPENSCHMIDT, J., LINS, E.: Informational value and the therapeutical application of selective angiography. Adv. Neurosurgery 3, 381-385 (1975)

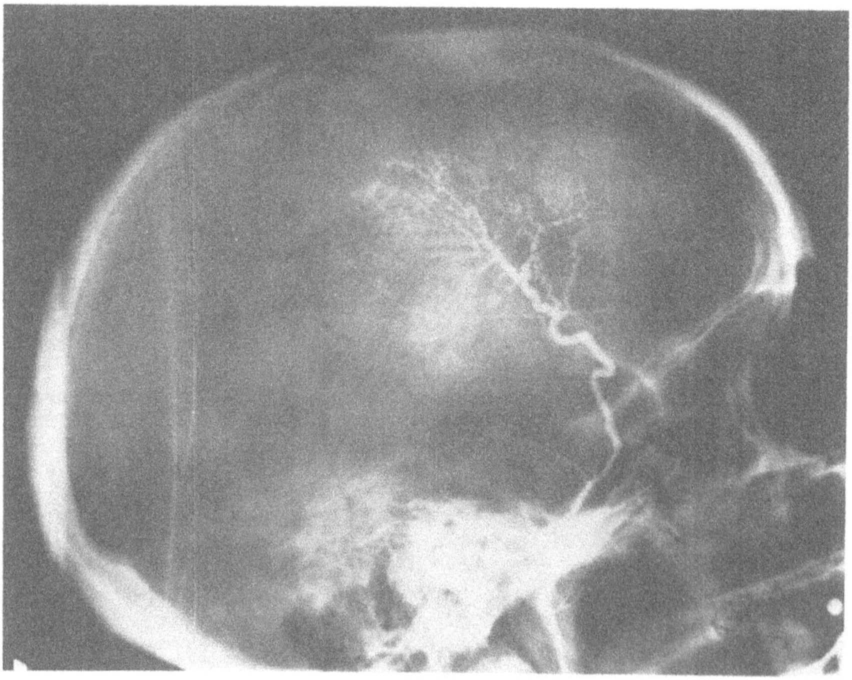

Fig. 1. Superselective arteriography of a fronto-lateral convexity meningioma

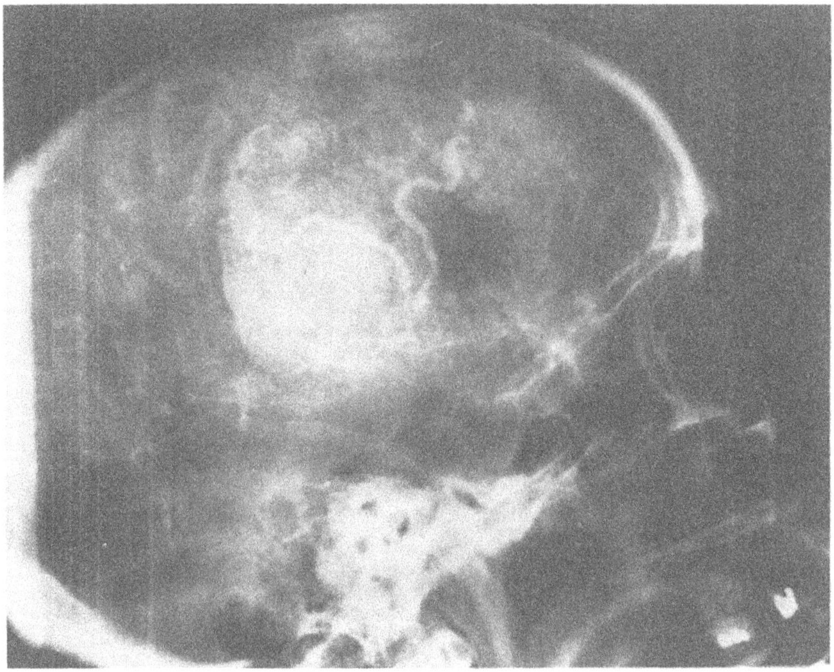

Fig. 2. Selective angiography of the internal carotid artery

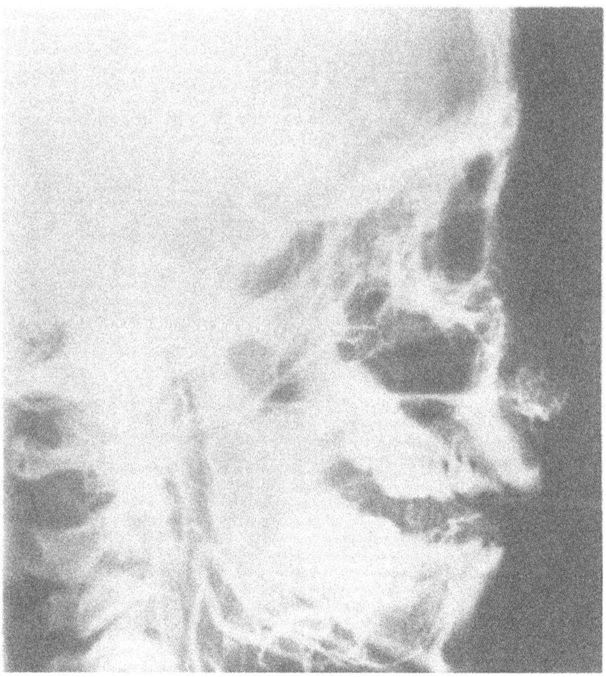

Fig. 3. Tumor metastasis of the right nasal lobe

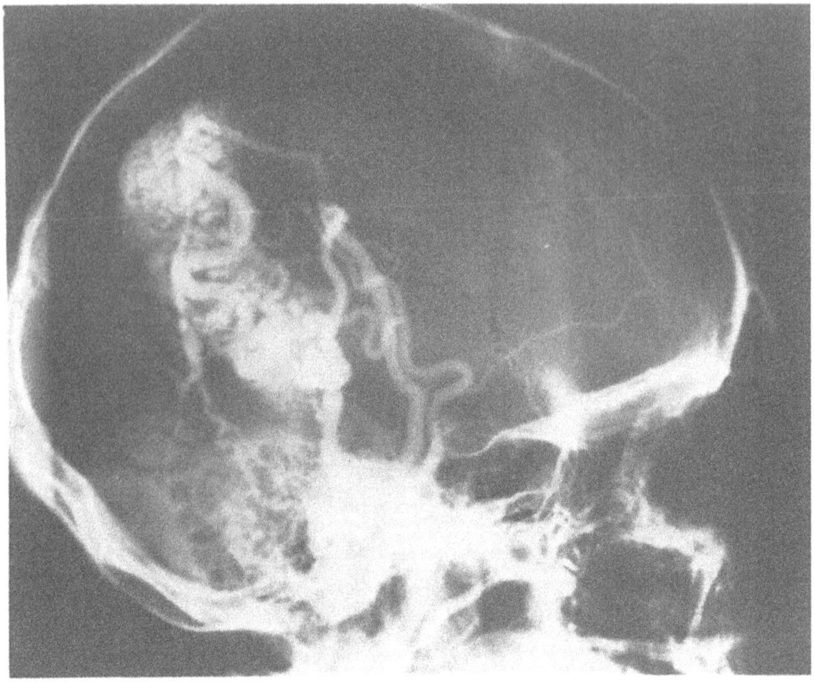

Fig. 4. Suberselective angiography of a parietal angioma

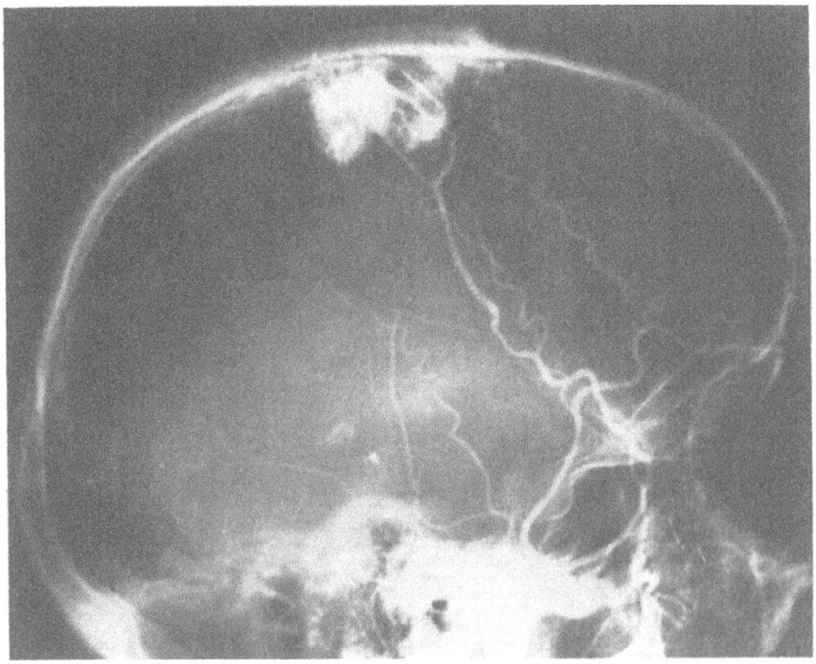

Fig. 5. Superselective arteriography of a parasagittal meningioma

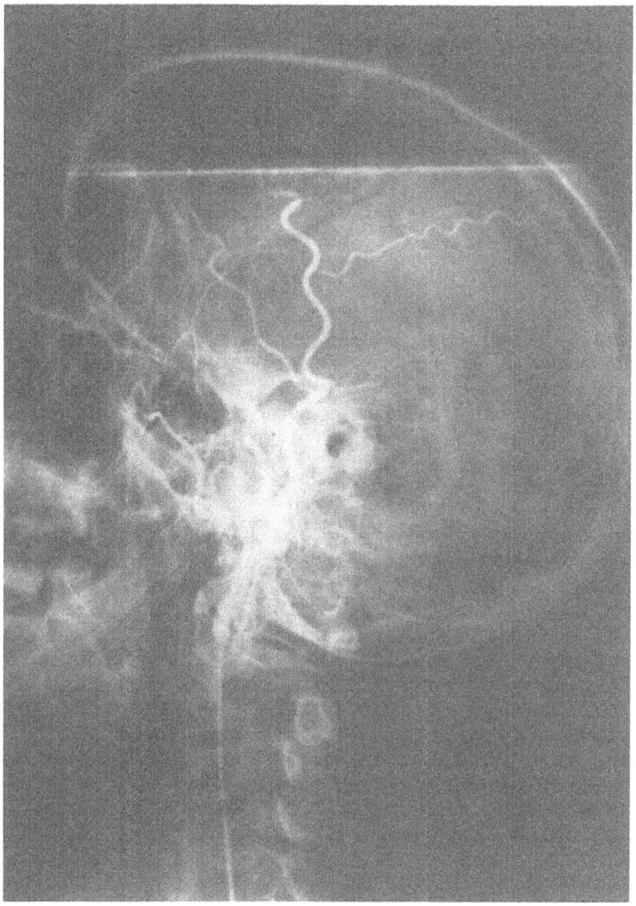

Fig. 6. Superselective arteriography of a parasagittal meningioma after embolization

Surgical Management of Deep-Seated Angiomas of the Brain

K.-A. BUSHE, E. HALVES, and N. SÖRENSEN

In 1974 at the Symposium on Cerebral Angiomas in Gießen (1,2), we made reference to 20 cases of deep-seated arteriovenous angiomas situated in or near to the midline. We had operated on 17, three of whom subsequently died. In two cases, this was due to the necessity of operating in a state of acute progressive hemorrhage. In the meantime significant progress in both neurosurgery and neuroradiology has expanded therapy of A-V malformations and made it safer.

Previously X-ray therapy was used in the treatment of so-called inoperable A-V malformations, but this was generally abandoned as unsuccessful. STEINER et al. (3), however, have revived it in a new form, using selective ionizing radiation from the stereotactic 60 gamma unit. Using this technique, it is possible to achieve up to 90% complete obliteration of the A-V malformation, provided both the malformation and its feeding arteries are irradiated. One disadvantage of this method is that there is a time lapse of between 7 and 19 months following irradiation, before the onset of obliteration, during which there is a constant threat of recurrent hemorrhage. Also, when treating large malformations in functionally important regions with high doses of radiation, this method runs the additional risk of causing serious neurological deficits. Nevertheless, it is a great step forward.

The latest technique in A-V malformation therapy is the Bragg peak proton beam, developed by KJELLBERG and co-workers (4). The high concentration of Bragg peak radiation, together with the stereotactic method, affords precise assessment of localization and extent of radionecrosis in the A-V malformation but has the same disadvantages as the latter method. It is also very expensive and only a few centers in the world can afford such equipment. Therefore, we cannot afford to forget our neurosurgical skills, which, together with modern technology, enable successful surgery of the so-called inoperable deep-seated angiomas.

I would now like to discuss briefly five cases of surgery on angiomas located in the basal ganglia. Prior to the availability of computer tomography (CT), we saw two cases of subependymal angiomas in the area of the trigone.

In a 6-year-old boy, we first tried to approach the angioma in the usual transventricular way. Despite precise angiographic localization and careful inspection during surgery, we were unable to locate the angioma due to its hidden site beneath the ependyma. To avoid further damage from surgical trauma, we abandoned this attempt. In a second operation we approached the dome of the angioma stereotactically, removing it transventricularly using the operating microscope. Although the thalamostriate veins had to be clipped, the postoperative course was without further complication. The boy subsequently showed no residual clinical signs.

In a 19-year-old girl, we were able to remove an angioma located in the same area, applying the experience gained from the previous case. The extirpation was much more difficult because of the very small ventricles. The postoperative course proceeded without complications, apart from slight extrapyramidal disorders. In the meantime, the patient has enjoyed a normal pregnancy and given birth to a healthy child.

In our experience, a combination of the stereotactic and open methods has proved satisfactory. The A-V malformation can be exposed with great accuracy through a small approach and clearly removed under the microscope. The other three cases suffered from apoplectiform onset and all showed signs of a massive intraventricular hemorrhage. The development was followed by repeated CT.

In the case of a 16-year-old girl, the following symptoms developed: headache, nausea, vomiting, and loss of consciousness. A few hours later she was in a coma. Angiography, carried out at her local hospital, suggested the presence of an angioma fed by the left posterior choroidal artery (Fig. 1). Four days after onset, CT showed blood within the left frontal horn, the cella media, and the left posterior horn (Fig. 2). A small increase of density was recorded in the supposed region of the angioma. Further CT controls followed. Twelve days after the acute onset (1 day before operation), only slight traces of the hemorrhage remained. At the same time we carried out air encephalography (Fig. 3) and angiography (Fig. 4), which showed that the malformation fed by the posterior choroidal artery was in direct relation to the left lateral horn. On the 13th day of illness, we extirpated a subependymal bean-sized angioma from the trigone of the left lateral ventricle. The girl recovered slowly after the operation.

While trying to crank up a diesel engine, a 53-year-old patient started to suffer from ventricular bleeding. Right brachial angiotomography in two planes demonstrated an A-V malformation, probably fed by the lateral posterior choroidal artery and emptying into the unshifted great vein of Galen. Computer tomography also showed a ventricular bleeding. A control, a week later, showed that the clot had disappeared almost entirely.

During surgery, using the same technique as before, we removed a walnut-sized clot lying on the ependyma. Upon opening the ependyma, we found and removed a pea-sized angioma, clipping the feeding vessels. The patient recovered so well that he was able to return to his job as a plumber. The temporary hemianopia has improved greatly.

An 11-year-old boy fell ill at school for no apparant reason, complaining of headache and vomiting. He soon lost consciousness, suffering from an extreme left-sided hemiparesis. On the day of onset a CT scan showed massive intraventricular bleeding. Angiography again revealed an A-V angioma within the trigone of the right lateral ventricle. Since there was no disappearance of the intraventricular clot at repeated CT scans, we operated on the boy 9 days after onset. A walnut-sized subependymal angioma was removed from the trigone. The seriously ill boy recovered rather quickly after surgery and was awake and cooperative within a week. The hemipareses improved with the help of physiotherapy so that the boy was able to walk alone. One year after surgery there still is a slight psychosyndrome and a left-sided hemiparesis. The boy has been admitted to a rehabilitation center.

Surgery was successful in four cases without severe neurological deficits. Only in the case of the 11-year-old boy did the massive intracerebral and intraventricular bleeding result in residual neurological disorders.

In our experience, it is best to delay operation, while carrying out constant neurological controls and CT scans until the ventricular bleeding has been arrested and the clot has disappeared. This is generally accompanied by an improvement of the overall clinical condition. Only in cases where the symptoms are well advanced and where there is no neurological improvement, as in the case of the 11-year-old boy, should an early operation be attempted. As this synopsis has proved, however, angiomas of the basal ganglia, mostly fed by the posterior choroidal artery, can be considered operable with no surgical mortality.

References

1. BUSHE, K.-A., BOCKHORN, J., SCHÄFER, E.R.: Macro- and microsurgery of central angiomas. In: Cerebral angiomas. PIA, H.W., GLEAVE, J. R.W., GROTE, E., ZIERSKI, J. (eds.). Berlin, Heidelberg, New York: Springer 1975
2. BUSHE, K.-A., Peterson, E., SCHÄFER, E.R.: Surgical indications for arterio-venous angiomas in functionally important regions and in case of spreading within the area of the ventricular system and the basal ganglia. In: Present limits of neurosurgery. Prague: Avicenum, Czechosloval Medical Press 1972
3. STEINER, L., BACKLUND, E.-O., GREITZ, T., LEKSELL, L., NOREN, G., RÄHN, T.: Radiosurgery in intracranial arterio-venous malformations II. A follow-up study. Excerpta Med. Int. Congr. Ser. 433 (1978)
4. KJELLBERG, R.N., POLETTI, C.E., ROBERSON, S. H., ADAMS, R.D.: Bragg peak proton beam treatment of arterio-venous malformations of the brain. Excerpta Med. Int. Congr. Ser. 433 (1978)

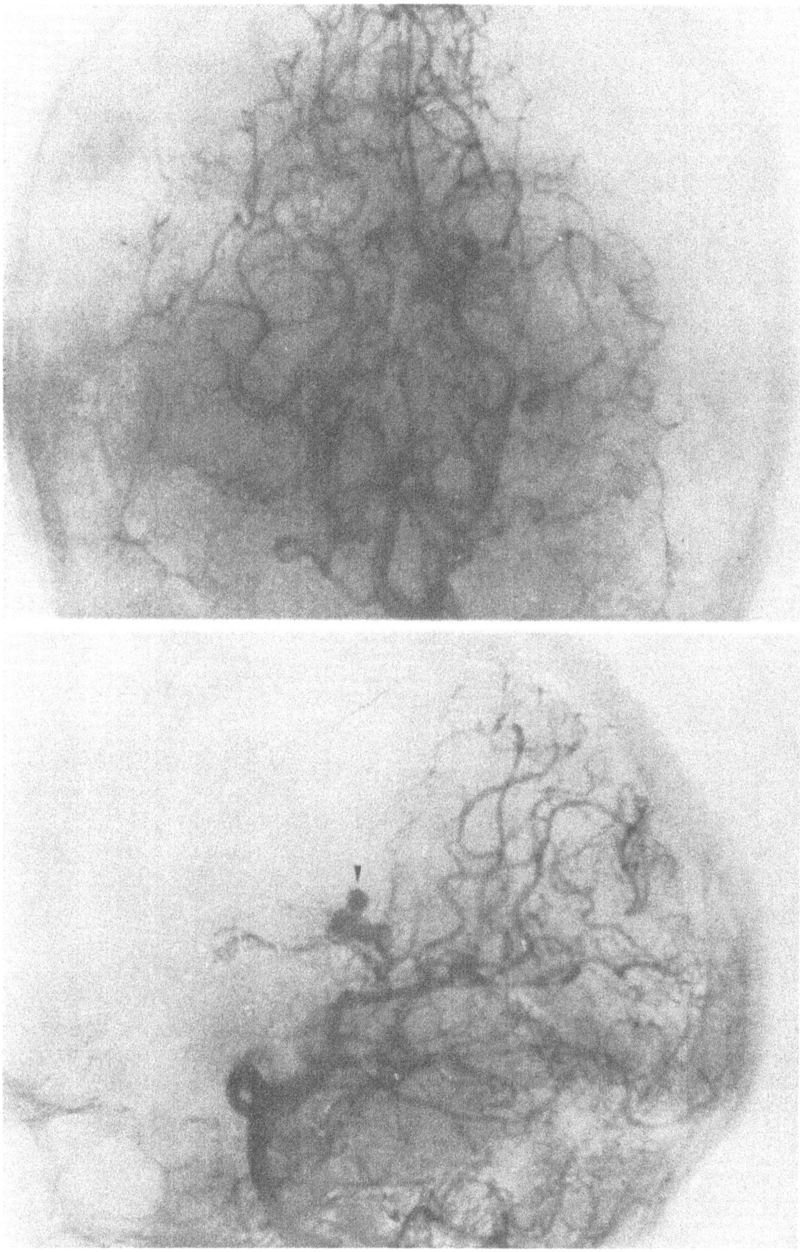

Fig. 1. Angioma, fed by the left posterior choroidal artery

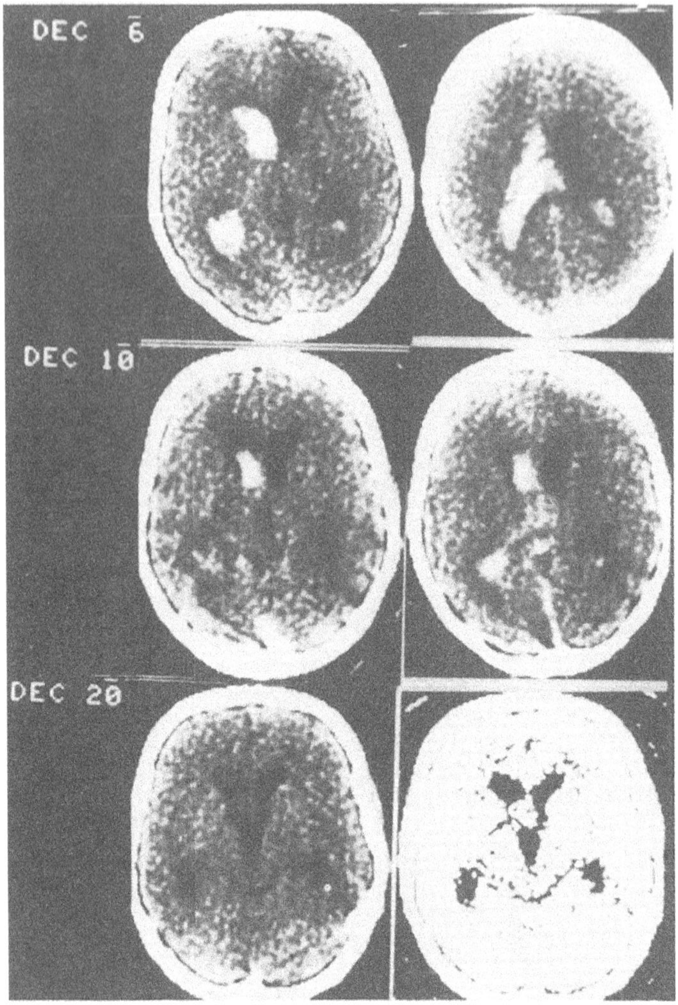

Fig. 2. Four days after acute bleeding the CT shows blood within the left frontal horn, the cella media, and the left posterior horn. A small increase of density is recorded in the supposed region of the angioma

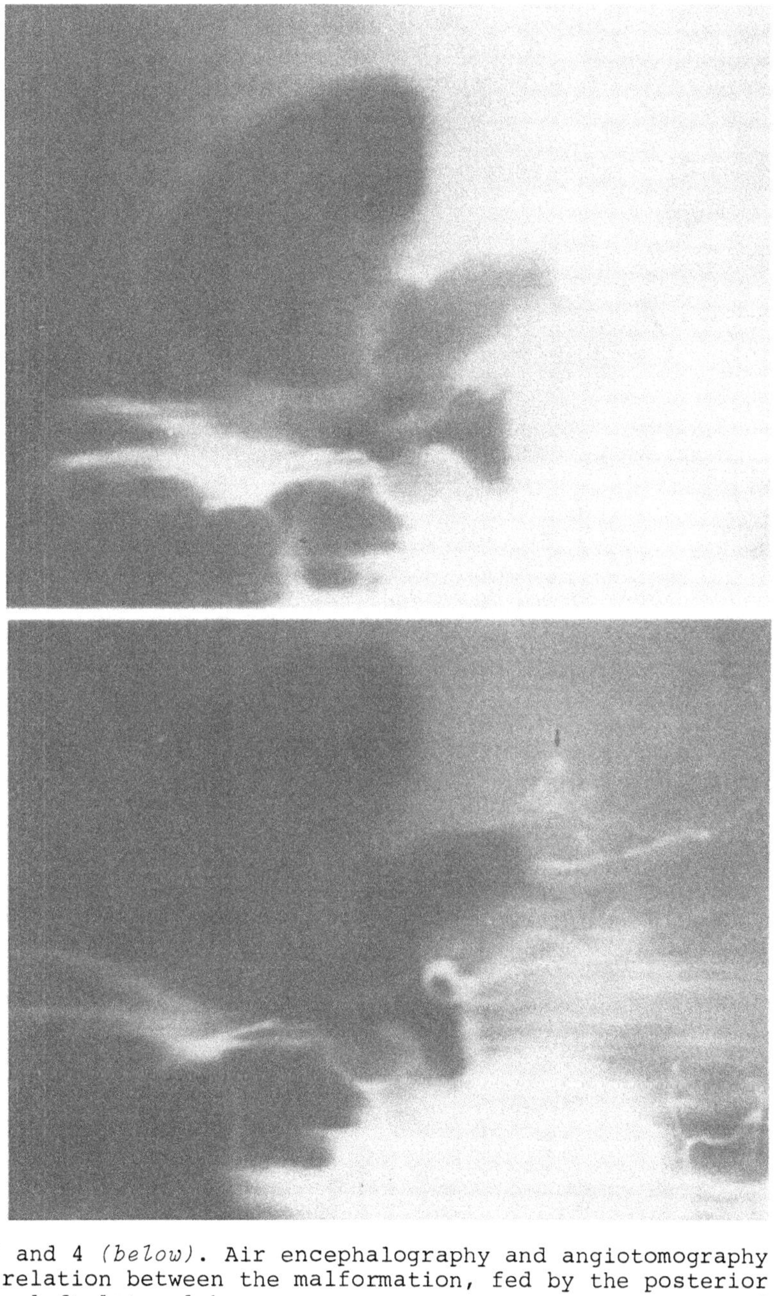

Fig. 3 *(above)* and 4 *(below)*. Air encephalography and angiotomography show a direct relation between the malformation, fed by the posterior artery, and the left lateral horn

Treatment of Intramedullary Angiomas

H. W. PIA

The operative treatment of spinal angiomas owes much to the crucial impulses toward improved and earlier diagnosis provided by selective spinal angiography and the technical adavances resulting from microsurgery and embolization. Indications and operations have been extended; however, many questions concerning the special indications and operative procedures, especially of the intramedullary and ventral angiomas, remain obscure or debatable.

This contribution is based on my personal experience with 231 spinal vascular anomalies and 197 patients (Table 1) and on close and stimulating cooperation with interested neurosurgeons in this field, especially with my close friend, the late RENÉ DJINDJIAN, the great pioneer of angiography and embolization of spinal angiomas.

Table 1. Spinal angiomas observed at the Neurosurgical University in Gießen, Germany, 1953 - 1977

Angiomas	No. of angiomas	No. of patients	Solitary angiomas	Complex angiomas No.	%
Vertebral	23	7	7	16	70
Extradrual	54	46	29	25	46
Intradural	72	63	55	17	24
Angioblastomas	12	11	4	8	67
	161	127	95	66	41
Lumbosacral vascular anomalies	70	70	70		
Total	231	197	164		

Of 161 true spinal angiomas in 127 patients, there were 72 intradural angiomas, as solitary angiomas in 54 and complex angiomas in 24, and an additional 12 angioblastomas, 8 of which were complex by the combination of true angioma with an angioblastoma. The intradural complex angiomas are combined extra-intradural and global angiomas with involvement of all continuous layers from skin to the cord itself.

In our material of 84 intradural angiomas there were

Dorsal extramedullary angiomas in 42%
Intramedullary angiomas in 18%
Extra- and intramedullary angiomas in 32%
global angiomas in 8% (Figs. 1 and 2).

Of 54 intramedullary or combined angiomas (58%) we found *intramedullary hematomas* in 6%-7%.

Our figures correspond with those of the Lariboisière/Paris group of R. DJINDJIAN + and HOUDART (Table 2): 60 cases (40%) were dorsal extramedullary angiomas and 90 (60%) intramedullary or combined-mixed angiomas. There are two main localizations of intramedullary or intra-extramedullary angiomas:

1) Cervical cord in the vast majority of cases
2) Dorsolumbosacral parts of the cord and dorsal part of the cord with the same incidence .

Table 2. Localization and arterial supply of spinal angiomas[a]

Site	Dorsal spinal angiomas	Anterior spinal angiomas	Combined supply	Total	%
Cervical	1	5	15	21	14
Upper dorsal D_1 - D_6	12	10	11	33	22
Lower dorsal-sacral and cauda equina	47	17	32	96	64
Total	60 (40%)	32 (21%)	58 (39%)	150	

a Material Service de Neurochirurgie et de Neuroradiologie de Lariboisière, Paris (R.HOUDART and R.DJINDJIAN †).

Diagnosis of Intramedullary Angiomas

The fate of patients with intramedullary angiomas depends completely on early diagnosis at the stage of a still reversible cord lesion. *From the clinical point of view*, the following symptoms and signs are highly suspicious:

1) *Early age* with maximum in the 2nd and 3rd decades
2) *Spinal subarachnoid hemorrhage* (50% of cases)
3) *Acute onset* and an *apoplectic or remittent course*
4) Associated malformations (30% of cases)
5) *Cervical localization* (almost always intramedullary angioma)

The morphologic intraoperative findings (Fig. 3) are often misleading. The differentiation between a huge dorsal or lateral isolated extramedullary and combined extra-intramedullary angioma can be impossible. In ventral angiomas the dorsal surface of the cord usually has a normal appearance. Subpial capillary angiomas are usually located extra- and intramedullary and may not be seen from the dorsal side. It may be impossible to differentiate between the feeding and draining vessels. Even such criterion as apparently angiomatous vessels entering or leaving the cord is not always absolutely reliable for recognizing the intramedullary angioma.

Selective spinal angiography with pictures in the anteroposterior and lateral projection and visualization of the inflow and outflow phase is absolutely necessary (Fig. 4a and b). Still, this absolute prerequisite has not been fulfilled in many cases in the past. *Myelography* with water-soluble contrast medium improved the early diagnosis of angiomas; however, the differentiation between an extra- or intramedullary localization or confirmation of such localization is not possible with this investigation.

Treatment

Even with optimal diagnostic conditions, the decision on which special procedure should be adopted demands the visualization of the cord in spite of the above mentioned difficulties. Without experience with these diagnostic procedures, no judgment on the operative indications is permitted.

Operative Procedures

Operative management (Table 3) as used in Paris since 1961 and in Gießen since 1954 reflects the possibilities of treatment and the development of preoperative approach in the last 20 years.

Table 3. Operative procedures in intramedullary angiomas

	No.	No. therapy	Palliative operations	Excision	Embolization
Paris	90	15	26	30	19
Gießen	49	4	25	19	1
Total	139	19 (14%)	51 (37%)	49 (35%)	20 (14%)

No therapy at all or explorative and/or decompressive laminectomy was not rare until recently in both departments; however, in total, such operations constituted only 14% of operative procedures.

Palliative Procedures

In one-half of the cases in our series and in one-third of the patients in Paris (in total almost 40%), palliative measures were used, which stresses the considerable difficulties that are encountered in the treatment of these angiomas.

Extra- and intradural ligatures of the main feeders were often used with the palliative measures in the department in Paris. For some time the results were regarded as quite satisfactory. Personally, I have never seen the disappearance of the angioma or interruption of the A-V shunt after sectioning the feeders in patients with "normal" angiomas. My experience is that the closure of the feeders alone results in development of new feeders out of the vessels that supplied the cord, resulting in deterioration of the steal syndrome.

Dorsal commissural myelotomy has been used in the last few years more often, similarly to the more active approach to intramedullary tumors. So far no definite conclusions about this procedure are possible.

Dividing the *arachnoidal adhesions and strangulations* and enlargement of the dural sac through suturing in a piece of *lyophilized dura* may be helpful. This procedure is at present all that we can do for patients with subpial capillary angiomas.

The complete excision of the angioma (Fig. 5) is the only logical operation. Only in such a way can the A-V shunt be eliminated and the permanent oxygen deficit and compression of the medulla removed. As logical as this may be, there are several handicaps that may render the excision impossible. Among them is the *size of the angioma,* which is sometimes larger than the cord itself. Try to imagine a cerebral angioma with the same relation of lesion to normal tissues. The other handicap is the *localization of the angioma,* particularly the ventral one. Other limiting factors are the degree of the cord damage with related *clinical picutre,* the duration of the disease, the patient's age, etc., and last but not least the *experience and attitude of the surgeon.*

In our series, patients in whom *total or partial excision* (Fig. 6) was performed constitute 35% of cases. Partial excision performed for extra-intramedullary angiomas in which the extramedullary part was removed was certainly not optimal, but it was quite satisfactory, and even today such an excision should be performed in particularly difficult cases.

Thanks to the microsurgical technique, *total extirpation* could be attempted. I recall the series of 12 cases of cervical angiomas reported by YASARGIL. Localized "encapsulated or cystic angiomas" in the center of the cord occurring in children or in adolescents with minimal neurological signs are the best indication for such total extipration. Old patients with far advanced neurological deficits or paraplegia are not qualified for extirpation of the lesion. The technique of removal is much less complicated than supposed. Combined angiomas and global angiomas are seldom, and the latter are never completely excisable.

Table 4. Operative procedures in intramedullary angiomas

		Normal	Improved	?	No. change	Worse	Dead
Total excision	9	3	2	1	2	1	1
Partial excision	10	2	3	2	2	-	-
Decompression	25	1	8	7	6	-	3
No treatment	5	1	-	-	1	3	-
Total	49	7	13	10	11	4	4

Table 5. Prognosis of spinal intradural angiomas

Type of angioma	No.	Normal	Better	Improved	Unchanged	Worse	Dead
Dorsal subarachnoid a.	35	7	10	9	5	3	1
Intramedullary a.	15	2	3	4	5	1	-
Intramedullary hematoma	6	-	1	2	1	1	(1)
Extra-intramedullary a.	27	3	10	3	5	3	3
Global a.	-	2	-	3	1	-	1

Our results (Tables 4 and 5) show that approximately 40% of patients improve, 40% of patients remain the same, and the minority of patients become worse after the operation. Mortality is connected with the sequelae of paraplegia and caused by pulmonary emboli or nephrogenic complications in older patients. Dramatic improvements from grade IV, i.e., condition with minimal residual motor function, to grade I, i.e., to normal motor function, are exceptional. In a "normal" case, the preoperative deficit should be minimal and should remain so. We do not think now that it is justified to attempt total extirpation in patients who were unable to stand up or to walk for many years have no chances for improvement. The type of angioma plays an important role as far as the results are concerned. Dorsal angiomas have, or course, the best prognosis, and angiomas combined with intramedullary hematomas the worst.

Embolization introduced and developed by R. DJINDJIAN in Paris and DOPPMAN in Washington unfortunately provided no solution for the most difficult or inoperable ventral and intramedullary angiomas. The two main arteries, the artery of the cervical enlargement and the artery of Adamkiewicz (the artery of lumbar enlargement), are the main feeders for the angiomas of that localization. Occlusion of these arteries amounts to a catastrophe with severe complications and even death, as happened in one of the patients (Figs. 7 and 8). The effect of embolization is similar to that of the ligature of feeders, i.e., transient and incomplete. It is too early to say if the embolization will retain its place as, for instance, the first procedure before an attempted excision or as the only procedure, for instance, in patients with severe spasms and paraplegia. There is no doubt that the technical progress has permitted a more active approach to intramedullary angiomas. However, the early diagnosis is the most important prerequisite.

References

1. DJINDJIAN, M.: Clinical symptomatology and natural history of arteriovenous malformations of the spinal cord. In: Spinal angiomas. Advances in diagnosis and therapy. PIA, H.W., DJINDJIAN, R. (eds.). Berlin, Heidelberg, New York: Springer 1978
2. DOPPMAN, J. L.: Embolization of spinal arteriovenous malformations. In: Spinal angiomas. Advances in diagnosis and therapy. PIA, H.W., DJINDJIAN, R. (eds.). Berlin, Heidelberg, New York: Springer 1978

3. PIA, H.W.: Operative treatment of arteriovenous malformations of the spinal cord. In: Neurological surgery. Internat. congr. series No. 433. Amsterdam, Oxford: Excerpta Medica 1977

4. PIA, H.W., DJINDJIAN, R.: Spinal angiomas. Advances in diagnosis and therapy. Berlin, Heidelberg, New York: Springer 1978

5. REY, A., DJINDJIAN, M., DJINDJIAN, R., HOUDART, R.: Surgical treatment of intramedullary and anterior spinal angiomas. In: Spinal angiomas. Advances in diagnosis and therapy. PIA, H.W., DJINDJIAN, R. (eds.). Berlin, Heidelberg, New York: Springer 1978

6. YASARGIL, M. G., DELONG, B., GUARNASCHELLI, H.: Complete microsurgical excision of cervical extramedullary and intramedullary vascular malformations. Surg. Neurol. 4, 211-224 (1975)

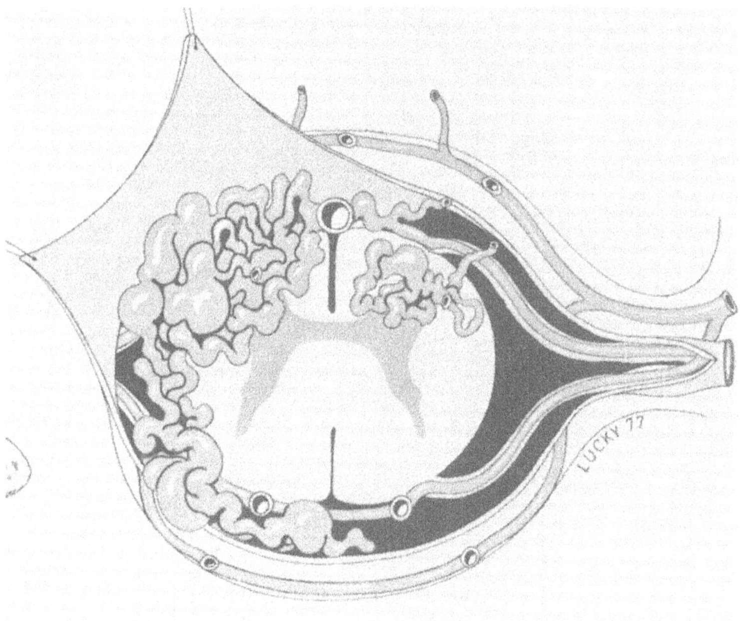

Fig. 1. Extra-intramedullary angioma

Fig. 2. Global angioma

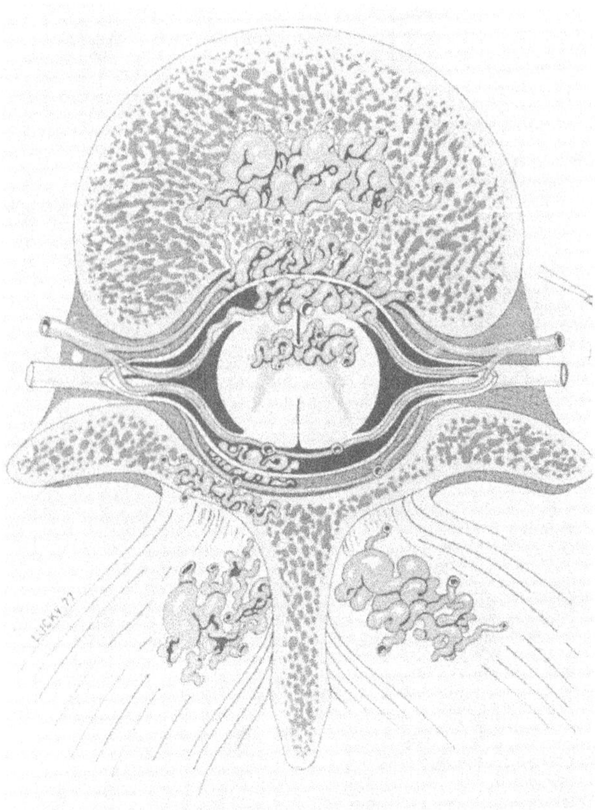

Fig. 3. Forms of intramedullary angiomas (after M. and R. DJINDJIAN)

▽

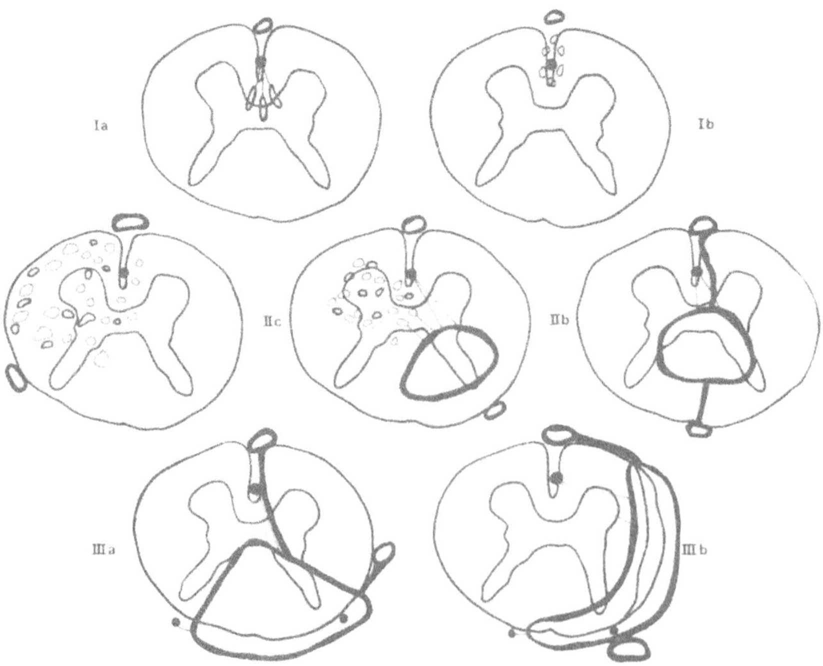

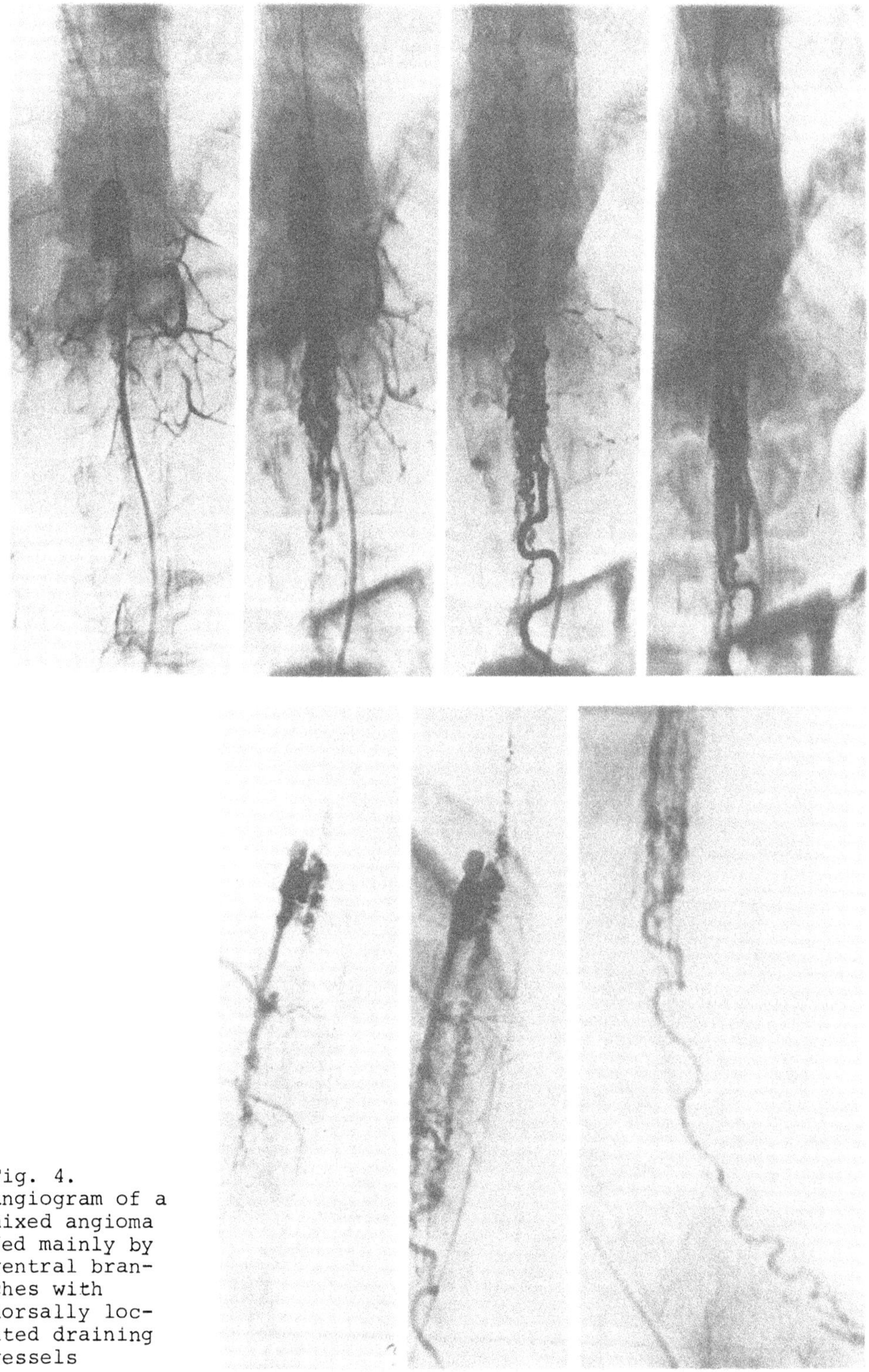

a

b

Fig. 4.
Angiogram of a mixed angioma fed mainly by ventral branches with dorsally located draining vessels

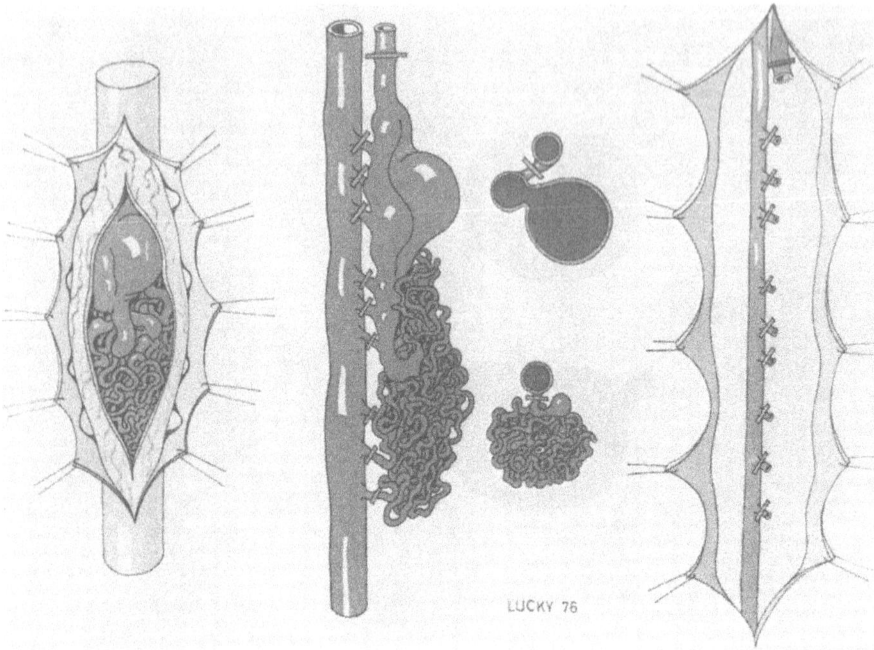

Fig. 5. Extirpation of an intramedullary angioma fed by anterior or spinal artery system

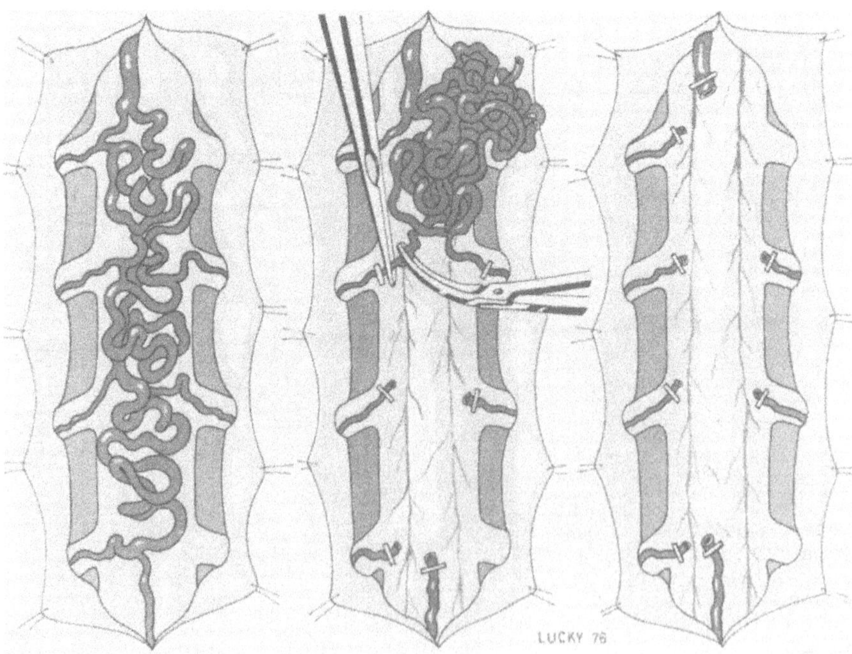

Fig. 6. Excision of a dorsal extramedullary angioma

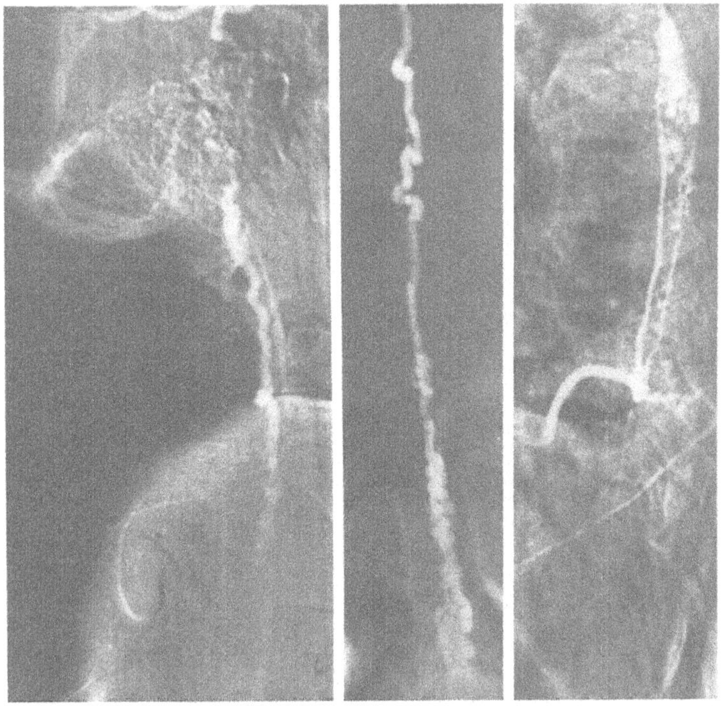

a

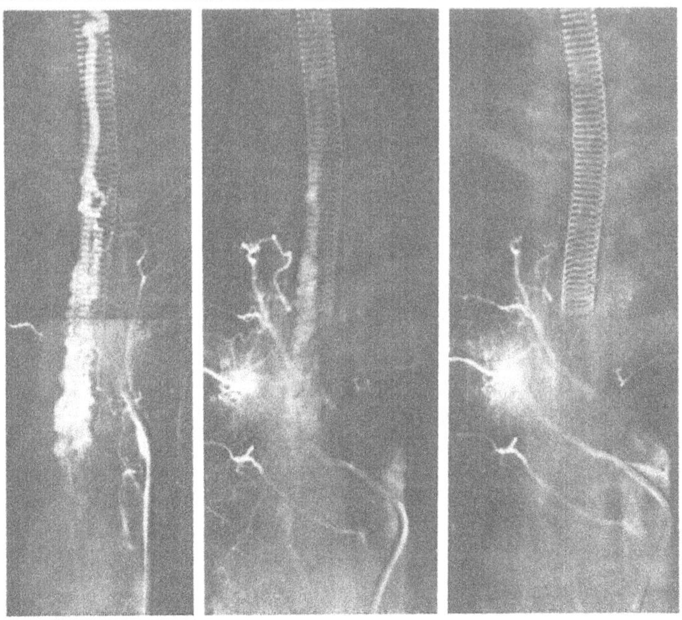

b

Fig. 7a - c. Huge extra- and intramedullary angioma of the dorselumbar region with draining vessels in the middle fossa. After embolization of seven feeders (a), there was no filling of the angioma on both sides (b)

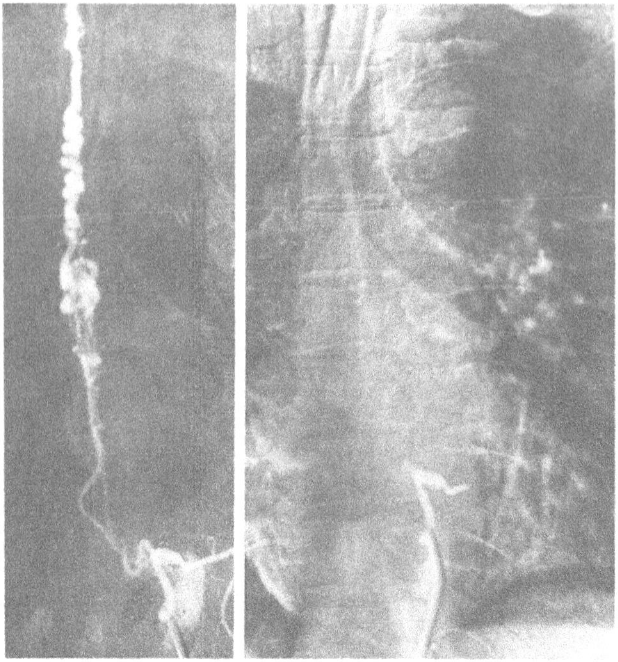

Fig. 7. c Two weeks later there was filling of angioma via the ascending branch of the artery of Adamkiewicz. Embolization of this artery and no opacification of the angioma

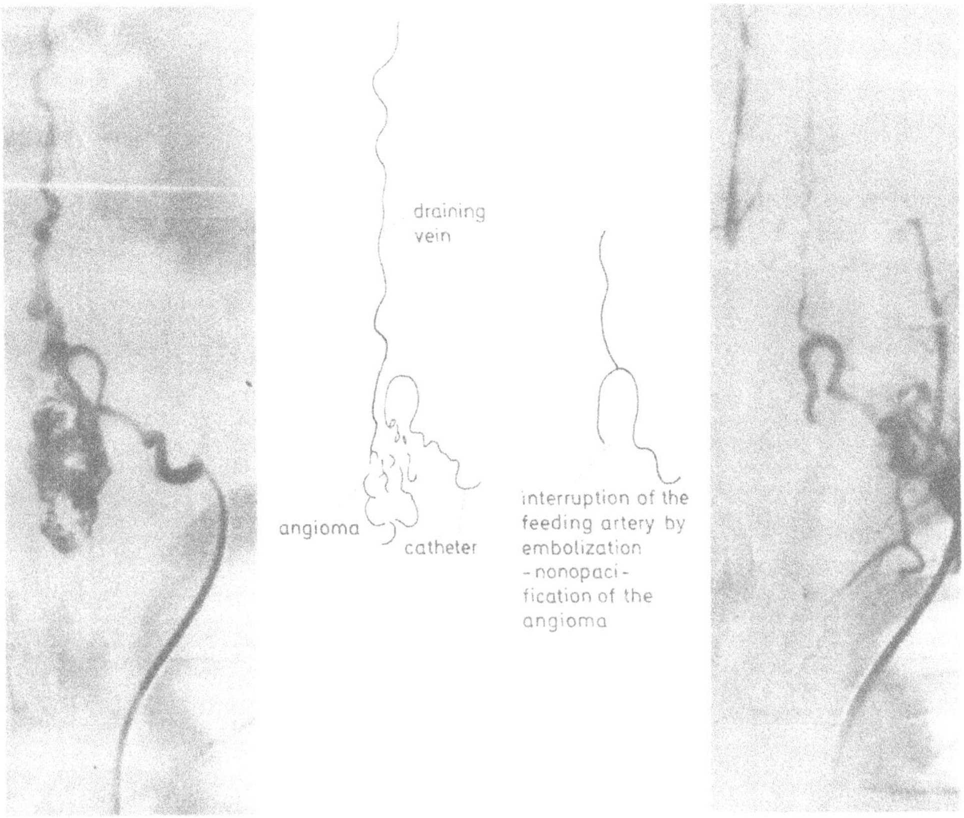

Fig. 8. Cervical intramedullary angioma embolized by R. DJINDJIAN

Results of Early Aneurysmorrhaphy in Good Risk Patients

W. E. HUNT and C. A. MILLER

Introduction

Over the last 3 decades there has been debate among neurosurgeons as to the optimal time for surgical repair of intracranial aneurysms. Many clinics have demonstrated that the risk of aneurysmorrhaphy should be under 3% when the aneurysm has never bled or when the patient has completely recovered from the last bleeding episode (2,3,5,9,11,12). This has caused many surgeons to delay aneurysmorrhaphy for a week or more to achieve minimal surgical mortality. This low surgical mortality, however, may be achieved at the cost of significant mortality and morbidity from rebleeding or from ischemic infarction during the period of medical therapy (7,9). The overall mortality in all series remains high, from 25% - 60% (6,8,12). It is not yet clear what the influence of various medical regimens may be on the Scylla and Charybdis or rebleeding versus infarction.

Materials and Approach

The experience with 556 intracranial aneurysms at The Ohio State University and Affiliated Hospitals has been analyzed in three series: the 12 years from 1954 - 1966, the 6 years from 1966 - 1972, and the 6 years from 1972 - 1978 (Table 1). It has been our policy throughout to operate early on patients with no neurological deficit, with our without meningismus (grades I and II), and to defer operation in patients with neurological deficit (grades III - V) except in the presence of life-threatening hematoma (Table 2). Significant vasospasms on angiography moves the patient into the next worse grade. A grade II risk may thereby be classified grade III and assigned to medical rather than surgical treatment.

Table 1. Grade at admission (1954 - 1978)

Grade	1954-1966	1966-1972	1972-1978	Total	Survival (%)
I	61	30	24	115	90
II	88	42	32	162	79
III	79	60	44	183	74
IV	35	12	24	71	46
V	12	2	11	25	8
Total	275	146	135	556	73

Table 2. Classification of patients with intracranial aneurysms according to surgical risk

Category	Critaria[a]
Grade O[b]	Unruptured
Grade I	Asymptomatic or minimal headache and slight nuchal rigidity
Grade Ia[b]	No acute meningeal or brain reaction, but with fixed neurological deficit
Grade II	Moderate to severe headache, nuchal rigidity, no neurological deficit other than cranial nerve palsy
Grade III	Drowsiness, confusion, or mild focal deficit
Grade IV	Stupor, moderate to severe hemiparesis, possibly early deceberate rigidity and vegetative disturbances
Grade V	Deep coma, deceberate rigidity, moribund appearance

a Serious systemic disease such as hypertension, diabetes, severe arteriosclerosis, chronic pulmonary disease, and severe vasospasm seen on arteriography result in assignment to the next less favorable category.

b Not included in the original 1968 classification.

Angiograms are made as soon as possible after admission, regardless of clinical status. Should the patient have no neurological deficit and no spasm, the aneurysmorrhaphy is done within 24 h regardless of the day posthemorrhage. If surgery is postponed due to neurological deficit, the next angiogram is done when the deficit has cleared. If it is postponed due to spasm, the next angiogram is done 7 - 10 days later. In some cases, persistent spasm has delayed operation for several weeks.

When a repeat angiogram is indicated, surgery is planned for the same day. If spasm is still present, operation is again postponed. In the past few years, virtually every patient has had an angiogram within 24 h prior to operation. The day of repeat angiography is largely governed by the clinical status. Most patients have had postoperative angiograms as well.

As a result of these policies, we have done 284 angiograms on 135 patients from January 1972 to March 1978. Twenty-nine (27%) patients met our criteria for operation within the 1st week posthemorrhage and 15 (11%) within the 2nd week. The results of these cases are reported herein.

Results

Over the 24-year period covered by this study, surgical mortality in grade I and grade O cases has remained very low (Table 3). It has been O in the last 29 patients admitted to the hospital in grades I or II and operated within 72 h of their most recent hemorrhage in the absence of vasospasm.

The surgical mortality in grade II risks has dropped from 22% in the initial 12-year series to O in the 1972-1978 period. This could be

Table 3. Outcome related to grade at operation (1954 - 1978)

Grade	Series	No.	Deaths	Survival
I	1954-1866	71	1	
	1966-1972	34	3	$\frac{154}{158}$ = 97%
	1972-1978	53	0	
		158	4	
II	1954-1966	58	13	
	1966-1972	66	6	$\frac{142}{161}$ = 88%
	1972-1978	37	0	
		161	19	
III	1954-1966	20	8	
	1966-1972	14	9	$\frac{23}{44}$ = 52%
	1972-1978	10	4	
		44	21	
IV	1954-1966	7	3	
	1966-1972	3	3	$\frac{4}{12}$ = 33%
	1972-1978	2	2	
		12	8	
V	1954-1966	0	0	
	1966-1972	1	1	$\frac{2}{6}$ = 33%
	1972-1978	5	3	
		6	4	
Total		381	56	$\frac{325}{381}$ = 85%

related to improved technique, but since delay of operation, due to immediate preoperative angiography, has occurred in a significant number of cases, the grade II risks, in the early years, doubtless included some cases that would not be operated today.

We have analyzed the entire series and compared our recent experience with our earlier experience. We note that, in spite of lower surgical mortality and a decrease in the rate of rebleeding, the overall mortality (based on all cases arriving at the hospital alive) has only fallen from 28% - 24%.

Discussion

ALVORD reports a 50% risk of dying within the first 3 weeks posthemorrhage (2,1). While there is no doubt that our regimen of medical therapy followed by surgery at an appropriate time improves in most reported series treated by medical means alone (7,9,12), we are dismayed that our reduction in surgical mortality has not produced much change in overall mortality. An attempt to determine the cause of death in the unoperated cases is, at present, underway.

Inasmuch as many of our patients have had more than one preoperative angiogram and virtually all of them have had a postoperative angiogram, we can demonstrate that the incidence of vasospasm in the first 72 h in good risk patients is quite low. However, vasospasm as shown by either serial angiography during the first 3 weeks or by postoperative angiography occurs at some time in virtually every case that has had a significant subarachnoid hermorrhage. This compares closely with the reports of others (10,13). There may, therefore, be an early window in time when operation can be tolerated better than at a later time when vasospasm has developed.

In the early years we postulated that the sole purpose of aneurysmorrhaphy was the prevention of rebleeding. However, it has become apparent that the hypotension and dehydration of medical regimen, intended to reduce the risk of rebleeding, may well increase the risk of infarction (7,9). It follows that aneurysmorrhaphy, by eliminating the danger of hemorrhage, permits a medical remigen more likely to prevent infarction. Specifically, maintenance of blood volume and elevation of blood pressure, ill-advised before the aneurysm is secured, are valuable in preventing the hemodynamic crisis that often occurs days after the initial hemorrhage (4).

Present practice is to estimate blood volume decrease due to bed rest, hyperosmolar diuretics, furosemide, and blood loss. As soon as the aneurysm is secured, this volume is replaced with crystalloids and blood and the blood pressure is elevated, if necessary with vasopressor agents. All of these patients have done well, although the severity of the spasm and brain swelling seen on postoperative angiograms has at times been startling when contrasted with the patient's excellent clinical course.

Conclusions

1) Early intervention in patients without neurological deficit and without vasospasm on angiography is the preferred course in such patients as meet these stringent criteria.
2) Either vasospasm or neurological deficit calls for delay of operation.
3) The problem of nonoperative deaths is as yet unsolved, but ischemic infarction seems to be a greater problem than secondary bleeding in the sicker patient.

References

1. ALVORD, E.C., Jr., LOESER, J.D., BAILEY, W.L., COPASS, M.K.: Subarachnoid hemorrhage due to ruptured aneurysms. Arch. Neurol. 27, 273-281 (1972)
2. ALVORD, E.C., Jr., THORN, R.B.: Natural history of subarachnoid hemorrhage: Early prognosis. Clin. Neurosurg. 24, 167-175 (1977)
3. HUNT, W.E., HESS, R.M.: Surgical risk as related to time of intervention in the repair of intracranial aneurysms. J. Neurosurg. 28, 14-19 (1968)
4. HUNT, W.E., KOSNIK, E.J.: Timing and perioperative care of intracranial aneurysm surgery. Clin. Neurosurg. 21, 79-89 (1974)
5. HUNT, W.E., MILLER, C.A.: The results in the timing of operations for aneurysm. Clin. Neurosurg. 24, 208-215 (1977)
6. JANE, J.A., WINN, H.R., RICHARDSON, A.E.: The natural history of intracranial aneurysms: Rebleeding rates during the acute and long-term period and implication for surgical management. Clin. Neurosurg. 24, 176-184 (1977)

7. MILLIKAN, C.H.: Cerebral vasospasm and ruptured intracranial aneurysm. Arch. Neurol. 32, 433-449 (1975)

8. McKISSOCK, W., PAINE, K.W.E., WALSH, L.S.: An analysis of the results of treatment of ruptured intracranial aneurysms. Report of 772 consecutive cases. J. Neurosurg. 17, 762-776 (1960)

9. POST, K.D., FLAMM, E.S., GOODGOLD, A., RANSOHOFF, J.: Ruptured intracranial aneurysms: Case morbidity and mortality. J. Neurosurg. 460, 290-295 (1977)

10. SAITO, I., NEDA, Y.: Significance of vasospasm in the treatment of ruptured intracranial aneurysms. J. Neurosurg. 47, 412-429 (1977)

11. SAMSON, D.S., HODOSH, R.M., CLARK, W.K.: Surgical management of unruptured asymptomatic aneurysms. J. Neurosurg. 46, 731-734 (1977)

12. TRAUPP, H., BJORKESTEN, G.: Results of a controlled trial of late surgical versus conservative treatment of intracranial arterial aneurysms. J. Neurosurg. 35, 20-24 (1971)

13. WEIR, B., GRACE, M., HANSE, J., ROTHBERG, C.: Time course of vasospasm in man. J. Neurosurg. 48, 173-178 (1978)

Management and Prognosis of Intraventricular Hemorrhage

W. I. STEUDEL, E. SCHNEIDER, and H. BECKER

Prior to the introduction of computer tomography (CT), intraventricular hemorrhage was mostly demonstrated by the pathologist or the neurosurgeon. For the first time CT permits direct observation of intracranial (10,16-18,22) bleeding in the patient (1,3-5,7,8,11-15,20,21,23-25). In head injuries and in spontaneous hemorrhages, CT has become practically indispensable. The present study describes the prognosis in relation to the extent and localization of intraventricular bleeding on CT and at surgery.

Patients and Methods

Among 10,000 CT examinations there were 60 patients with intraventricular bleeding of various etiology (among 610 patients with intracranial hemorrhages). The incidence of intraventricular hemorrhage in 369 patients is 5.7% in traumatic (21) and in 241 patients 16.2% in spontaneous (39) cases. Etiology, age, and sex distribution are seen in Table 1. The level of consciousness was classified into five grades (modified from HUNT, 1968): *grade 1*, no disturbance; *grade 2*, somnolence, the patient can be aroused to a normal level of awareness; *grade 3*, stupor, the patient may be aroused to some degree but cannot reach or sustain a normal level of consciousness; *grade 4*, coma, the patient cannot be aroused even by painful stimuli; *grade 5*, deep coma, the patient no longer has any reaction to painful stimuli and has dilated pupils and areflexia. CT was first performed with the SIRETOM prototype (matrix size 80·80; 4000 examinations) and later with the SIRETOM I (matrix 128·128; 6000) from 1974 - 1978. The CT findings were classified (according to PIA, 1972) into CSF-blood mixture and clotted blood with partial or total filling of the ventricular system.

Results

CT Findings. Clotted blood and CSF-blood mixture can be distinguished in CT. Freshly *clotted blood* is shown with density values of +40 - 80 units in the SIRETOM. Density values of +20 - +40 units are measured for the *CSF-blood mixture.* The CSF-blood mixture discernable in CT is frequently found in the occipital horns according to the (supine) position of the patient during the examination and displays a surface reflection. We have not been able so far to detect CSF-blood mixtures below the specified density values.

Traumatic Hemorrhages. Of 21 patients with traumatic hemorrhages, 20 were comatose at the time of CT examination, 8 of whom were deeply comatose (Table 2). Only one patient could still be aroused by stimuli. CT showed partially clotted blood in ten cases, a CSF-blood mixture in 12 cases, and a combination of both in one of these. Patients

Table 1. Intraventricular hemorrhages

Etiology	No.	Sex	Median age	Interval from 1st symptom to death (days) median (range)	Surviving patients
Trauma	21	F=5 M=16	41	3 (1-13)	4
Hypertension	11	F=6 M=5	50	2 (1-4)	3
Hemorrhagic disorders	4	M=4	53	5 (1-9)	2
Aneurysm	9	F=6 M=3	34	42 (1-155)	-
Angioma	1	M=1	36		1
Tumor	4	F=2 M=2	53	6 (3-7)	-
Unknown	10	F=5 M=5	47	9 (1-25)	2

Table 2. Level of consciousness and CT findings in 21 traumatic intraventricular hemorrhages

Level of consciousness	CT findings		
	CSF-blood mixture	Clotted blood partial	total
I normal			
II somnolence	●		
III stupor			
IV coma	●●OOO OOOO	●OOO	
V deep coma	OO	OOOOO O	

O, patient; ●, surviving patient.

with traumatic intraventricular hemorrhages with clots in several ventricular parts survived the accident only by a few hours. Only one patient with clotted blood in the right ventricle and an epidural hematoma that was removed survived. In 9 of 21 patients, intracranial hematomas (three epidural, two subdural, five intracerebral) were removed. Only the above-mentioned patient recovered (Fig. 1).

Three patients had minimal symptoms for several hours after the accident. They were only examined with CT after onset of unconsciousness. Since an intracerebral hematoma was found, the intraventricular penetration probably occurred secondarily. In these cases the hematoma was operated on; these patients also died, although one survived hemorrhage for 2 weeks.

Hypertensive Hemorrhages. Of 11 patients known hypertension three had no disturbance of consciousness or somnolence (Table 3). Eight patients were comatose (four of these in deep coma). The three patients who were not comatose showed a tiny hemorrhage in one part of the ventricular system and survived. In the other eight patients, a complete intraventricular bleeding was shown twice in the occipital horns. These patients survived the bleeding by only a few days (Table 1). Surgery was not performed in these cases (Fig. 2).

Table 3. Level of consciousness and CT findings in 11 hypertensive intraventricular hemorrhages

Level of concsiousness	CT findings		
	CSF-blood mixture	Clotted blood Partial	Total
I normal		●●	
II somnolence	●		
III stupor			
IV coma	O	OO	O
V deep coma	O	OOO	O

O, patient; ●, surviving patient.

Aneurysm and Angioma Hemorrhages. In the nine aneurysm hemorrhages, the origin was the anterior communicating artery in five cases, the middle cerebral artery in three, and the posterior communicating artery in one case. All patients were comatose (Table 4). In eight patients the third ventricle was filled with clotted blood and in five of these the fourth ventricle as well.

Table 4. Level of consciousness and CT findings in nine patients with aneurysms

Level of consciousness	CT findings		
	CSF-blood mixture	Clotted blood Partial	Total
I normal			
II somnolence			
III stupor			
IV coma	OO	OOOOO	O
V deep coma		OO	O

O, patient.

The operation of two of these (comatose) patients did not have any influence on the prognosis. In four patients with an anterior communicating artery aneurysm, the intraventricular hemorrhage occurred secondarily. Moderate enlargement of the ventricles occurred in two patients, and marked enlargement occurred in one who died despite insertion of a ventricular drain (Fig. 3). One patient with a right temporo-occipital angioma and a complete filling of the left lateral ventricle with clotted blood, who was somnolent on admission, recovered.

Tumor Hemorrhages. Four patients with brain tumors showed clotted blood in the ventricular system. In two cases, there was a glioblastoma multiforme and in the other two cases multiple metastases. Surgery was not undertaken.

Hemorrhages in Hemorrhagic Disorders. An intraventricular hemorrhage occurred four times in connection with anticoagulant treatment; these patients were somnolent on admission. CT showed an intracerebral hematoma in two cases and an extensive intracerebellar hematoma combined with a clot located in the fourth ventricle; this patient died. In one case the intracerebral hematoma was removed and in another case of an acute hydrocephalus a shunt operation was performed; these patients recovered.

Hemorrhages of Unknown Etiology. In ten cases, the etiology remained unclear. Two of these patients with an intraventricular hemorrhage in which only parts of the ventricular system were involved survived (Table 1). Neither of these patients were comatose at the time of CT examination.

Discussion

Catamnestic studies of intraventricular hemorrhages are possible using computer tomography (8,14). Our study shows (as has been known for a long time) that patients do not survive extensive intraventricular hemorrhages. Hemorrhages with unilateral or partial intraventricular involvement and with CSF-blood mixture may be survived. Our findings support the classification of intraventricular hemorrhages into hematocephalus totalis et partialis and hemorrhagia intraventricularis (18,19). The point of penetration of the intracerebral hematoma into the ventricle could be verified by CT in 23 of 39 spontaneous hemorrhages. The most common site is the region of the basal ganglia as is already well-known (Fig. 4). CT findings are usually clear cut. In some cases, however, it cannot be definitely decided whether the hemorrhage is intraventricular or subependymal (2,9,20,21).

Angiography should be performed in every spontaneous hemorrhage in which there is a chance of survival. To establish the etiology prior to surgical intervention (e.g., the presence of an angioma or aneurysm), WALSHE et al. (25) pointed out that the diagnostic lumbar puncture has thus become superfluous. Surgical treatment of intracerebral hematomas depends mainly on the clinical picture and the size and localization of the hematoma (18,19,23,25). In patients with hydrocepahlus, shunt procedures can be of particular value (23).

Summary

Sixty patients with intraventricular hemorrhage were examined and the extent of the bleeding compared to the clinical course. With the help of computer tomography it is possible to distinguish between intraventricular clotted blood and CSF-blood mixture. Of these 21 cases involving traumatic hemorrhages, all but one patient with clotted blood in the ventricle died. Operative treatment of intra- or extracerebral hematomas only changed the prognosis in one case. Of the other three surviving patients, CT showed only CSF-blood mixtures. Operative procedures were also ineffective for aneurysms, as all patients who were comatose upon admission died. However, the angioma patient who had an extensive ventricular hemorrhage recovered. Of the other 29 cases of intraventricular hemorrhages eight patients survived. All of the latter had only partially filled ventricles and were not comatose at the time of examination. The clinical course of intraventricular bleeding is largely related to the extent and degree of clotting. Operative procedures did not essentially reduce the mortality rate in comatose patients.

References

1. BAKER, H.L., Jr., CAMPBELL, J.K., HOUSER, O.W., REESE, D.F., SHEEDY, P.F., HOLMAN, C.B., KURLAND, R.L.: Computer assisted tomography of the head. An early evaluation. Mayo Clin. Proc. 49, 17-27 (1974)
2. BECKER, H., GRAU, H., HACKER, H.: Endokranielle Verkalkungen in der Computer-Tomographie. - Ein Vergleich zum Röntgenbild. Fortschr. Röntgenstr. 126, 509-512 (1977)
3. DORNDORF, W.: Schlaganfälle - Klinik und Therapie. Stuttgart: Thieme 1975
4. GRUMME, Th., LANKSCH, W., WENDE, S.: Diagnosis of spontaneous intracerebral hemorrhage by computerized tomography. In: Cranial computerized tomography. LANKSCH, W., KAZNER, E. (eds.), pp. 284-290. Berlin, Heidelberg, New York: Springer 1976
5. HEIDRICH, R.: Subarachnoid haemorrhage. In: Hdb. of clinical neurology. VINKEN, P.J., BRUYN, G.W. (eds.), Vol. 12, pp. 68-185. Amsterdam: North-Holland 1972
6. HUNT, W.E., HESS, R.M.: Surgical risk as related to time of intervention in the repair of intracranial aneurysms. J. Neurosurg. 28, 14-20 (1968)
7. KAZNER, E., LANKSCH, W., STEINHOFF, H., WILSKE, J.: Die axiale Computer-Tomographie des Gehirnschädels - Anwendungsmöglichkeiten und klinische Ergebnisse. Fortschr. Neurol. Psychiatr. 43, 487-574 (1975)
8. KRICHEFF, I.J., LIN, J.P., CHASE, N.E.: Computer assisted tomography in intracerebral hematomas and head trauma. In: Advances in cerebral angiography. SALAMON, G. (ed.). Berlin, Heidelberg, New York: Springer 1975
9. LANKSCH, W., MEESE, W., KAZNER, E.: CT findings in closed head injuries with special reference to contusions. In: Cranial computerized tomography. LANKSCH, W., KAZNER, E. (eds.). pp. 318-328. Berlin, Heidelberg, New York: Springer 1976
10. LUYENDIJK, W.: Intracerebral haematoma. In: Hdb. of clinical neurology. VINKEN, P.J., BRUYN, G.W. (eds.), Vol. 11, pp. 660-719. Amsterdam: North-Holland 1972
11. MARSHALL, W.H., EASTER, W., ZATZ, L.W.: Differentiation of hemorrhage from other dense lesions in computer tomography of the brain. International symposium on computer assisted tomography in nontumoral disease of the brain, spinal cord and eye. Bethesda, 11-15. October 1976

12. MINAUF, M., SCHACHT, L.: Zentrale Hirnschäden nach Einwirkung stumpfer Gewalt auf den Schädel. II. Mitteilung. Läsionen im Bereich der Stammanglien. Arch. Psychiatr. Nervenkr. 208, 162-176 (1966)

13. NEW, P.F.J., SCOTT, W.R., SCHNUR, J.A., KENNETH, R.D., TAVERAS, P.M.: Computerized axial tomography with the EMI scanner. Radiology 110, 109-123 (1974)

14. O'CONNOR, L., HYSHAW, C., WINTER, J., BENTSON, J., WILSON, G., NEWTON, Th.H.: Intraventricular hemorrhage: Correlation of CT scan findings with clinical, angiographic and autopsy findings. Wiesbaden: Symposium Neuroradiologicum 4-10, Juni 1978

15. PAXTON, R., AMBROSE, J.: The EMI scanner. A brief review of the first 650 patients. Br. J. Radiol. 47, 530-565 (1974)

16. PETERS, G.: Klinische Neuropathologie. Stuttgart: Thieme 1970

17. PEUSNER, P.H., GARCIA-BUNUEL, R., LEEDS, N., FINKELSTEIN, M.: Subependymal and intraventricular hemorrhage in neonates. Early diagnosis by computed tomography. Radiology 119, 111-114 (1976)

18. PIA, H.W.: The surgical treatment of intracerebral and intraventricular haematomas. Acta Neurochir. Wien 27, 149-164 (1972)

19. PIA, H.W.: Die operative Behandlung der spontanen Massenblutungen des Gehirns. Dtsch. Ärzteblatt 12, 423-430 (1975)

20. PRESSMAN, B.D., KIRKWOOD, J.R., DAVIS, D.O.: Computerized transverse tomography of vasailar lesions of the brain. Part. I: arteriovenous malformations. Am.J. Roentgenol. 124, 208-224 (1975)

21. SCOTT, W.R., NEW, P.F.J., DAVIS, K.R., SCHNUR, J.A.: Computerized axial tomography of intracerebral and intraventricular hemorrhage. Radiology 112, 73-80 (1974)

22. SELLIER, K., UNTERHARNSCHEIDT, F.: Mechanik und Pathomorphologie der Hirnschäden nach stumpfer Gewalteinwirkung auf den Schädel. Hefte Unfallheilkd. 76, 1 (1973)

23. STEINER, L., BERGVALL, U., ZWETNOW, N.: Quantitative estimation of intracerebral and intraventricular hematoma by computer tomography. Acta Radiol. (Suppl.) (Stockh.) 36, 143-154 (1975)

24. VERMESS, M., DI CHIRO, G., NEWBY, N.R., HERDT, J.R.: Positional shift of intraventricular blood clots demonstrated by computed tomography. Radiology 118, 341-342 (1976)

25. WALSHE, T.M., KENNETH, R.D., FISCHER, C.M.: Thalamic hemorrhage: A computed tomographic - clinical correlation. Neurology 27, 217-222 (1977)

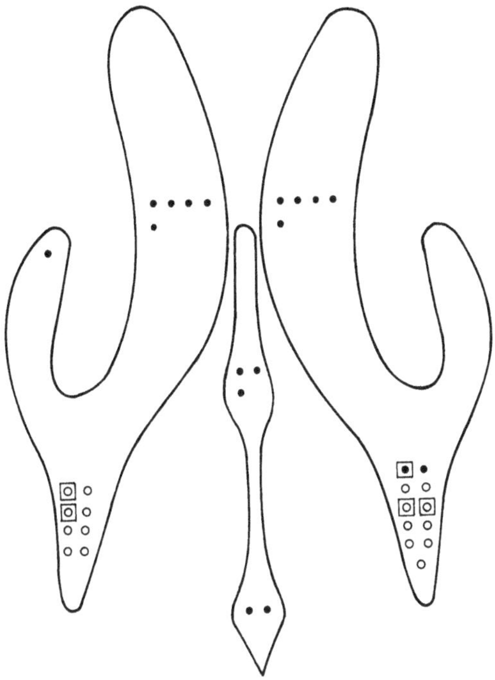

Fig. 1

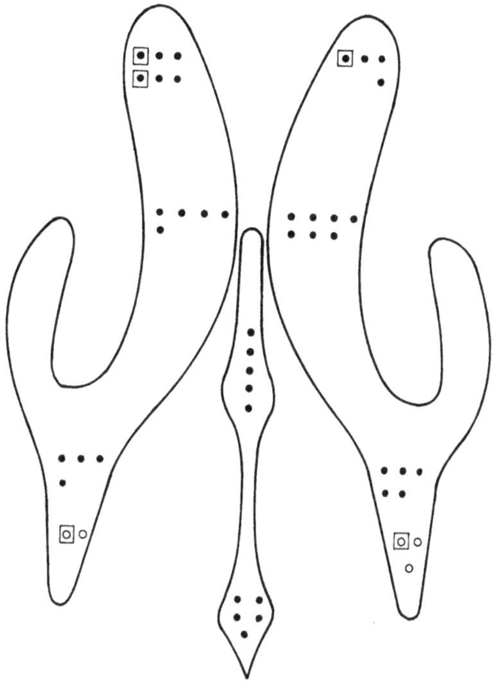

Fig. 2

Fig. 1. Distribution of the blood in the ventricular system (frontal horns, cella media, posterior and temporal horns, third and fourth ventricle) in 21 traumatic intraventricular hemorrhages. ●, clotted blood; o, CSF-blood mixture; □, surviving patient

Fig. 2. Distribution of intraventricular blood in 11 patients with hypertension. Abbreviations see Fig. 1

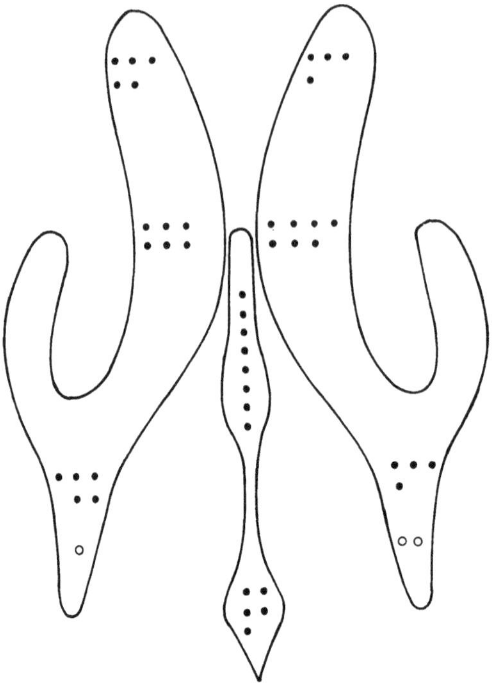

Fig. 3

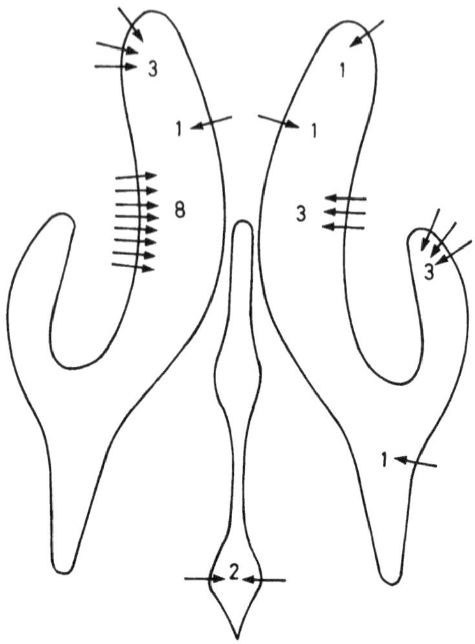

Fig. 4

Fig. 3. Distribution of intraventricular blood in nine patients with aneurysms. Abbreviations see Fig. 1

Fig. 4. The point of penetration of the intracerebral hematoma into the ventricle in 23 of 39 spontaneous intraventricular hemorrhages

Specialized Neurosurgical Techniques

The Anterior Transcallosal Approach to Brain Tumors

R. L. HARPER and G. EHNI

Introduction

The interhemispheric or transcallosal approach to lesions occupying or encroaching upon the third and anterior lateral ventricles is the subject of infrequent reports. Experience in 34 cases with a wide range of pathology suggests this is a safe and anatomically sensible approach, deserving preference over the more widely used transcortical technique. Specifically, it avoids the inherent disadvantages of the transcortical route - removal of brain, restrictive operative field, especially with normal ventricular size, and the risk of epilepsy.

In 1913 BRUNNER made a posterior transcallosal approach for a suspected tumor (2). Beginning in 1921 DANDY used both posterior and anterior transcallosal incisions successfully (4,5,6). More recently, BALDWIN and then MILHORAT and BALDWIN working with primates emphasized the excellent exposure obtained via an interhemispheric, transcallosal approach (1,12). EHNI, LONG and CHOU, SCARFF, and SHUCART and STEIN have all reported excellent clinical results by this route (8,11,13,14,15,16).

Material and Approach

The anterior transcallosal route was utilized in 34 patients, including 20 adults and 14 children. The lesion was in the third ventricle in 14 cases, a lateral ventricle in 16, and in both lateral and third in five cases. There were 27 tumors with ten histologic types represented. Seven of these tumors proved to be malignant. Seven patients had hematomas, hydrocephalus, an arachnoid cyst, and lateral ventriculomegaly of unknown cause.

In the past, identification of appropriate candidates for transcallosal surgery required angiography to demonstrate a mass within the concavity of the midline arteries and air to demonstrate a mass within the ventricle or its wall. Currently computer tomography plus angiography usually fulfills these roles, although air is still occasionally useful. These studies eliminate masses lying on the underside of the first part of the anterior cerebral arteries or those beneath and elevating the third ventricle. Also, the venous phase of the angiogram demonstrates the least traumatic side of approach based on the pattern of veins draining into the sagittal sinus. Either lateral ventricle may be entered from either side of the falx within equal facility via the transcallosal approach.

With the patient supine, a coronal incision is made with a deeper limb on the side of approach. A bone flap of generous size and low on the supraorbital ridge is made. This provides room to retract the hemisphere in cases with relatively small ventricles and also permits subfrontal exploration if indicated. A single burrhole is placed in the midline just above the frontal sinus, followed by a pair of holes either side of the sagittal sinus just anterior to the coronal suture. The bone over the sinus is removed with a narrow rongeur and a bone cut between the frontal burrhole and the lateral coronal burrhole is made without risk to the sinus. Lateral holes are placed and a large flap is turned. The dural flap is cut with a pedicle just up to the sagittal sinus to insure a perfectly sagittal view between the hemispheres. Employing magnification one, or occasionally two of the smaller veins entering the sinus anteriorly are taken and the hemisphere retracted from the falx. An occasional adhesion is cut and a self-retaining retractor placed. Care must be taken that the cingulate gyrus isn't mistaken for the corpus callosum by noting the latter's characteristic white transverse fibers. The pericallosal arteries are then found. The presence of apparent anastomosis between arteries usually indicates one is not between but lateral to the pericallosals. The corpus callosum, often thinned by hydrocephalus, is divided 2-3 cm back from the genu between the pericallosals by blunt dissection. From this midline incision one gently slants the incision to enter the ventricle of choice. The other side is easily accessible by blunt fenestration of the septum pellucidum or through a corpus callosum incision slanted oppositely. Placing the retractor over the edge of the corpus callosum incision immediately brings the intraventricular landmarks in view. The foramen of Monro is easily identified by the course of the thalamostriate vein and the choroid plexus. Great care must be taken to avoid damage to even one fornix, as the competence of the other fornix is not insured and bilateral injury will cause severe impairment of recent memory. Lesions within the lateral ventricle are immediately obvious, those within the third ventricle are usually easily seen through a dilated foramen of Monro. Further access to third ventricle masses may be gained by incising the postero-inferior margin of the foramen of Monro, or by incising the roof of the third ventricle in the midline (3). The excellent exposure and subsequent resection allowed by such maneuvers is obvious in Figs. 1 and 2. Drains in the ventricular cavity are rarely needed.

Results

Eight deaths occurred. Six were 13 days to 15 months after operation for malignant tumors. The deaths of two patients with benign tumors involved fluid mismanagement in a neonate in one case, and inadvertent bilateral occlusion of the anterior cerebral arteries in another case. There were three cases of transient hemiparesis contralateral to the retracted hemisphere, and one instance of permanent paresis from clipping of a pericallosal artery.

Of the 26 cases with benign lesions, only one failed to function socially and intellectually at preoperative levels or better. The exception involved a left thalamic hematoma, the excision of which resulted in aphasia (Table 1).

Discussion

The effects of complete cerebral commissurotomy have been recently reviewed by DIMOND and by GESCHWIND (7,10). With complete callosal section, transfer of information between hemispheres is subtly impaired, although the usual clinical sequence of neurologic examination may be

Table 1. Pathology and surgical results

Lesion	Ventricular location	No. cases	hydro-cephalus	Shunt	Excision
1) Colloid cyst	Third	5	5	0	5-Total
2) Astrocytoma I or II	Third	3	2	2	3-Partial
	Lateral	2	2	0	1-Partial 1-Total
3) Malignant gliomas	Third	2	1	1	2-Partial
	Lateral	4	3	1	3-Partial
4) Oligodendro-glioma	Third	1	1	1	1-Total
	Lateral	2	1	0	1-Total 1-Partial
5) Cranio-pharyngioma	Third	2	2	0	2-Partial
6) Ependymoma	Lateral	1	1	0	1-Partial
7) Epidermoid	Third	1	0	0	1-Total
	Lateral	1	1	1	1-Partial
8) Arachnoid Cyst	Third	1	1	1	1-Partial
9) Hematoma	Lateral caudate	2	0	0	2-Total
	thalamus	1	1	0	1-Total
10) Sarcoma	Diffuse	1	0	0	1-Partial
11) Teratoma	Third and lateral	1	1	0	1-Partial
12) Ganglio-glioma	Both lateral	1	1	0	1-Total
13) Ventriculo-megaly	Right lateral	1	1	0	Negative exploration
14) Congenital hydrocephalus	Third and lateral	2	2	2	Sump ventricu-lostomy

normal. Anterior section of the corpus callosum analogous to the surgical approach described has rarely been reported and the function of the anterior fibers is poorly understood. GAZZANICA et al. did study one patient with surgical section of the anterior one-third of the corpus callosum, but could find only a questionable defect of transfer of olfactory information (9). The few patients in our series subjected to formal psychometrics were normal, and almost all with benign lesions resumed previous activities, including graduate education and executive level functions. SHUCART and STEIN found no defects by their tests for callosal functions (14).

A more serious deficit is loss of recent memory due to injury to the fornices. One intact patient, a child, transiently had such a postoperative deficit, but of four with this deficit preoperatively, none recovered the capability of recent memory even with 15 years follow up. Dissection around the fornices should be done with the utmost caution.

References

1. BALDWIN, M., OMMAYA, A.K., FARRIER, R., McDONALD, F.: Mesial cerebral incision. J. Neurosurg. 20, 679-686 (1963)
2. BRUNNER, C.; quoted by RORSCHACH, H.: Zur Pathologie und Operabilität der Tumoren der Zirbeldürse. Beitr. Z. Klin. Chir. 83, 451-474 (1913)
3. BUSCH, E.: A new approach for the removal of tumors of the third ventricle. Acta Psychiatr. Neurol. (Kbh) 19, 57-60 (1944)
4. DANDY, W.E.: An operation for the removal of pineal tumors. Surg. Gynecol. Obstet. 33, 113-119 (1921)
5. DANDY, W.E.: Diagnosis, localization, and removal of tumors of the third ventricle. Bull. Johns Hopkins Hosp. 33, 188-189 (1922)
6. DANDY, W.E.: Congenital cerebral cysts of the cavum septi pellucidi (fifth ventricle) and cavum vergae (sixth ventricle). Arch. Neurol. Psychiatry 25, 44-66 (1931)
7. DIMOND, S.G.: The disconnection syndromes. Mod. Trends Neurol. 6, 35-57 (1975)
8. EHNI, G.: Transcallosal removal of brain tumors. 16 mm motion picture. 14 minutes. American College of Surgeons Film Library and Baylor College of Medicine, 1969
9. GAZZANIGA, M.S., RISSE, G.L., SPRINGER, S.P., CLARK, E., WILSON, D.H.: Psychologic and neurologic consequences of partial and complete cerebral commissurotomy. Neurology 25, 10-15 (1975)
10. GESCHWIND, N.: The clinical syndromes of the cortical connections. Mod. Trends Neurol. 1, 29-40 (1970)
11. LONG, D.M., CHOU, S.N.: Transcallosal removal of craniopharyngiomas within the third ventricle. J. Neurosurg. 39, 563-567 (1973)
12. MILHORAT, T.H., BALDWIN, M.: A technique for surgical exposure of the cerebral midline: Experimental transcallosal microdissection. J. Neurosurg. 24, 687-691 (1966)
13. SCARFF, T.B., REYAL, D.H., LYONS, T.A.: Transcallosal approach to the third ventricle in children. Abstracted in: Neurosurg. 2, 154 (1978)
14. SHUCART, W.A., STEIN, B.M.: Experience with the transcallosal approach to the anterior ventricular system. J. Neurosurgery (to be published)
15. STEIN, B.M., FRASER, R.A.R., TENNER, M.S.: Tumors of third ventricle in children. J. Neurol. Neurosurg. Psychiatry 35, 776-788 (1975)
16. STEIN, B.M.: Transcallosal approach to third ventricular tumors. In: Current techniques in operative neurosurgery. SCHMIEDECK, H.H., SWEET, W.H. (eds.), pp. 247-256. New York: Grune & Stratton 1977

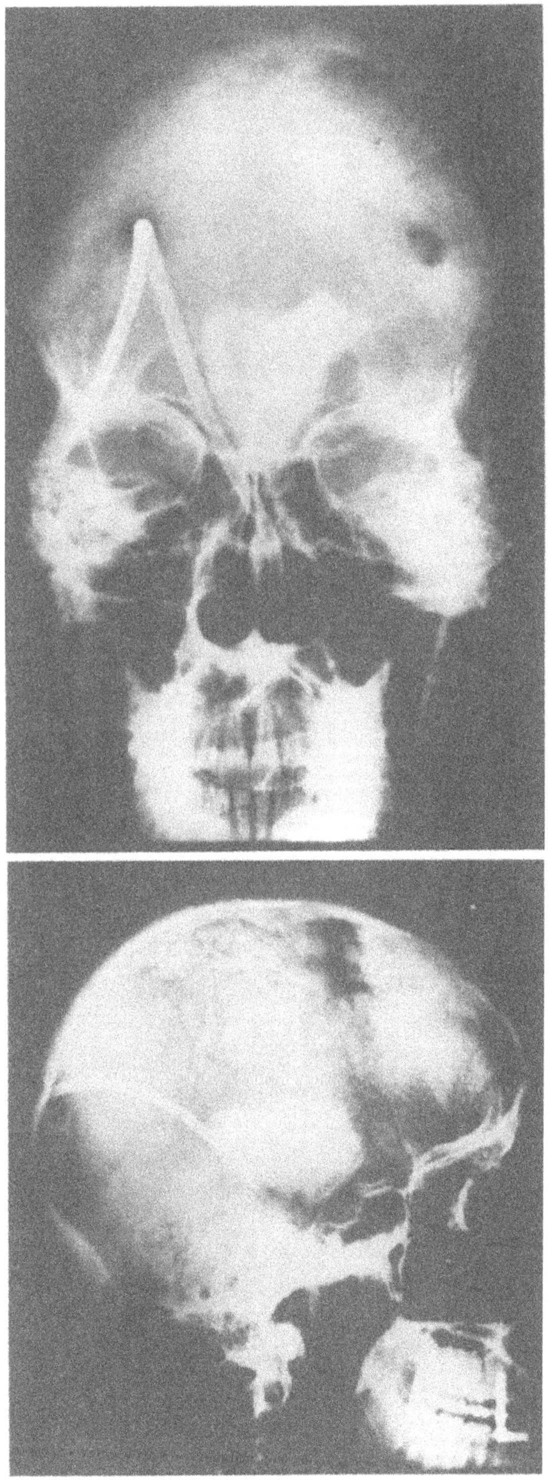

Fig. 1.
Enlarging calcified mass over 10 years with Torkildsen's shunt

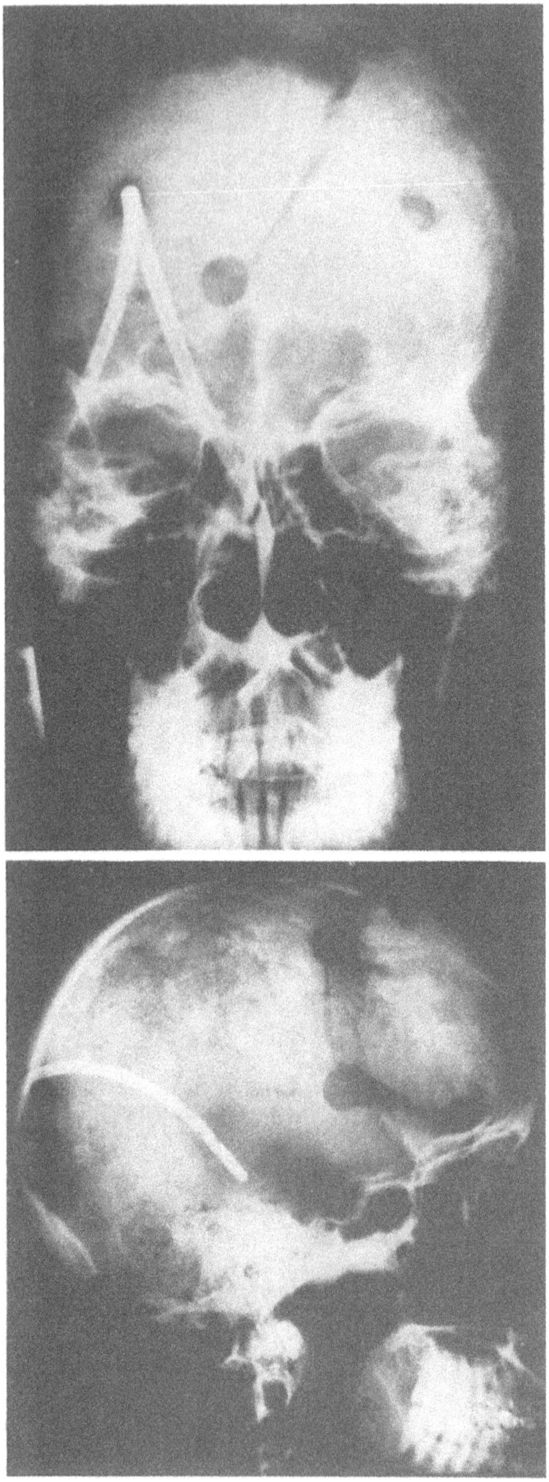

Fig. 2. Same patient. Complete resection of oligodendroglioma of third ventricle. Doing well 15 years later

Experience with the Direct Surgical Approach in 52 Tumors of the Pineal Region

M. SCHÄFER, C. LAPRAS, and H. RUF

Introduction

Since 1964 we have been trying a direct surgical approach in certain tumors of the pineal region. We first used DANDY's transcallosal and van WAGENEN's transventricular temporal approach. However, results were not satisfying, and we looked for another approach to the pineal region with more practicability and better visibility of the deep-seated structures (4,8). Since 1971 we have been performing the right occipital approach, first published by POPPEN in 1966 (5) (Table 1).

Table 1. Direct surgery (55/52 patients)

	No. of cases
Occipital supra-tentorial	7
Cysts without solid tumor	5
Cystic astrocytomas	2
Transventricular temporal	2
Total removal	2
Transcallosal	9
Total removal	3
Partial removal	6
Occipital transtentorial	37
Total removal	26
Partial removal	8
Biopsy	3

Material and Method

Diagnostic Procedures

Most of the patients with pineal tumors had signs of increased intracranial pressure and visual troubles, such as vertical visual paresis (Parinaud's syndrome) or pupillary motor failure. Very rarely, angiography showed local abnormalities. If during lumbar pneumencephalography (PEG) air did not enter into the aqueduct, ventriculotomography with positive contrast medium (Dimer X, BYK-Gulden, Konstanz, West Germany) was performed. Since computer tomography (CT) was available, no further neuroradiologic examinations were necessary. CT has proved to be the best management for showing the localization and extension of the lesion. After intravenous injection of contrast medium (1 ml/kg Telebrix 380, BYK-Gulden, Konstanz, West Germany), one could distinguish very well between cystic and solid tumors with or without calcifications (11,12). Lateral extension of a pineal tumor into the thalamus in particular would be a contraindication for direct surgery (Fig. 1).

Between 1964 and 1978, 52 patients with space-occupying lesions of the pineal region were operated on by a direct approach in the two above-mentioned neurosurgical centers. Three patients had two interventions because of recurrent tumors (Table 2).

Table 2. Pathology of space-occupying lesions of the pineal region (7)

	No.
Pinealomas	14
Pineocytomas	5
Pineoblastomas	9
Germinomas (atypical teratoma)	7
Teratomas	6
Gliomas	17
Glioblastomas	2
Astrocytomas	9
Spongioblastomas	2
Ependymomas	3
Oligodendroglioma	1
Meningeoma	1
Sarcoidosis (granuloma)	1
Plexuspapilloma	1
Cysts	5
Total	52

Operative Technique (right Occipital Approach)

In all cases with obstructive hydrocephalus, we insert a left occipital or right frontal ventriculoatrial shunt 10-14 days before operating the tumor directly (4). We operate on the patient in a sitting position, the head slightly turned to the left and anteflected.

Central venous pressure and arterial pressure are continuously monitored. Positive end-expiratory pressure (PEEP) is performed to avoid air embolism. For the early detection of such complications a capnograph is used routinely.

We perform a large right occipital craniotomy, overlying the midline and the transverse sinus. After opening the dura, the occipital lobe is mobilized, lifted laterally, and fixed by a self-retractor. Then the tentorium is broadly incised parallel to the straight sinus. The upper cerebellum (culmen), quadrigeminal plate, and after opening of the arachnoidea, the tumor are visible. Tumor dissection always has to start with the superior cerebellar veins, running up to the caudal tumor pole. In this way, the upper cerebellum will move down, and there is more space for the extirpation of the tumor. Arterial feeding vessels coming from the two posterior choroidal arteries are coagulated. Tumor removal can now be carried out, beginning from the inferior side. When the cavum of the third ventricle is visible and CSF leaks out, the lateral wall of the neoplasm can be dissected. Finally, its origin just below the vein of GALEN should be removed by bipolar coagulation.

Results

We observed the same predominance of males in germinomas and teratomas as described by other authors (7,13) (Tables 3, 4).

Table 3. Sex ratio (30 males and 22 females)

Pineal tumors and cysts	Male	Female	Total
Pineocytomas	2	3	5
Pineoblastomas	4	5	9
Germinomas	6	1	7
Teratomas	6	0	6
Cysts	2	3	5

Table 4. Average age of 52 patients

Pineal tumors	14 years
Pineocytomas	17 years
Pineoblastomas	14 years
Germinomas	13 years
Teratomas	12 years
Cysts	6 months
Gliomas	22 years

There were four deaths during the 1st postoperative months. Two of these cases were large invasive tumors (glioblastomas) so that only a biopsy was performed. One case had been operated on in a comatose state, after 8 years shunt and X-ray therapy. One other patient with a germinoma included in our early series had been operated on by a transcallosal approach. Necropsy showed infarction of both thalami because of damage to the deep veins (Table 5).

Table 5. Mortality during 1st year after operation (ten cases)

	No.
Before 3 months	4
After 3 months	6
Before X-ray therapy	2
After X-ray therapy	8
After biopsy (partial removal)	8
After total (?) transcallosal removal (pineoblastoma)	1
After total occipital trans-tentorial removal (pineoblastoma)	1
Histiopathology of 10 cases	
Pineoblastomas	5
Malignant teratomas	2
Germinoma	1
Astrocytoma	1
Benign teratoma (partial removal, X-ray before surgery)	1

Between 1 and 2 years after the operation there were three deaths, all after X-ray therapy; one was a pineoblastoma and two were astrocytomas grade II. After 2 years, three more patients died: one had an astrocytoma after X-ray therapy and three operations; one had a pineoblastoma after X-ray therapy for spinal metastasis of 2.5 years; and one had a nontumoral cyst with shunt after surgery, mental retardation, no further shunt revision for 5 years (Table 6).

Table 6. Histopathologic findings (time of observation more than 2 years)

Diagnosis	No. of cases	Dead	Alive
Cysts	5	1	4
Pineocytomas	5	1	4
Pineoblastomas	9	7	2
Germinomas	7	2	5
Teratomas	6	3	3
Gliomas	17	6	11
Others	3	0	3

The overall mortality over 14 years is 38%. Most of these patients had malignant tumors, such as gliomas or pineoblastomas (Tables 7 and 8).

Table 7. Results of partial or total removal

Surg. approach	Partial	Total	Dead	Alive
Transventr.-temp.	0	2	0/0	0/2
Transcallosal	6	3	6/2	0/1
Occipital supratent.	0	4	0/1	0/3
Occipital transtent.	11	26	8/3	3/23

Of 35 total removal, 29 patients alive and six deaths.

Table 8. Results of total removal (35 cases)

Deaths (over 14 years)	6
Postoperative death (1 month)	1
Secondary death	5
Patients alive (29/35)	
Pineocytomas (4)	4
Pineoblastomas (4)	1
Germinomas (6)	5
Teratomas (3)	3
Gliomas (10)	9
Cysts (5)	4
Others (3)	3
Total	29

Of 35 patients whose neoplasms were removed completely according to macroscopic inspection, 29 are still alive. The survival rate in cases with totally removed tumors is much better than in cases with partially removed ones, even with subsequent X-ray therapy.

In three males we observed a precocious puberty (9). One of these had a germinoma and two others had pineocytomas. One of the patients with a pineocytoma had high choriogonadotropin and α-fetoprotein levels, which were normalized immediately after the operation.

Discussion

As criteria for the indication for the direct surgical approach in tumors of the pineal region, neuroradiologic findings are of particular importance (1). Since CT has become available, the strict midline location can be clearly detected (8,10). Lateral extension of a tumor with infiltration into the thalamus is a contraindication for the direct approach. In our experience with 41 cases, the right occipital approach with incision of the tentorium has proved to be the safest and most effective way to remove a pineal neoplasm (3,4,8). Preoperative shunting in cases of increased ICP is recommended. We routinely perform postoperative X-ray therapy in all pineal tumors except pineocytomas; however, gliomas are included. Additional radiation to the spinal axis is given in pineoblastomas, germinomas, and malignant teratomas. However, shunting and X-ray therapy alone are not adequate treatment for tumors of the pineal region. Many of them are not sensitive to radiation, and secondary surgery would be difficult and dangerous.

With a mortality rate of 5%, we feel that direct surgery is just as justified in tumors of the pineal region as in the case of pituitary adenomas or craniopharyngeomas.

Summary

The authors report a consecutive series of 52 tumors of the pineal region operated on by a direct surgical approach. The first nine cases were operated by a transcallosal approach (2) and two others by a transventricular temporal approach (12). Since 1971, encouraged by POPPEN, the right occipital approach has been performed. Of 41 patients, only three died as a consequence of the operation. Most of the cases had a preoperative ventriculoatrial shunt. Neuroradiologic findings are of particular importance for the indication of the direct approach. Operative techniques and results are demonstrated.

References

1. CAPDEVILLE, J.: Les tumeurs de la région pinéale. Thesis, Lyon 1974
2. DANDY, W.E.: An operation for the removal of pineal tumours. Surg. Gynecol. Obstet. 33, 113-179 (1921)
3. JAMIESON, K.G.: Excision of pineal tumors. J. Neurosurg. 35, 550-553 (1971)
4. LAPRAS, C., DECHAUME, J.P., DERUTY, R.: Traitement des tumeurs de la région pinéale. Lyon Chir. 69, 196-198 (1973)
5. POPPEN, J.L.: The right occipital approach to a pinealoma. J. Neurosurg. 25, 706-710 (1966)
6. POPPEN, J.L., MARINO, R.: Pinealomas and tumors of the posterior portion of the third ventricle. J. Neurosurg. 28, 357-364 (1968)
7. RUSSELL, D.S., RUBINSTEIN, L.J.: Pathology of tumors of the nervous system, 3rd ed. London: Edward Arnold 1+72
8. SCHÄFER, M., LAPRAS, C., THOMALSKE, G.: Sarcoidosis of the pineal gland. J. Neurosurg. 47, 630-632 (1977)
9. SCHMIDEK, H.: Pineal tumors. New York: Masson 1977
10. THOMALSKE, G., GRAU, H., SCHÄFER, M.: The significance of cranial computer tomography for the diagnosis of certain expansive lesions of the midline. In: Cranial Computerized Tomography. LANKSCH, W., KAZNER, E. (eds.), pp. 104-109. Berlin, Heidelberg, New York: Springer 1976
11. THOMALSKE, G., BECKER, H., SCHÄFER, M.: Diagnostic différentiel des tumeurs intraventriculaires par la tomodensitométrie. Neuro-Chirugie 23, 1, 81-91 (1977)
12. Van WAGENEN, W.P.: A surgical approach for the removal of certain pineal tumours. Surg. Gynecol. Obstet. 53, 216-220 (1931)
13. ZÜLCH, K.J.: Biologie und Pathologie der Hirngeschwülste. In: Handbuch der Neurochirurgie. Vol. III, pp. 57-59. OLIVECRONA, H., TÖNNIS, W. (eds.). Berlin, Göttingen, Heidelberg: Springer 1956

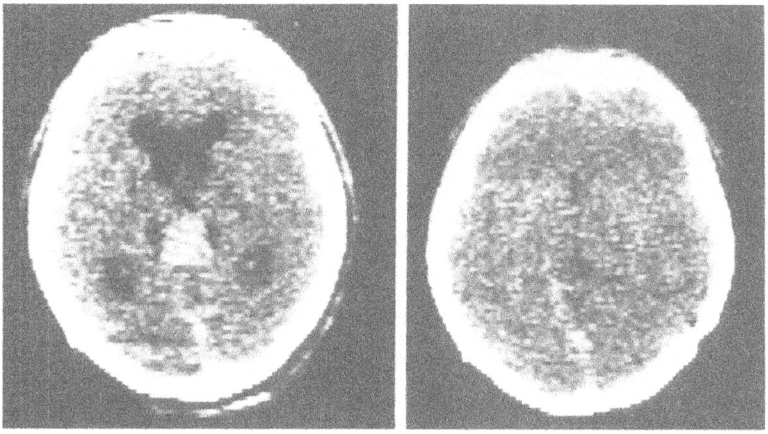

Fig. 1. F.E., 42, female. CT image: pineocytoma with obstructive hydrocephalus (*left*). Same patient. CT control, 1 year after the operation (*right*). (We are indebted to Prof. Dr. H. HACKER, Director of the Department for Neuroradiology at the University Clinic in Frankfurt/Main for the CT examinations)

Transmaxillary Approach to Intraorbital Tumors

J. MENZEL and H. J. DENECKE

Surgery of intraorbital tumors confronts the surgeon with several problems. The most important of all is the decision about the approach to the tumor. Tumors localized anteriorly, laterally, and inferiorly to the optic globe are in the domain of ophthalmologists. However, in the majority of cases, the retrobulbar space is inaccessible for the ophthalmologist. For that reason other specialties such as general surgery, neurosurgery, and rhinosurgery have tried to find different approaches.

KRÖNLEIN (5) reached the retrobulbar space by the lateral approach. After transient resection of the zygoma the periorbital capsule was incised, the lateral rectus muscle divided, and the retrobulbar space explored. This technique has been improved several times, especially by DENECKE (3) who reached the retrobulbar space by the infratemporal approach. For the neurosurgeon the best way to reach retro-orbital tumors is the transfrontal approach as proposed by NAFFZIGER (6). But it is also well-known that this approach is associated with all the risks of an intracranial operation. Besides, it is very difficult to reach tumors localized under the optic nerve, and often additional damage to the levator palpebrae and superior rectus muscles occurs.

Rhinosurgeons used the transethmoidal route, which allowed only a small field. About 70% of all retrobulbar tumors are localized in the lower half of the retrobulbar space (1). These tumors are accessible via the transmaxillary route. This approach was first used in 1926 by SEIFFERT (7) in cases of retrobulbar abscesses. HIRSCH (4) practiced this approach to remove fat in cases of malignant exophthalmos. DENECKE and SEIFFERT (2) used the transmaxillary route for the extirpation of retrobulbar tumors.

The procedure starts with a CALDWEELL-LUC operation of the maxillary sinus (Fig. 1). An incision 3 cm long is made in the buccal mucosa which is pushed upward to the infraorbital nerve (Fig. 2). The anterior wall of the maxillary sinus is removed, the mucosa incised, and the floor of the orbit resected widely enough (Fig. 3). Care must be taken not to injure the infraorbital nerve and artery and not to remove the anterior infraorbital bony part. The periorbital capsule is slit (Fig. 4). For the visualization of the tumor, a long-armed speculum is introduced. Fat should not be removed to prevent enophthalmos. In some cases digital palpation is helpful in finding the tumor and in localizing the optic nerve. The tumor is removed under microscopy. After extirpation of the tumor, the periorbital capsule should be sutured. Reconstruction of the bony floor of the orbit is not necessary. The operation is finished with a fenestration of the maxillary sinus to the nose. The tamponade is removed 48 h after the operation.

We have operated on five patients using the transmaxillary approach. The most important parameters are presented in Table 1. Age varied from 10-50 years. Four patients were male, one female. Leading symptoms were exophthalmos in all and reduced vision in two cases. One patient suffered from restriction of ocular motility. Histologic examination revealed hemangioma cavernosum in three and cystic intraorbital tumor in two cases.

Table 1. Summary of the most important clinical parameters of five patients with retrobulbar tumors

Age, sex	Symptoms	Operation	Pathology	Postoperative course
50 years, male	Exophthalmos, ocular motility restricted	Transmaxillary approach	Hemangioma cavernosum	Uneventful, full recovery of ocular motility
11 years, male	Exophthalmos, reduced vision	Transmaxillary approach	Hemangioma cavernosum	Uneventful, full recovery of vision
10 years, female	Exophthalmos	Transmaxillary approach	Hemangioma cavernosum	Uneventful
40 years, male	Exophthalmos	Transmaxillary approach	Cystic intraorbital tumor	Uneventful
45 years, male	Exophthalmos, reduced vision	Transmaxillary approach	Cystic intraorbital tumor	Uneventful, partial recovery of vision

Exophthalmos disappeared in all cases postoperatively. Vision returned completely in one case and partially in the other case. No additional injuries to nerves, muscles, or vessels occurred. Rhinologic complications were not observed.

In conclusion, we believe that the transmaxillary route is an alternative approach to retrobulbar tumors, especially in those localized in the lower half of the orbit. Tumor of the optic nerve, those with intracranial extension, and those in the upper half of the orbit are not accessible by this method. The question of whether the neurosurgeon or the rhinosurgeon performs the operation is decided in our team as follows. The maxillary sinus is operated by the rhinosurgeon, who also resects the orbital floor. The intraorbital part of the operation is performed by the neurosurgeon. The rhinosurgeon finishes the procedure in the manner described.

References

1. BENEDICT, W.: Surgical treatment of tumors and cysts of the orbit. Am. J. Ophthalmol. 32, 763-772 (1949)
2. DENECKE, H.J.: Erfahrungen bei der permaxillären Entfernung von retrobulbär gelegenen Orbitalcavernomen und -cysten. Arch. Otorhinolaryngol. N.Y. 164, 416-420 (1954)

3. DENECKE, H.J.: Der infratemporale Zugangsweg zur Orbita und zur Fossa pterygoidea. Fortschr. Kiefer Gesichtschir. 14, 241-242 (1970)

4. HIRSCH, C.: Chirurgische Entlastung bei malignem Exophthalmus. Arch. Otorhinolaryngol. N.Y. 51, 325-332 (1950)

5. KRÖNLEIN, R.U.: Zur Pathologie und operativen Behandlung der Dermoidcysten der Orbita. In: Laupp'sche Buchhandlung, Klinische Chirurgie, Vol. IV. Tübingen: 1889

6. NAFFZIGER, H.C., JONES, O.W., Jr.: The surgical treatment of progressive exophthalmos following thyroidectomy. J.A.M.A. 99, 638-648 (1932)

7. SEIFFERT, A.: Zur operativen Behandlung retrobulbärer Eiterungen von der Oberkieferhöhle aus. Passow Schäfers Beitr. 23, 112-124 (1926)

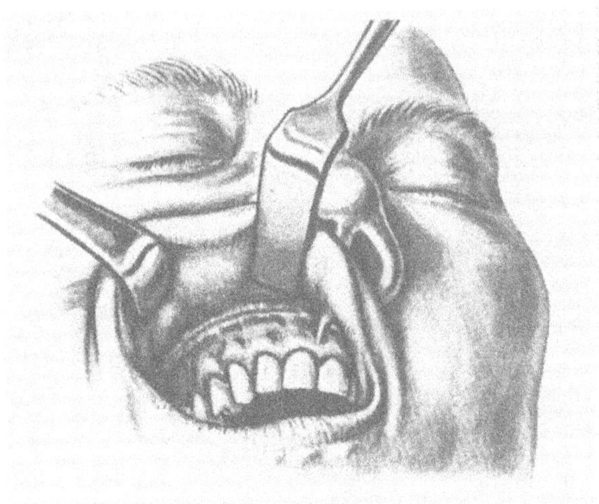

Fig. 1. Incision in the buccal mucosa

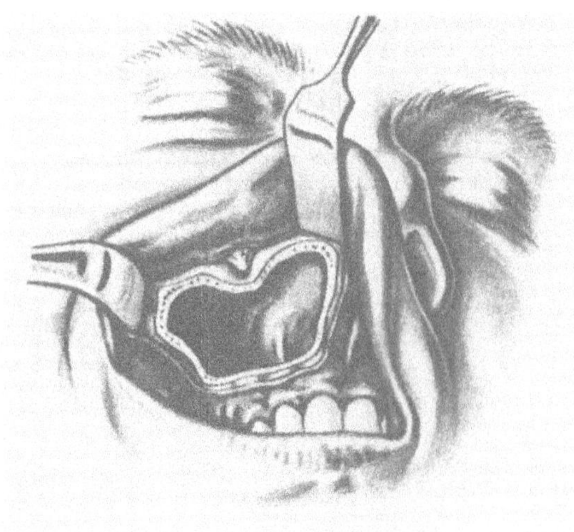

Fig. 2. The anterior wall of the maxillary sinus is resected and the periorbital capsule slit

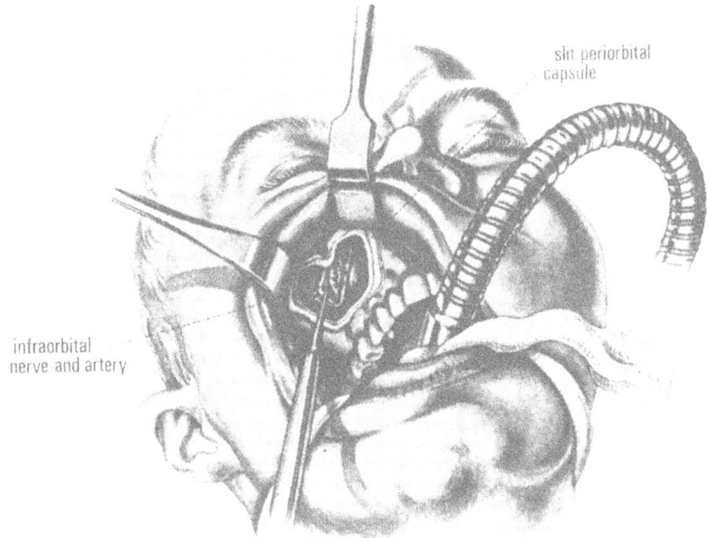

Fig. 3. The floor of the orbit is resected and the periorbital capsule slit

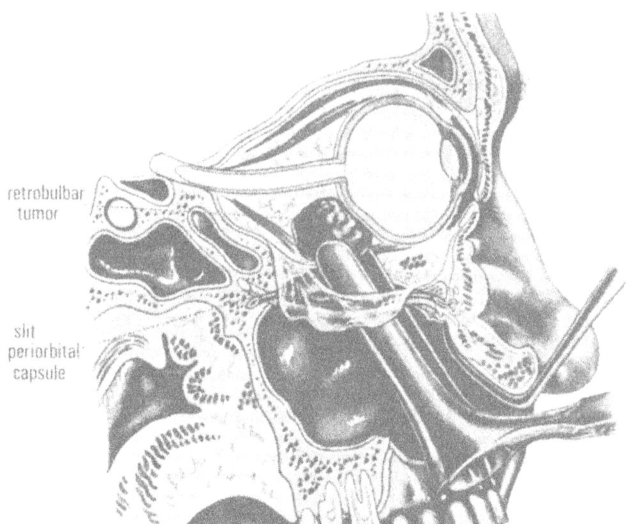

Fig. 4. The long-armed speculum is introduced; the retrobulbar tumor is presented

Concerning the Question of Total Tumor Removal in Medulloblastoma in View of New Postoperative Techniques in Radiotherapy

E. B. BONGARTZ, H.-E. NAU, M. BAMBERG, C. BAYINDIR, and W. GROTE

Of all intracranial neoplasms of childhood, the medulloblastoma is the most common (16,27). It is a highly radiosensitive tumor. Its tendency to spread via the cerebrospinal fluid is well known. Since 1930, the irradiation of the whole cerebrospinal axis has become a well-established principle in the treatment of medulloblastoma (1-6,9,11,12, 18,24). Improved operative techniques succeeded in lowering the surgical mortality. Nevertheless, the results of this treatment with respect to long-term survival have been very disappointing. The previously poor prognosis for children sufferung from medulloblastoma has led us to develop a joint neurosurgical-radiotherapeutic scheme of treatment.

Clinical Material and Methods

Thirty patients with medulloblastoma were treated from 1969-1977 in the departments of neurosurgery and radiotherapy in Essen. Because of different radiation techniques, these patients were divided into two groups. The first group of 12 patients was treated between 1969 and 1973 with telecobalt or telecesium γ-rays. Only in five cases was the complete nervous system irradiated. Between 1974 and 1977, the second group of 18 patients was treated with the linear accelerator applied to the complete nervous system. There were 26 males and 10 females with an average age of 8.7 years (Fig. 1).

Twenty-six patients (90%) were admitted to the hospital with a history of less than 3 months. Headache, vomiting, and vertigo were the first complaints in all but three patients. Two patients complained of ataxia and one of seizures.

Papilledema was found in 17 patients, and disturbed synergia was observed in 19 patients. Other symptoms were cranial nerve palsy (18 patients), reflex disturbances (3 patients), inertia (2 patients), speech disorders (2 patients), and impaired memory (1 patient).

Computer tomography confirmed its superior value in demonstrating posterior fossa tumors. In all patients investigated with this method, the tumor could be visualized whereas pneumencephalography or ventriculography, carried out in 25 cases, showed normal findings in two patients. Radionuclide brain scans were performed in 17 patients. Eight of these showed negative results. However, routine investigations, such as plain skull films, electroencephalography, and cerebrospinal fluid cytology, are also very important studies.

Total tumor removal was carried out in 16 patients. Subtotal extirpation was performed in eight patients, partial removal in five, and a biopsy in one patient. Three patients died during the early postoperative period, resulting in a surgical mortality of 9%. In these patients a macroscopic total tumor removal was performed. They were operated before 1973 and were not included in this study because no postoperative irradiation followed. The purpose of the operation was to unblock the cerebrospinal fluid pathway and to remove tumor for tissue verification. We tried to remove as much tumor as possible without increasing the neurological deficit. In almost all cases, an additional shunt was necessary to prevent the development of an occlusive hydrocephalus, which might be caused by local tumor recurrence or brain edema during radiotherapy. After the operative treatment, all patients were submitted to radiotherapy as soon as possible.

Since 1974 we have treated our patients with photons of a 5.7-MeV linear accelerator according to a specially developed irradiation technique. During treatment the patient is positioned prone in a plaster body cast. Face, eyes, and the anterior part of the neck are shielded with a block of Lipowitz metal (Fig. 2). At first, the spinal cord and dural sac are irradiated with a small vertical field 40 cm long. Subsequently, the whole brain is irradiated by two opposing parallel portals. To avoid "hot spots" (dose inhomogeneities), the junction of brain and spinal fields is moved daily in four steps from position 1 to 4 (Fig. 2). We give a tumor dose of 36 Gy (3600 rad) to the cerebrospinal axis over 5 weeks, followed by a booster dose of 14 Gy to the posterior fossa with smaller portals over 2 weeks. The dose distribution of this radiation technique was measured by using an Alderson phantom human and thermoluminescent dosimeters (Fig. 3).

Results

The first group of 12 children received irradiation of the primary tumor with up to 40 Gy of telecobalt or telecesium γ-rays. Only in five cases was the spine irradiated sequentially in separate fields with a dose of 20 Gy. None of these young patients survived for more than 3 years. In nine of them local recurrences developed first. Spinal metastases were seen in five patients within 7-34 months after diagnosis (Fig. 4).

The 18 patients of the second group were treated with the linear accelerator according to the described technique (Fig. 5). After a follow-up period of 1-5 years, 12 patients are living and six died of local recurrence after 6-20 months. Spinal metastases were seen in only two cases; in one case during the 1st week after the beginning of radiotherapy and in the other case at autopsy, 2 months after a local recurrence (Table 1). During radiotherapy blood counts were performed twice a week. Because a large proportion of the bone marrow was irradiated, leukopenia or thrombocytopenia were seen frequently (Table 2). In two cases, radiotherapy had to be interrupted for two weeks because of myelosuppression (Table 1). One year after completion of radiotherapy, the peripheral leukocyte and thrombocyte counts have been totally restored to the preoperative level in all patients.

The 12 surviving patients were followed up by the departments of neurosurgery and radiotherapy. Eight children are doing well at school, with average or better performances. Three patients are living at home and are able to take care of themselves but show dyssynergia, dysphasia, or differences or reflexes. One young boy attends a special school, as he developed amaurosis of both eyes in the 1st week after the beginning of radiotherapy (Table 3). No growth disturbances were observed after radiotherapy. Only a slight increase of the alkaline phosphatase level was noticed in five patients (21).

Table 1. Survival and recurrence rates of the six dead patients

Age at diagnosis	Sex	Extent of surgery	Shunt	Survival time (months)	Comments
10	M	Total	Yes	6	Spinal metastases in the 1st week after the beginning of radiotherapy, extended radiation treatment time, desmoplastic variant
20 1/4	M	Total	Yes	8	Local recurrence after 3 months with amaurosis of both eyes, permanent vomiting during radiotherapy
6 1/2	M	Partial	Yes	10	Local recurrence after 8 months, spinal metastases were found at autopsy, desmoplastic variant
8 1/2	M	Partial	Yes	13	Radiotherapy discontinued because of staphylococcemia wound infection, local recurrence after 10 months
13	M	Total	Yes	14	Extreme leukopenia and thrombocytopenia local recurrence after 10 months
3	M	Total	Yes	20	Local recurrence after 20 months, desmoplastic variant

Table 2. Blood count changes during irradiation of the spinal cord

Findings	No. of cases	%
Leukopenia total	16/18	88.9
$< 3000/mm^3$	7/18	38.9
$> 3000/mm^3$	9/18	50.0
No leukopenia	2/18	11.1
Thrombocytopenia total	11/18	61.1
$< 10000/mm^3$	6/18	33.3
$> 10000/mm^3$	5/18	27.8
No Thrombocytopenia	7/18	38.9

Table 3. Performance of 12 patients living with no evidence of disease (NED)

Age at diagnosis	Sex	Extent of surgery	Shunt	Survival time (months)	Comments
8 3/4	F	Total	Yes	16	Attends school, in top third of the class
9 1/2	M	Total	No	22	Attends school, average performance, dyssynergia
15	F	Biopsy	Yes	23	Attends high school, average performance
8 1/2	M	Total	Yes	25	Attends school, in lower third of the class, nystagmus, reflex differences
2	M	Partial	Yes	25	Amaurosis of both eyes, developed during the first weeks of radiotherapy, no mental debility
15 1/4	F	Subtotal	Yes	26	Living at home, takes care of herself, dyssynergia, dysphasia, reflex differences
13 1/4	F	Subtotal	No	26	Attends high school, average performance, dyssynergia, reflex differences
15 3/4	F	Total	Yes	33	Living at home, takes care of herself, slight dyssynergia and headache
24	F	Subtotal	No	35	Living at home, takes care of herself, postoperative pareses of n. facialis and n. trigeminus
6 3/4	M	Subtotal	Yes	37	Attends school, in top third of the class
15 1/2	M	Total	Yes	41	Training for technician, normal mental development
7 1/2	M	Subtotal	Yes	57	Attends school, average performance
	1				

Discussion

The cerebellar medulloblastoma as originally defined by BAILEY and CUSHING (1a) in 1925 is by general agreement an embryonic tumor predominantly found in males (16,18,20). Its cells are largely primitive or poorly differentiated and nowadays is recognized as arising only in the cerebellum. Especially in the 1st decade, the majority originate in the midline whereas in adults they are more likely to occupy a lateral lobe.

The bad prognosis for very young children below the age of 2 years is well-known. No clear evidence exists relating age at diagnosis to prognosis; however, the long-term survival seems to be better in the younger children (3,11).

Neurosurgeons and radiotherapists generally agree that operative tissue verification should be performed before irradiation. It has been mentioned that attempts at radical surgical resection should be avoided (6). Like other authors, we tried to remove as much tumor as possible without increasing the preoperative neurological deficits (20,24,26). Our study does not support the opinion that results following gross subtotal or total tumor removal are superior to those of partial excision or biopsy (4,11,15,22). Our material shows no marked difference in survival between patients in whom tumor removal was macroscopically total, subtotal, or only partial. We think that the question of the extent of tumor removal should not be answered in general because it depends on the operative findings.

In almost all patients a shunt system was applied to assure a free passage of cerebrospinal fluid in case of obstruction of the posterior fossa by local tumor recurrence or radiotherapy-induced brain edema. According to the opinion of GUTIERREZ (10), HOVIND (13), and LORBER (17), *extracranial medulloblastoma metastases* caused by shunting systems are the exception rather than the rule. The desmoplastic variant of the medulloblastoma frequently arises in the cerebellar hemispheres of adults. One of the characteristic patterns of this type of medulloblastoma is the reticulin-free island. It is assumed that the desmoplastic variant has a more favorable prognosis (7,23). Three of our patients with this tumor type died within 20 months. This experience is shared by BLOOM et al. (4). An attempt to correlate prognosis to a histologic malignancy scale did not succeed. Our results obtained by surgery and consecutive irradiation are in agreement with the results of other investigators. Up to now the application of chemotherapeutic agents showed different results (8,14,19); its indication and timing are also still under discussion. Important is the statement that by combining surgery, radiotherapy, and chemotherapy, complications and risks, i.e., intracerebral hematomas and transverse myelitis, will increase exponentially (25).

Conclusions

The results of treatment for medulloblastoma by surgery alone are very disappointing; however, since the application of radiotherapy, the long-term survival statistics justify the impression that medulloblastoma is a radiocurable tumor. There was no marked correlation between the length of survival and the extent of surgery. Surgery is determined only by the size and localization of the tumor. It is not yet clear whether better results can be obtained by the application of chemotherapeutic agents or radiosensitizers.

References

1. BAILEY, P.: Further notes on the cerebellar medulloblastoma. The effect of roentgen therapy. Am. J. Pathol. 6, 126-136 (1930)

1a. BAILEY, P., CUSHING, H.: Medulloblastoma cerebelli. A common type of midcerebellar glioma of childhood. Arch. Neurol. Psychiat. (Chic.) 14, 192-224 (1925)

2. BAMBERG, M., SCHMITT, G., BONGARTZ, E.B., NAU, H.E., SCHERER, E.: Irradiation techniques and clinical results in the treatment of medulloblastomas. 12th International Cancer Congress. Buenos Aires, 5-11 October 1978

3. BLOOM, H.J.G.: Medulloblastoma: Prognosis and prospects. Int. J. Radiat. Oncol. Biol. Phys. 2, 1031-1033 (1977)

4. BLOOM, H.J.G., WALLACE, E.N.K., HENK, J.M.: The treatment and prognosis of medulloblastoma in children. A study of eighty-two verified cases. Am. J. Roentgenol. 105, 43-62 (1969)

5. BONGARTZ, E.B., BAMBERG, M., NAU, H.E., SCHMITT, G., BAYINDIR, C.: The optimum therapy in medulloblastoma. 6th Congress of the European Society for Paediatric Neurosurgery. Rotterdam, 30 August - 2 September 1978

6. CHANG, C.H., HOUSEPIAN, E.M., HERBERT, C., Jr.: An operative staging system and a megavoltage radiotherapeutic technic for cerebellar medulloblastomas. Radiology 93, 1351-1359 (1969)

7. CHATTY, M., EARLE, K.M.: Medulloblastoma: report of 201 cases with emphasis on relationship of histological variants to survival. Cancer 28, 977-983 (1971)

8. CRAFTS, D.C., LEVIN, V.A., EDWARDS, M.S., PISCHER, T.L., WILSON, C.B.: Chemotherapy of recurrent medulloblastoma with combined procarbazine, CCNU, and vincristine. J. Neurosurg. 49, 589-593 (1978)

9. CUTLER, E.C., SOSMAN, M.C., VAUGHAN, W.W.: The place of radiation in the treatment of cerebellar medulloblastoma. Report of twenty cases. Am. J., Roentgenol. 35, 429-453 (1936)

10. GUTIERREZ, F.: Personal communication. 6th Meeting of the International Society for Paediatric Neurosurgery. Jerusalem, 24-27 September 1978

11. HARISIADIS, L., CHANG, C.H.: Medulloblastoma in children. A correlation of staging and results of treatment. Int. J. Radiat. Oncol. Biol. Phys. 2, 833-841 (1977)

12. HOPE-STONE, H.F.: Radiotherapy in modern clinical practice. London: Crosby Lockwood Staples 1976

13. HOVIND, K.H.: Personal communication. 6th Meeting of the International Society for Paediatric Neurosurgery. Jerusalem, 24-27 September 1978

14. HOVIND, K.H., GLOMSTEIN, A., SORTLAND, O.: The timing of cytostatic medication in the treatment of medulloblastoma. 6th Meeting of the International Society for Paediatric Neurosurgery. Jerusalem, 24-27 September 1978

15. KING, G.A., SAGERMAN, R.H.: Late recurrence in medulloblastoma. Am. J. Roentgenol. 123, 7-12 (1975)

16. KRAUS, M., KOOS, W.: Hirntumoren im Kindes- und Jugendalter. Wien. Klin. Wochenschr. 79, 934-943 (1967)

17. LORBER, J.: Personal communication. 6th Meeting of the International Society for Paediatric Neurosurgery. Jerusalem, 24-27 September 1978

18. McFARLAND, D.R., HORWITZ, H., SAENGER, E.L., BAHR, G.K.: Medulloblastoma - a review of prognosis and survival. Br. J. Radiol. 43, 198 - 214 (1969)

19. MEALEY, J., HALL, P.V.: Medulloblastoma in children. J. Neurosurg. 46, 56-64 (1977)

20. MILES, J., BHANDARI, Y.S.: Cerebellar medulloblastomata in adults: Review of 18 cases. J. Neurol. Neurosurg. Psychiatry 33, 208-211 (1970)

21. PROBERT, J.C., PARKER, B.R., KAPLAN, M.S.: Growth retardation in children after megavoltage irradiation of the spine. Cancer 32, 634-636 (1973)

22. RAIMONDI, A.J., TOMITA, T.: Medulloblastoma in childhood: Comparative results of partial and total resection. 6th Congress of the European Society for Paediatric Neurosurgery. Rotterdam, 30 August - 2 September 1978

23. RUBINSTEIN, L.J.: Tumours of the central nervous system, pp. 130-153. Washington, D.C.: Armed Forces Institute of Pathology, 1972

24. SHELINE, G.E.: Radiation therapy of tumors of the central nervous system in childhood. Cancer 35, 957-964 (1975)

25. SHUT, L., BRUCE, D.A., D'ANGIO, G.J.: Complications for combined therapy for CNS tumors. 6th Meeting of the International Society for Paediatric Neurosurgery. Jerusalem, 24-27 September 1978

26. SMITH, R.A., LAMPE, I., KAHN, E.A.: The prognosis of medulloblastoma in children. J. Neurosurg. 18, 91-97 (1961)

27. ZÜLCH, K.J., CHRISTENSEN, E.: Pathologische Anatomie der raumbeengenden intrakraniellen Prozesse. In: OLIVECRONA, H., TÖNNIS, W. (Eds.). Handbuch der Neurochirurgie, Vol. 3. Berlin, Göttingen, Heidelberg: Springer 1956

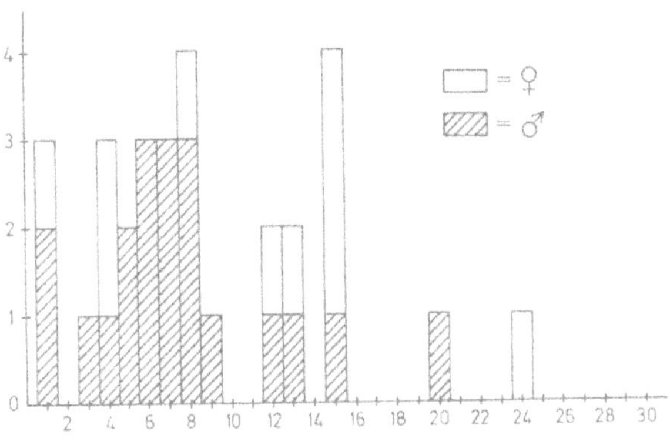

Fig. 1. Age and sex of the patients sufferung from medulloblastoma

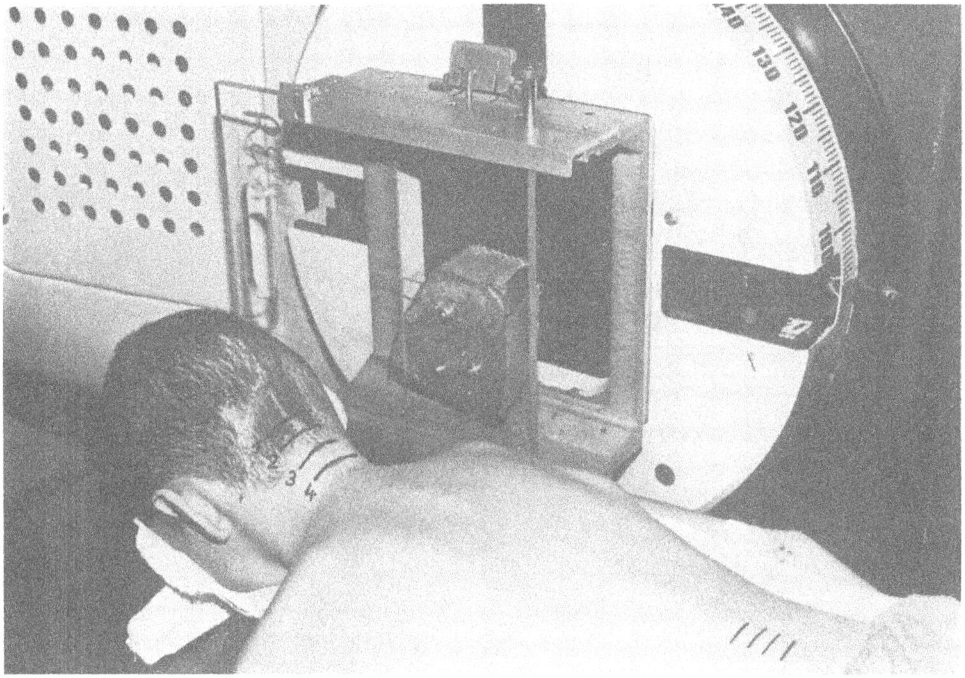

Fig. 2. Patient in plaster body cast. Face, eyes, and anterior part of the neck are shielded with a block of Lipowitz metal

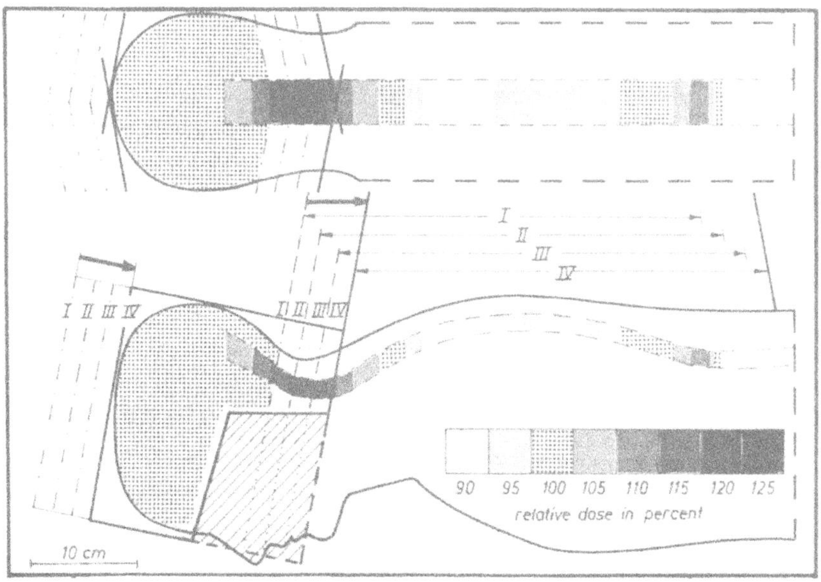

Fig. 3. Relative dose in brain and spinal cord in an Linac, X 5.7 MeV, irradiation technique for medulloblastomas in Essen

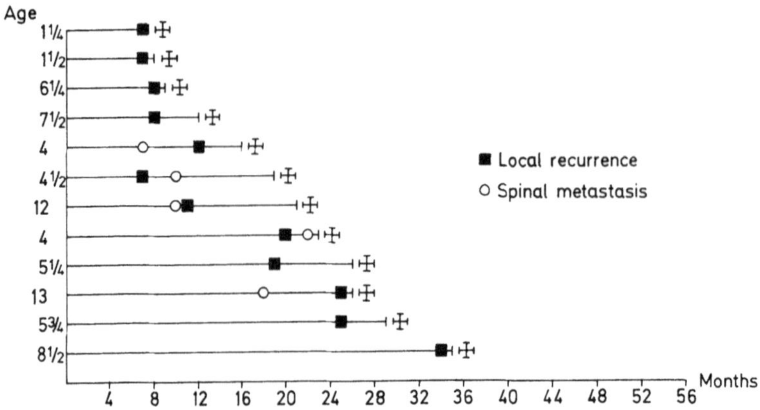

Fig. 4. Survival rates of the 12 patients in the first group (1969 - 1973)

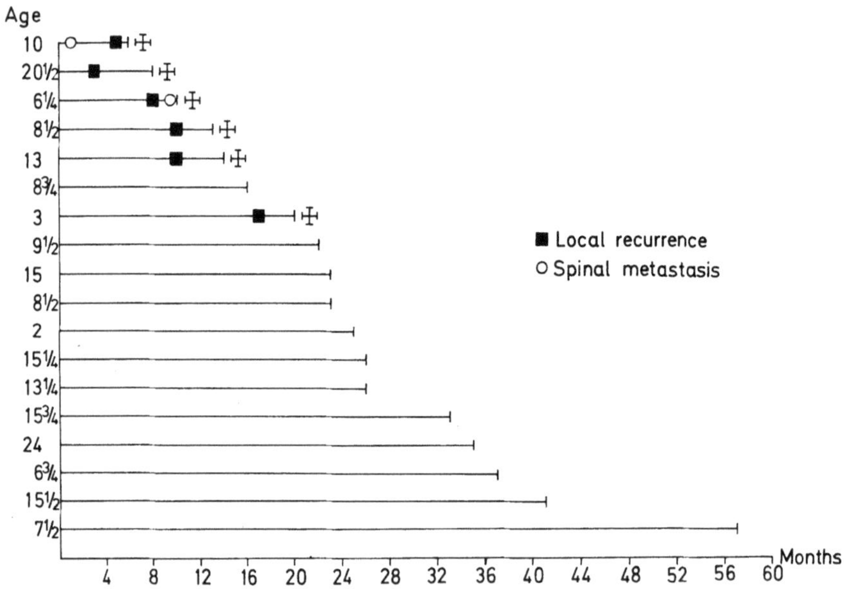

Fig. 5. Survival rates of the 18 patients in the second group (1974 - 1977)

Early Neurosurgical Repair in Craniofacial Dysmorphism

H. J. HOFFMAN and E. B. HENDRICK

Introduction

The craniofacial dysmorphic states have come under increasing scrutiny in recent years because of the interest of plastic surgeons and neurosurgeons in the reconstructive surgery of these anomalies (8) and the interest of the geneticist (1) in the etiology of these disorders. Furthermore, modern neurosurgical techniques have led to the improved treatment of many of these conditions with the resulting cosmetic repair allowing patients in the childbearing age to have offsprings with similar disorders, particularly where the disorder is due to an autosomal - dominant gene.

Several investigators (2,5,7,9) now agree that the cause of the craniofacial dysmorphic states is synostosis occurring in the sutures of the cranial base, in particular the frontosphenoidal and frontoethmoidal sutures in the floor of the anterior cranial fossa. As a result of this synostotic process in the base, there is secondary synostosis of the cranial vault sutures, including the coronal suture.

The ventral portion of the frontal lobes estabilishes the size and alignment of the floor of the anterior cranial fossa, which in turn determines the extent and direction of facial growth. Thus, patients with synostosis of these basal skull sutures have not only a foreshortened cranium but also severe midface hypoplasia, shallow orbits, and proptosis. Simply opening the coronal suture does nothing for the synostotic process in the base of the skull, and the face consequently remains hypoplastic.

Furthermore, the time of surgery is critical. The human brain grows more rapidly during the first 6 months of life than it does during the remainder of childhood. It is this rapid growth of brain that determines growth and shape of the overlying skull vault. Thus, to achieve a good cosmetic result without repeated and complex surgical procedures, the basal sutures must be opened early in infancy and preferably before the age of 3 months.

Hydrocephalus is a common concomitant of these craniofacial dysmorphic states and may well be due to the synostosis-producing compression of the venous sinuses. Whenever hydrocephalus is present, it magnifies the bizarre appearance of these patients as we see in disorders, such as craniotelencephalic dysplasia (4) and Kleeblattschädel (6). Furthermore, untreated hydrocephalus combined with craniosynostosis no doubt accounts for the severe mental retardation that some of these untreated patients display. In our experience, adequate treatment of the craniosynostosis will often lead to spontaneous resolution of the hydrocephalus.

Table 1. Craniofacial dysmorphism

Syndrome	Genetics			Craniofacial findings	Associated findings
	Sporadic	Autosomal dominant	Autosomal recessive		
Crouzon	Yes (25%)	Yes	No	Craniosynostosis involving coronal sutures, basal skull sutures frequently associated with maxillary hypoplasia, shallow orbits, proptosis	Hydrocephalus rare
Saethre-Chotzen	No	Yes	No	"	Ptosis, brachydactyly; soft tissue syndactyly; often asymmetric; hydrocephalus rare
Apert	Yes (95%)	Yes	No	"	Osseous and soft tissue, syndactyly of digits 2,3,4 of hands and soft tissue syndactyly of digits 2,3,4 of feet; shortened upper extremities; hydrocephalus common
Carpenter	No	No	Yes	"	Polysyndactyly of the feet, soft tissue syndactyly of hands; hydrocephalus rare
Pfeifer (Noack)	Yes (occasional)	Yes	No	"	Partial soft tissue syndactyly of hands and feet; broad thumbs and great toes; hydrocephalus rare
Summitt	No	No	Yes	"	Variable syndactyly, obesity, gynecomastia
Baller-Gerold	No	No	Yes	"	Radial aplasia
Lowry	No	No	Yes	"	Fibial aplasia
Gorlin-Chaudry-Moss	No	No	Yes	"	Hypertrichosis, anomalies of eyes, teeth, heart and external genitalia

Herrmann-Opitz	Yes	Yes	No	"	Brachysyndactyly of hands, absent toes; soft tissue syndactyly of 2,3,4 fingers
Herrmann-Pallister-Opitz	Yes	Yes	No	"	Severe symmetrically malformed limbs, cleft clip and palate, radial aplasia; microcephaly
Sakati-Nyhan-Tisdale	Yes	Yes	No	"	Polysyndactyly, short limbs, congenital heart disease, ear anomalies
7P-	Yes	Yes	No	"	Deletion of band P21 on chromosome 7 Simian crease; hypogenitalism; naevus flammeus on forehead
Weiss	No	No	Yes	"	Medially deviated great toes, occasional mild syndactyly
Fairbanks	Yes	Yes	No	"	Short legs, failure of tooth eruption
Cranio-telence-phalic Dysplasia	Yes	Yes	?[a]	Craniosynostosis with protruding frontal region (? variant of Crouzon)	Isolated or may be associated with Apert's syndrome, encephalocele; hydrocephalus
Kleeblatt-schädel	Yes	Yes	No	Craniosynostosis with trilobular-shaped skull (? variant of Crouzon)	Isolated or may be associated with thanatrophic dwarfism or Apert's syndrome; hydrocephalus

a Two personally cases in two siblings.

Material and Approach

The craniofacial dysmorphic states are categorized according to genetic patterns and associated anomolous variants (Table 1). There are at least 17 different types of craniofacial dysmorphisms, among which Crouzon's syndrome and Apert's syndrome are the most common. All of these patients have relatively similar facies directly related to the craniosynostosis, and the early neurosurgical treatment is basically the same in all these disorders.

During the past 13 years, we have treated 13 infants with a variety of types of craniofacial dysmorphic states, and in the majority of cases we have been able to produce excellent results. These 13 patients consisted of nine females and four males who ranged in age at the time of initial surgery between 10 days and 6 months, with a mean age of 4 weeks.

Crouzon's syndrome and Apert's syndrome accounted for seven and three patients, respectively. Our series also included one patient with Chotzen's syndrome, one patient with Kleeblattschädel, and one patient with craniotelencephalic dysplasia. Hydrocephalus was present in seven of these patients and in four required a shunting procedure.

All 13 patients had synostosis of both coronal sutures and of the accompanying basal skull sutures. In only four patients was the synostosis confined to these sutures, however. Synostosis of one or more additional sutures was present in two patients, and total craniosynostosis was found in seven patients. A maternal family history was documented in one case of Chotzen's syndrome and one case of Crouzon's syndrome.

With the exception of our patient with Kleeblattschädel of 13 years ago, all patients were treated initially by a bilateral lateral canthal advancement (3). In this procedure, the supraorbital margins are first freed up; the lateral extent of the supraorbital margin is then advanced to normal position and held in this position by a strut of bone, which is fastened posteriorly to parietal bone over silastic. This allows for the expanding frontal lobe to carry forward the supraorbital margin as well as the overlying frontal bone. As a result, the anterior cranial fossa expands and carries the facial structures forward in a normal fashion.

Results

Seven of the 12 patients who had bilateral lateral canthal advancement as neonates have required no further surgery. The follow-up on this particular group of patients has ranged from 3 months to 8 years with an average of 2.9 years. All of these patients have had an excellent cosmetic result (Fig. 1 - 3).

In three cases where neonatal lateral canthal advancement proved inadequate, a simple repeat of this procedure later achieved excellent results. Two patients have required a combined neurosurgical-plastic surgical procedure and have had a final good result. One patient with severe craniotelencephalic dysplasia died at the age of 8 months due to an associated gross cerebral anomaly.

Discussion

The craniofacial dysmorphic states are due to synostosis of the basal skull sutures in the anterior cranial fossa. Bilateral lateral canthal advancement allows the expanding frontal lobe to properly shape the anterior cranial fossa and prevent the midface hypoplasia, which gives these patients their characteristic deformed appearance. Since the human brain grows so quickly during the early months of infancy, it is imperative that proper correction of the craniosynostosis be carried out early in infancy to allow this rapid growth of brain to be taken advantage of.

Accompanying hydrocephalus must be properly diagnosed; if it is not relieved by surgical correction of the craniosynostosis, then a by-pass shunting procedure should be undertaken to prevent the brain damage that will otherwise result. Assuming there are no associated cerebral anomalies - only one such case has come to our attention - these children will then demonstrate normal mentation.

Conclusion

Early neurosurgical intervention in patients with craniofacial dysmorphism allows the growing brain to shape the skull and the attached face. The craniofacial dysmorphic states are becoming increasingly common because of recognition and heredity. Proper and early neurosurgical management of these patients can prevent the bizarre appearance that these children may exhibit as well as prevent the brain damage that many of these children displayed in the past due to inadequate treatment.

References

1. COHEN, M.M.: Genetic perspectives on craniosynostosis and syndromes with craniosynostosis. J. Neurosurg. 47, 886-898 (1977)
2. ENLOW, D.H., AZUMA, M.: Functional growth boundaries in the human and mammalian face. Birth Defects Xl/7, 217-230 (1975)
3. HOFFMAN, H.J., MOHR, G.: Lateral canthal advancement of the supraorbital margin. A new corrective technique in the treatment of coronal synostosis. J. Neurosurg. 45, 376-381 (1976)
4. JABOUR, J.T., TAYBI, H.: Craniotelencephalic dysplasia. Am. J. Dis. Child. 108, 627-632 (1964)
5. MOSS, M.L.: New studies of cranial growth. Birth Defects. Xl/7, 283-295 (1975)
6. MULLER, P.J., HOFFMAN, H.J.: Cloverleaf skull syndrome case report. J. Neurosurg. 43, 86-91 (1975)
7. SEEGER, J.F., GABRIELSON, T.O.: Premature closure of the frontosphenoidal suture in synostosis of the coronal suture. Radiology 101, 631-635 (1971)
8. TESSIER, P.: Osteotomies totales de la face syndrome de Crouzon; syndrome d'Apert. Oxycephalies. Scaphocephalies. Turricephalies. Ann. Chir. Plast. 12, 273-286 (1967)
9. TESSIER, P.: Relationship of craniostenoses to craniofacial dysostoses and to faciostenoses. A study with therapeutic implications. Plast. Reconstr. Surg. 48, 224-237 (1971)

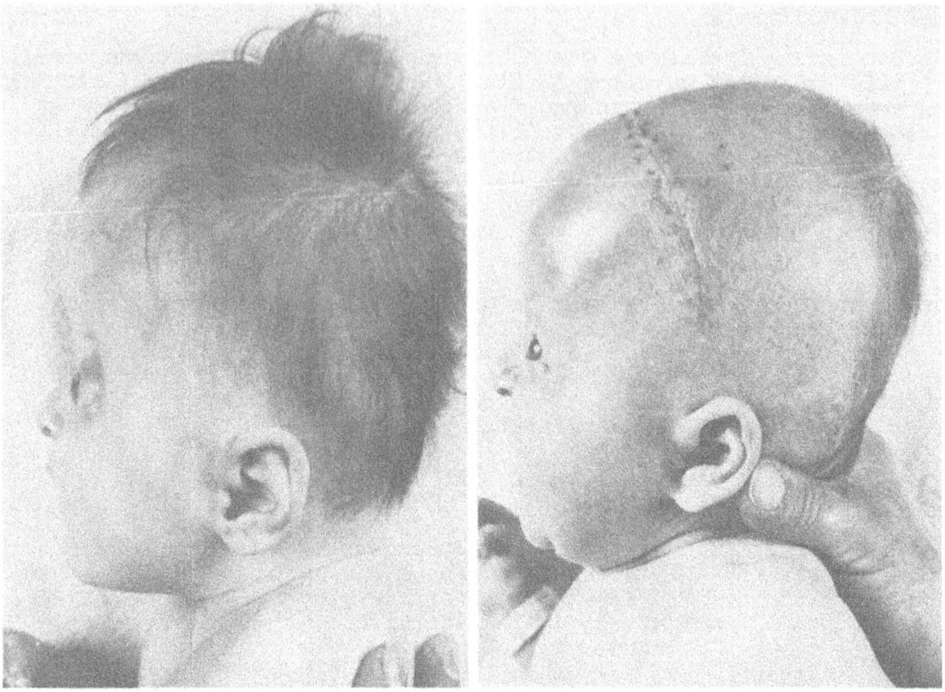

Fig. 1. Lateral view of infant with Apert's syndrome at age 4 months *(left)*. Same child 2 weeks postoperatively showing immediate improvement in appearance *(right)*

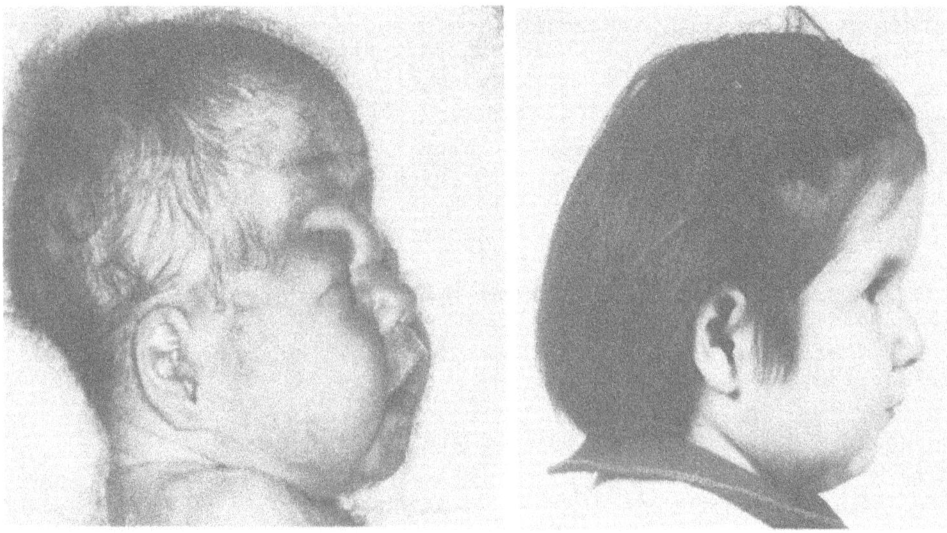

Fig. 2. Lateral view of neonate with Crouzon's syndrome *(left)*. Same child at age 3 years following correction at age 4 weeks *(right)*

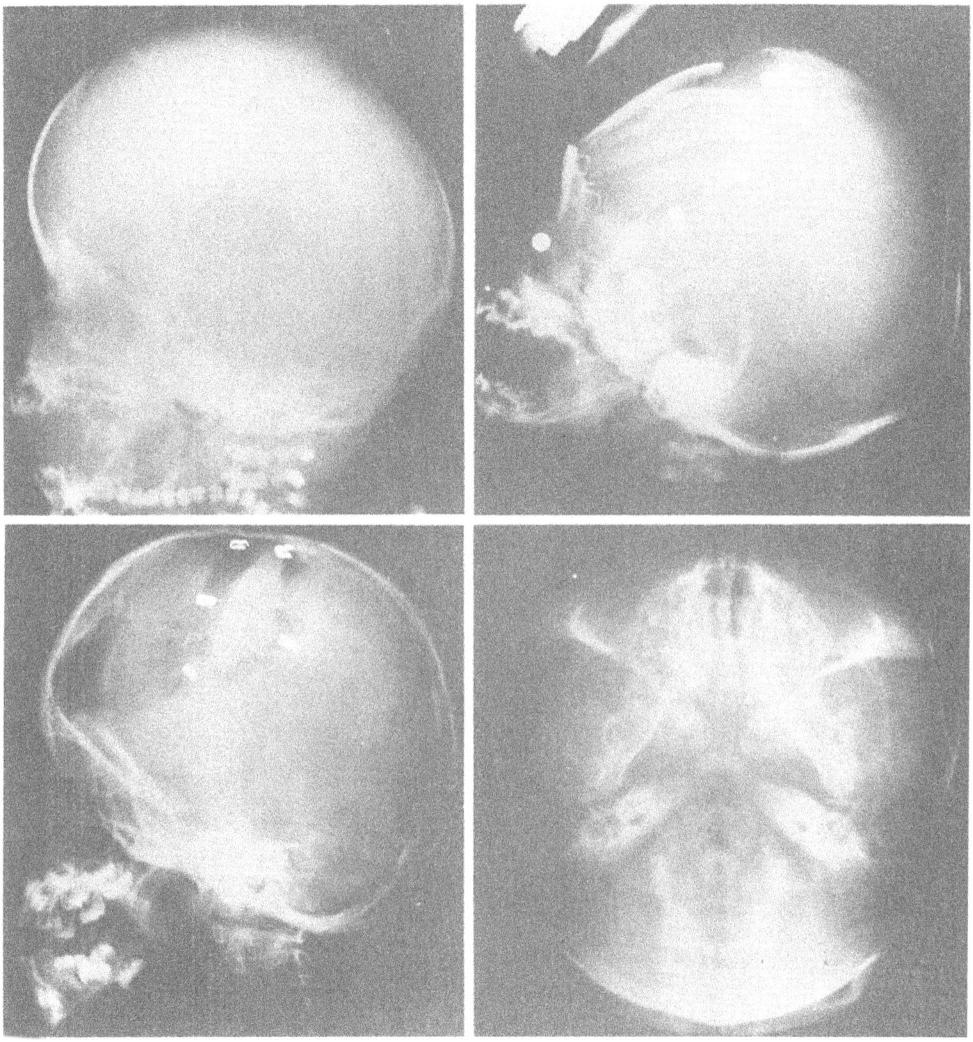

a,c b,d

Fig. 3. a Lateral skull X-ray in neonate with Crouzon's syndrome. b Same child immediately postoperatively. c Same child at age 3 years. Note normal skull configuration. d Basal skull X-ray of same patient as neonate

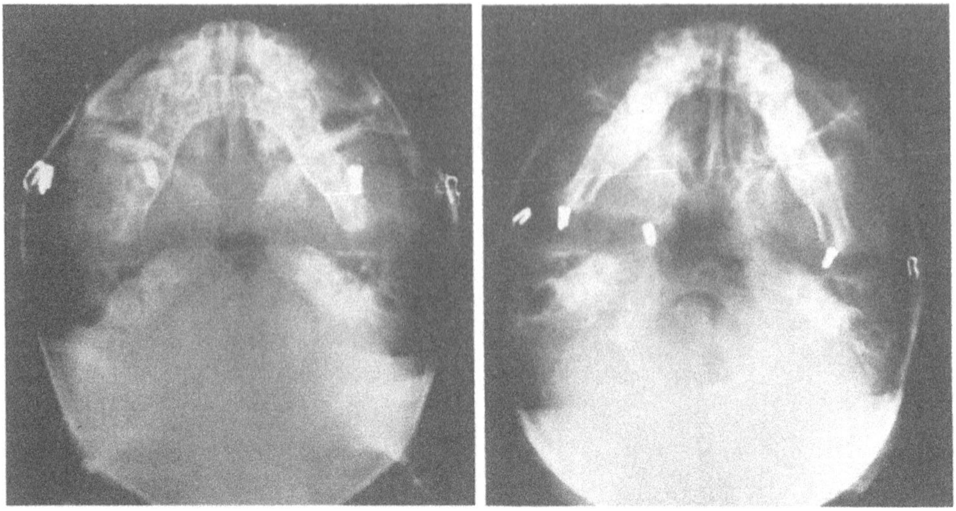

e,f

Fig. 3. e Same child immediately postoperatively. f Same child at age 2 years showing normal basal skull configuration

Surgical Treatment of Amenorrhea-Galactorrhea

J. S. Brodkey, O. H. Pearson, and A. Manni

The association of amenorrhea and galactorrhea with pituitary tumors has been known for many years (1), but only occasionally did such patients come to the attention of the neurosurgeon. The recent development of the sensitive radioimmunoassay for prolactin (3) marked a major advancement, and it was soon shown that the most common hormone secreted in excess by pituitary tumors was prolactin. Furthermore, it rapidly became apparent that small pituitary tumors called microadenomas, which hypersecreted prolactin and produced amenorrhea and galactorrhea in the young woman, were often the cause of infertility (4,6).

Along with the advancement in the diagnosis of these pituitary tumors, several new concepts developed with regard to treatment. Transsphenoidal microsurgery improved the chances for removing the tumor and restoring normal endocrine status with little morbidity or mortality (2). At the same time, it was demonstrated that bromocriptine could suppress prolactin levels and subsequently restore fertility (5). It remains to be determined which of these two treatments, medical or surgical, is most appropriate for the restoration of fertility in the patient harboring a small pituitary adenoma. In actual fact, only close study and long follow-up of these patients will answer this question.

Material and Approach

This report covers 29 patients, aged 18-41, followed an average of 3.3 years and up to 9 years after the removal of a prolactin-secreting adenoma. Clinically all the patients had amenorrhea and galactorrhea. Two patients had minor visual field abnormalities that were attributed to chiasmal compression, but there were no changes in visual acuity.

Endocrine evaluation included the usual thyroid and adrenal studies. Prolactin and growth hormone were studied with an extensive protocol requiring several days for completion. Basal levels of prolactin were always greater than 25 ng/ml, and the larger tumors usually had higher values. Overnight prolactin and growth hormone levels were drawn every 2 h. The normal three- to fivefold increase of prolactin between 2:00 a.m. and 4:00 a.m. was not seen in any tumor patient. Also, the normal increases to thorazine and thyrotropin-releasing hormone (TRH) were not seen. However, one-half of the tumor patients did suppress prolactin levels with L-dopa. All patients but the initial two had such dynamic tests performed and, of course, TRH has only been available in the last 2 years.

Preoperative study of these patients included extensive X-ray testing. By far, the most helpful test has been thin section polytomography, which all patients had. During the early part of the series, pneumoencephalograms (PEGs) were done on all patients, a total of 22. The X-ray studies have been helpful in telling ahead of time which side of the sella to explore first to find the tumor, but we have not hesitated to operate on patients with normal X-ray studies who we were sure harbored a tumor by other criteria. In fact, 3 of these 29 patients with tumors had normal X-ray studies. We have not found the PEG to be helpful enough to warrant its routine use and have thus stopped doing the test.

We have classified the tumors found at operation as follows: The *microadenomas* were contained totally within the sella and did not involve more than one-half of the sella. *Large adenomas* involving more than one-half of the sella, often both sides of the sella, were much larger than a normal gland. *Adenomas with extension* were those that extended outside of the sella. The worst problem that one encounters at surgery is extension laterally into the cavernous sinus. It has been impossible to diagnose this extension preoperatively with current radiologic techniques. The problem is that, as one works with these tumors that extend laterally into the cavernous sinus, careful and total removal is almost impossible.

Tumor left in the cavernous sinus may be a problem not solvable by surgery, but tumor hopefully should not be left within the sella. There are several ways to avoid this possibility. One is to obtain as many frozen sections during the operation as is necessary to define the tumor and normal gland. The other method, to avoid leaving tumor in the sella, is to remove a strip of normal gland adjacent to the tumor to be certain that one has not left any tumor. This has often amounted to performing a hemihypophysectomy, removing one-half of the gland on the side of the tumor, leaving the remainder of the gland attached to the pituitary stalk. It has been estimated that 20%-30% of a pituitary is all that is needed to avoid hypopituitarism. In many of these cases, we purposely entered the subarachnoid space, identified the pituitary stalk, and removed the residual pituitary on one side in one large piece using microscissors.

Results

Table 1 shows the results in these 29 patients. There were no major complications and no deaths. Only two patients required cortisone postoperatively. Both of these patients had very large tumors and probably had very little pituitary reserve. It is apparent that the results depend on the size of the tumor. The small microadenomas were all cured in the sense that in every case prolactin levels were reduced to normal. The amenorrhea was resolved and each of the five patients who wished to become pregnant were able to do so. In the cases of those with larger tumors, the results were not as good. Three patients were treated with bromocriptine to achieve pregnancy when surgery had failed. Two of these patients had tumors with extension and one had a large adenoma. These treatments with bromocriptine worked two of three times and accounted for one pregnancy in the group with extension and one of the pregnancies in the group with large tumors.

Twelve of the 29 patients reverted to normal dynamics postoperatively in the sense that the prolactins were not only reduced to normal levels but responded normally to thorazine and TRH, and there was a normal sleep rise. The interesting question is whether the patients who reverted to normal prolactins and resolved the amenorrhea but retained abnormal dynamics were really cured or whether they will recur in time. To this date only one patient has relapsed. This patient had a micro-

Table 1. Postoperative results in prolactin secreting adenomas

	Normal Prolactin	Normal Dynamics	Resolve Amenorrhea	Resolve Galactorrhea	Pregnancies
Microadenomas	11/11	8/11	11/11	10/11	5/5[a]
Large adenomas	6/11	4/11	5/11	8/11	3/7
Adenomas with extension	2/7	0/7	1/7	2/7	1/3
Total	19/29	12/29	17/29	20/29	9/15

a Five patients pregnant of five who desired to become pregnant.

adenoma following the removal of which prolactins became normal, galactorrhea and amenorrhea resolved, but the dynamics remained abnormal. Nineteen months postoperatively, menses became irregular, galactorrhea resumed, and the prolactin rose to 50, twice the normal level. The lesson to be learned from this case is that resolution of clinical symptoms and reduction of basal prolactin levels to normal is no guarantee that the tumor will not recur. Perhaps the persistence of the abnormal dynamics was a sign that the tumor was not totally removed.

Discussion

Is the medical or surgical treatment the most appropriate in this group of patients? Surgery has the theoretical advantage that it may be possible to totally cure the patient forever and always. However, this ability would seem to depend upon the size of the tumor found at operation, which does not seem to be totally predictable preoperatively. Only time and long follow-up of these patients will tell whether we have really cured those patients whom we believe are now cured. We will also be interested in learning whether failure of resolution of the abnormal dynamics postoperatively is predictive of a possible recurrence.

Conclusion

Twenty-nine patients with amenorrhea, galactorrhea, and pituitary tumors were operated upon by the transsphenoidal route. While at least 17 of these patients were seemingly cured clinically, only 12 patients had restoration of normal prolactin dynamics to thorazine and TRH stimulation and overnight levels. One of these patients with abnormal dynamics has now relapsed. To achieve optimal surgical results and to prevent relapse, the surgeon should, insofar as possible, make every effort to totally remove the tumor.

References

1. FORBES, A.P., HENNEMAN, P.H., GRISWOLD, G.C., et al.: Syndrome characterized by galactorrhea, amenorrhea and low urinary FSH: Comparison with acromegaly and normal lactation. J. Clin. Endocrinol. Metab. 14, 265-271 (1954)
2. HARDY, J.: Transsphenoidal surgery of hypersecreting pituitary tumors. In: Diagnosis and treatment of pituitary tumors. In: KOHLER, P.O., ROSS, G.T. (eds.), p. 179-194. Amsterdam: Excerpta Medica 1973
3. HWANG, P., GUYDA, H., FRIESEN, H.A.: A radioimmunoassay for human prolactin. Proc. Natl. Acad. Sci. U.S.A. 68, 1902-1906 (1971)
4. KLEINBERG, L., NOEL, C.L., FRANTZ, A.G.: Galactorrhea: A study of 235 cases, including 48 with pituitary tumors. N. Engl. J. Med. 296, 589-600 (1977)
5. LUTTERBECK, P.M., PRYOR, J.S., VARGA, L., WENNER, R.: Treatment of non puerperal galactorrhea with ergot alkalid. Br. Med. J. 3, 228 (1971)
6. NASR, H., MOZAFFARIAN, G., PENSKY, J., PEARSON, O.H.: Prolactin secreting pituitary tumors in women. J. Clin. Endocrinol. Metab. 35, 505 (1972)

Concepts in Neurosurgical Treatment of Pituitary Adenomas

R. FAHLBUSCH and F. MARGUTH[1]

Concepts in the neurosurgical treatment of pituitary adenomas are based on microsurgical technique, computer tomography of the skull, and advances in endocrinologic diagnosis and treatment (6).

The endocrinologic classification of the 200 patients with pituitary adenomas operated on in the last 2.5 years was as follows: 56 adenomas produced prolactin (PRL), 62 growth hormone (GH), and 13 adrenocorticotropic hormone (ACTH). Sixty-nine, i.e., one-third, of all adenomas were endocrinologically inactive (Table 1). The transsphenoidal operation was performed in 170 intrasellar adenomas and tumors with symmetric extension into the suprasellar space. The transcranial approach was indicated in 24 larger assymetric adenomas. Both approaches in short intervals were used in six patients. Three patients with inoperative large adenomas had shunt operations and were irradiated.

Table 1. 200 surgically treated patients with pituitary adenomas (1976 - Aug. 78)

Hormone excess	No. patients	Trans-sphenoidal	Trans-cranial	Both	+ Shunt
PRL	56	48	7	1	2
GH	62	60	-	2	-
ACTH	13	12	-	1	-
"Inactive"	69	50	17	2	1
Total	200	170	24	6	3

The small intrasellar and endocrine active adenomas can be identified only by the microsurgical transsphenoidal operation, which we owe to GUIOT (11,12) and HARDY (14,15). The approach is performed by us with the head in the same position as originally described by CUSHING: the surgeon's head is behind the patient's head. We prefer the sublabial paraseptal-submucosal midline approach to the sphenoid sinus.

1 The authors would like to express their thanks for the good and continous cooperation of: P.C. SCRIBA, K. HORN, R. LANDGRAF, C.R. PIKKARDT, K. v. WERDER (Endokrinologische Arbeitsgruppe, Medizinische Klinik Innenstadt, Dir.: K. BUCHBORN) and H.K. RJOSK (I. Frauenklinik, Dir.: J. ZANDER), all of the Ludwig-Maximilians University in München.

Adenomas smaller than 10 mm in diameter are called *microadenoma* (14), although there is no clear anatomic delineation from the macroadenomas. The anterolateral localization is preferred by GH-producing adenomas (Fig. 1). In nearly 20% of the patients with Cushing's disease, an extraglandular herniation of the adenoma into the cavernous sinus was observed. Microprolactinomas were often found mediolaterally but also in the posterolateral and other parts of the sella in the majority of cases, the pituitary was displaced to the sellar periphery.

The removal of the pituitary adenoma with preservation of "normal" pituitary tissue, which is called selective adenomectomy, can be demonstrated endocrinologically by unchanged or improved pituitary functions and the elimination of the hormone excess.

Selective adenomectomy was indicated in women with hyperprolactinemic amenorrhea and prolactin-producing adenomas who wished to become pregnant. After selective removal of 56 microprolactinomas PRL levels normalized in 55% of the patients (the MILAN-MUNICH cooperative study, 8). Similar results were obtained by others (2,13,16). The highest PRL level that could be normalized by us was 10.100 μU/ml. Normal PRL levels are below 650 μU/ml for women and 500 μU/ml for men; for comparison: 20 μU/ml MRC standard are 1 ng/ml VLS-PRL (NIH). Most of the patients who did not normalize completely had postoperative PRL levels only slightly above normal.

The best operative results were obtained in microprolactinomas under 5 mm in diameter, located mediolaterally with PRL levels not above 2500 μU/ml (Fig. 2). All these eight patients had normal postoperative PRL levels, which is in agreement with HARDY's (15) results. These eight patients were operated on because there was no desire for pregnancy or because bromocriptine was not well tolerated. It is still under discussion whether the patients with the smallest microprolactinomas should be treated medically (1,9) or surgically (15,30). In general, our patients with PRL levels under 3000 to 5000 μU/ml and under 5 mm are treated with bromocriptine, which is decided for every patient together with our endocrinologists and gynecologists (28): 10 of 22 patients became pregnant without complications (23,24). Sellar enlargement and impairment of vision during pregnancy (1,22) can only be expected in the larger adenomas. Thirty-two of these patients were operated on, 18 had normal menses and seven became pregnant. After additional bromocriptine therapy, all patients had normal PRL levels and all had their menses; three further patients became pregnant.

The results in 80 acromegalic patients operated on since 1974 also show that the smaller the adenoma and the lower the GH levels the greater the possibility or normalizing GH levels (Table 2). Normalization means GH levels under 5 ng/ml under the oral glucose tolerance test, which was observed in 87% of the intrasellar but only in 41% of the suprasellar adenomas. This in in agreement with the large series of HARDY (14), KAUTZKY (17), and LÜDECKE (19). To improve the results in patients with extremely elevated GH levels above 50-100 ng/ml and/or a smaller but firm tumor, additional cryotherapy was performed successfully. Open transsphenoidal cryotherapy, used routinely 6-8 years ago in our acromegalic patients, is no longer practiced in every patient because of its higher complication rate and panhypopituitarism following the radical procedure in more than half of the patients (5).

The question of radical adenomectomy in the sense of hypophysectomy or selective adenomectomy was also posed in Cushing's disease some years ago (19). Since we were able to demonstrate 2 years ago (20,21)

Table 2. GH results in 80 acromegalic patients (OP 74 - 6.78)

Tu. localization		GH normal	%
Intrasellar (No. = 63)	A	47/53	87
	B	8/10	
Suprasellar (No. = 17)	A	7/14	41
	B	0/ 3	
		62/80	77.5

Group A = transsphenoidal selective adenomectomy (No. = 67).
Group B = open transspenoidal cryotherapy (No. = 13).

that selective adenomectomy without replacement therapy was possible and that no remission occurred over a period of now 7 years, 17 patients with ACTH-dependent Cushing's disease of hypothalamopituitary origin were operated on. In eight patients, no pathologic sellar configuration was observed in the sellar tomograms. In 15 patients, selective adenomectomy was performed leading to complete clinical and endocrinologic remission in 13 patients. In the two other patients, no adenoma could be identified. One elderly patient was hypophysectomized - he had a hyperplastic anterior pituitary - followed by complete clinical remission. In a younger female, bilateral adrenalectomy had to be performed (Table 3). According to these results, also published recently by others (25,26), transsphenoidal selective adenomectomy has to be recommended as the first step and choice of therapy for Cushing's disease. Nelson's tumor, operated in 10 of 16 patients, can probably be prevented by treating Cushing's disease in this way, including the larger and invasively growing tumors with Cushing's disease (two patients).

Table 3. Indications for the transcranial operation of pituitary adenomas

ACTH-dependent Cushing's disease	
17 patients with normal (No. = 8) or slightly enlarged sella (No. = 9)	
Microadenomectomy	15/17
Remission	13/15
No remission	2/15
Hypophysectomy with remission	1/17
Sellar exploration	1/17

Normalization of GH and PRL levels occurred immediately after the adenomectomy (4,5,7,27). This was investigated in 50 acromegalics and 50 patients with prolactinomas by perioperative hormone measurements. With the exception of one single macroprolactinoma, acutely normalized GH and PRL levels remained normal over a period of 1-4 years. In larger adenomas, however, no normalization of extremely elevated GH and PRL levels will occur.

In many of these large tumors, the transsphenoidal operation was performed, but in about 15% of all pituitary adenomas the transcranial operation was indicated (Fig. 3), which is in agreement with GUIOT (11,12). Operation is necessary in the case of retrosellar, subfrontal, or parasellar extension, for example, or in the case of adenoma growth mainly outside the sella. In this case as well as in cases with capsule perforation, the sella is too small in comparison with the large suprasellar tumor part. Perforation can be suspected if only moderate visual deterioration stands in contrast to the large suprasellar tumor extension.

Computer tomography (CT) of the skull could also demonstrate pituitary adenomas (3,18) consisting of two nodules, located in the supra- and parasellar region, which could be completely removed only by the transcranial operation. CT is also very helpful for follow-up. If remaining tumor can be demonstrated, which occurs in about 15%-20% of the patients, additional therapy may be indicated (Table 4).

Table 4. Additional therapy in patients with pituitary adenomas

Procedure/adenoma	Inactive GH PRL ACTH
Two operations: transsphenoidal and transcranial	Assymmetric large adenoma for complete removal (CT, hormone excess)
Radiotherapy	Invasive adenoma high mitoses rate remaining adenoma (CT, hormone excess)
Cryotherapy	Large, firm, invasive adenoma GH > 50-100 ng/ml Primary: Microadenoma > 5 mm
Medical therapy	PRL < 5000 μU/ml GH ↑: Secondary post OP:PRL ↑

In a 16-year-old male, a macroprolactinoma was removed incompletely by the transsphenoidal approach. As expected, PRL levels decreased only from 10,000 μU/ml to 4000 μU/ml but fell into the normal range under bromocriptine therapy. However, residual supra- and parasellar tumor could still be seen in CT. After withdrawal of bromocriptine, the PRL levels increased. Since the chiasm syndrome also did not improve, a second transcranial operation was performed, after which PRL levels fell nearly into the normal range and are now normal under bromocriptine therapy with normal CT results over a period of 2 years. Both forms of operations in short intervals have been performed in seven patients with prolactinomas and in eight with other adenomas.

The effect of postoperative radiation could be demonstrated in 12 macroprolactinomas (29) over a period of 20-30 months, in which PRL levels decreased from 100%-20%, depending on when radiation had been started (Fig. 4).

Conclusions

Various therapeutic procedures have to be planned prospectively to obtain the best results for patients with pituitary adenomas. For additional therapy, a second transcranial operation may be indicated if no complete adenoma removal is possible as demonstrated by CT and/ or still remaining GH, PRL, and ACTH excess. Radiotherapy is indicated mainly in cases of invasive adenoma with a high mitosis rate and cryotherapy in large hormonally active adenomas and in acromegalic patients if the GH levels are above 50-100 ng/ml. Medical therapy has to be recommended as a secondary treatment to normalize (GH and) PRL levels postoperatively and as primary treatment in microprolactinomas under 5 mm in diameter and PRL levels under 3000-5000 μU/ml.

References

1. BERGH, T., NILLIUS, S.J., WIDE, L.: Bromocriptine treatment of 42 hyperprolactinaemic women with secondary amenorrhea. Acta Endocrinol. (Kbh.) 88, 435-451 (1978)
2. CHANG, R.J., KEYE, W.R., YOUNG, J.R., WILSON, C.B., JAFFE, R.B.: Detection, evaluation, and treatmentoof pituitary microadenomas in patients with galactorrhea and amenorrhea. Am. J. Obstet. Gynecol. 128, 356-363 (1977)
3. FAHLBUSCH, R., GRUMME, Th., AULICH, A., WENDE, S., STEINHOFF, H., LANKSCH, W., KAZNER, E.: Suprasellar tumors in the CT Scan. In: Cranial computerized tomography. LANKSCH, W., KAZNER, E. (eds.), pp. 114-127. Berlin, Heidelberg, New York: Springer 1976
4. FAHLBUSCH, R., RJOSK, H.K., v. WERDER, K.: Perioperative prolactin levels in patients with prolactinomas. Acta Endocrinol. (Kbh.) (Suppl.) 208, 46-47 (1977)
5. FAHLBUSCH, R., RJOSK, H.K., WERDER, K., v.: Operative treatment of prolactin-producing pituitary adenomas. In: Treatment of pituitary adenomas. In: Treatment of pituitary adenomas. FAHLBUSCH, R., WERDER, K. v. (eds.), pp. 225-237. Stuttgart: Thieme 1978 a
6. FAHLBUSCH, R., MARGUTH, F.: Developments in surgical treatment of pituitary adenomas. Neurosurg. Rev. 1/2, 5-13 (1978 b)
7. FAHLBUSCH, R.: Endokrine Funktionsstörungen bei cerebralen Prozessen. Stuttgart: Thieme 1978 c
8. FAHLBUSCH, R., GIOVANELLI, M., CROSIGNANI, P.G., FAGLIA, G., RJOSK, H.K., v. WERDER, K.: Differentiated therapy of microprolactinomas: Significance of transsphenoidal adenomectomy. In: Pituitary microadenomas, FAGLIA, G., GIOVANELLI, M.A. (eds.). London, New York, San Franzisco: Academic Press 1979 (in press)
9. FRIESEN, H.G., TOLIS, G.: The use of bromocriptine in the galactorrhea-amenorrhea syndromes: the Canadian cooperative study. Clin. Endocrinol. Suppl. 6, 91-99 (1977)
10. GIOVANELLI, M., GAINI, S.M., TOMEI, G., MOTTI, E.D.F., BECK-PECCOZ, P., PARACCHI, A., DE CAMILLI, P.: Transsphenoidal microsurgery of hypersecreting pituitary tumors. In: Treatment of pituitary adenomas, FAHLBUSCH, R., WERDER, K. v. (eds.), pp. 372-379. Stuttgart: Thieme 1978
11. GUIOT, G.: Transsphenoidal approach in surgical treatment of pituitary adenomas: General principles and indications in nonfunctioning adenomas. In: Diagnosis and treatment of pituitary tumors. KOHLER, P.O., ROSS, G.T. (eds.), pp. 159-178. Amsterdam, New York: Exerpta medica, American Elsevier 1973
12. GUIOT, G.: Considerations on the surgical treatment of pituitary adenomas. In: Treatment of pituitary adenomas. FAHLBUSCH, R., WERDER, K.v. (eds.), pp. 202-218. Stuttgart: Thieme 1978

13. GUITELMAN, A., APARICIO, N.J., MANCINI, A., ENCINAS, M.T., Levalle, O., SCHALLY, A.V.: Correlation of serum prolactin and LH response to stimulation with LH-RH before and after extirpation of pituitary adenomas with clinical outcome. J. Clin. Endocrinol. Metab. 45, 810-813 (1977

14. HARDY, J.: Transsphenoidal surgery of hypersecreting pituitary tumors. In: Diagnosis and treatment of pituitary tumors. KOHLER, P.O., ROSS, G.T. (eds.), pp. 174-194. Amsterdam, New York: Exerpta Medica, American Elsevier 1973

15. HARDY, J., BEAUREGARD, H., ROBERT, F.: Prolactin-secreting pituitary adenomas: Transsphenoidal microsurgical treatment. In: Profress in prolactin physiology and pathology. ROBYN, C., HARTER, N. (eds.), pp. 361-370. Amsterdam: Elsevier North Holland/Biomedical Press 1978

16. JAQUET, P., GRISOLI, F., GUIBOUT, M., LISSITZKY, J.-C., CARAYON, P.: Prolactin secreting tumors. Endocrine status before and after surgery in 33 women. J. Clin. Endocrinol. Metab. 46, 459-466 (1978)

17. KAUTZKY, R., LÜDECKE, D., NOWAKOWSKY, H., SCHRADER, D., STAHNKE, N., LUCKE, Ch., SOLBACH, H.G., WIEGELMANN, W.: Transsphenoidal operation in acromegaly. In: Treatment of pituitary adenomas. FAHLBUSCH, R., WERDER, K. v. (eds.), pp. 219-225. Stuttgart: Thieme 1978

18. KAZNER, E., FAHLBUSCH, R., LANKSCH, W., ROTHE, R., SCHERER, U., STEINHOFF, H., GRUMME, Th., LANGE, S., MEESE, W., AULICH, A., WENDE, S.: Computerized tomographie in diagnosis and follow-up of pituitary adenoams. In: Treatment of pituitary adenomas. FAHLBUSCH, R., WERDER, K. v. (eds.), pp. 101-114. Stuttgart: Thieme 1978

19. LÜDECKE, D., KAUTZKY, R., SAEGER, W., SCHRADER, D.: Selective removal of hypersecreting pituitary adenomas. Acta Neurochir. (Wien) 35, 27-41 (1976)

20. MÜLLER, O.A., FAHLBUSCH, R.: Differentid therapy in patients with Cushing's disease. Acta Endocrinol. (Kbh.) (Suppl.) 215, 23-24 (1978 a)

21. MÜLLER, O.A., BAUR, X., FAHLBUSCH, R., MADLER, M., MARGUTH, F., UHLIG, C., SCRIBA, P.C., BAYER, J.M.: Diagnosis and treatment of ACTH-producing pituitary tumors. In: Treatment of pituitary adenomas. FAHLBUSCH, R., WERDER, K. v. (eds.), pp. 343-351. Stuttgart: Thieme 1978 b

22. NELSON, P.B., ROBINSON, A.G., ARCHER, D.F., MAROON, J.C.: Symptomatic pituitary tumor enlargement after induced pregnancy. J. Neurosurg. 49, 283-297 (1978)

23. RJOSK, H.K., FAHLBUSCH, R., HUBER, H., WERDER, K. v.: Growth of prolactin-producing pituitary adenomas during pregnancy. In: Treatment of pituitary adenomas. FAHLBUSCH, R., WERDER, K. v. (eds.), pp. 395-400. Stuttgart: Thieme 1978

24. RJOSK, H.K., FAHLBUSCH, R., HUBER, H., WERDER, K. v.: Growth of prolactinomas during pregnancy. In: Pituitary microadenomas. FAGLIA, G., GIOVANELLI, M.A. (eds.). London, New York, San Franzisco: Academic Press (in press)

25. SALASSA, R.M., LAWS, E.R., CARPENTER, P.C., MORTHCUTT, R.C.: Transsphenoidal removal of pituitary microadenomas in Cushing's disease. Mayo Clin. Proc. 53, 24-28 (1978)

26. TYRELL, J.B., BROOKS, R.M., FITZGERALD, P.A., COFOID, P.B.: Cushing's disease. Selective trans-sphenoidal resection of pituitary microadenomas. N. Engl. J. Med. 289. 753-758 (1978)

27. WERDER, K. v., FAHLBUSCH, R.: Perioperative GH and PRL levels in acromegalic and hyperprolactinemic patients. Eur. J. Clin. Invest. 7, 233 (1977)

28. WERDER, K. v., FAHLBUSCH, R., LANDGRAF, R., PICKARDT, C.R., RJOSK, H.K., SCRIBA, P.C.: Treatment of patients with prolactinomas. J. Endocrinol. Invest. 1, 47-58 (1978 a)

29. WERDER, K. v., GOTTSMANN, M., BRENDEL, C., LANDRAF, R., LIEVEN, H. v., RJOSK, H.K., FAHLBUSCH, R.: Treatment of prolactinomas: efficacy of radiotherapy. Acta Endocrinol. (Kbh.) (Suppl.) 215, 1 (1978 b)

30. WILSON, C.B., DEMPSEY, L.C.: Transsphenoidal microsurgical removal of 250 pituitary adenomas. J. Neurosurg. 48, 13-22 (1978)

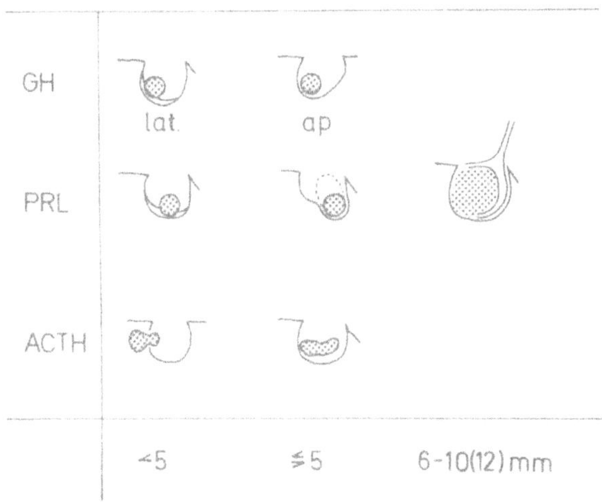

Fig. 1. Typical localization of microadenomas

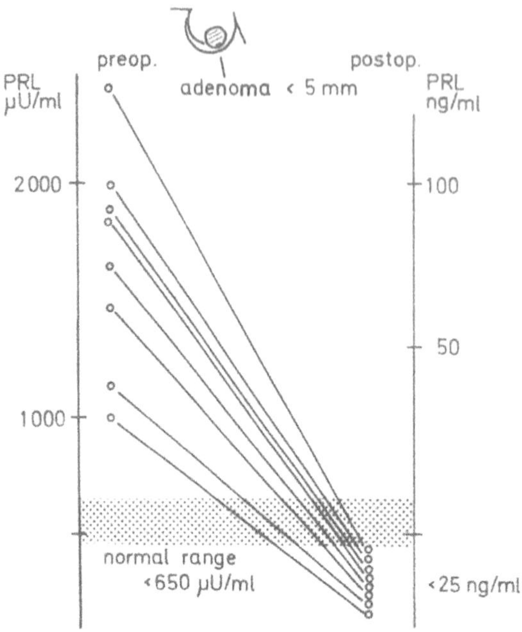

Fig. 2. PRL levels of eight patients with hyperprolactinemic amenorrhea before and 6 weeks after selective transsphenoidal adenomectomy

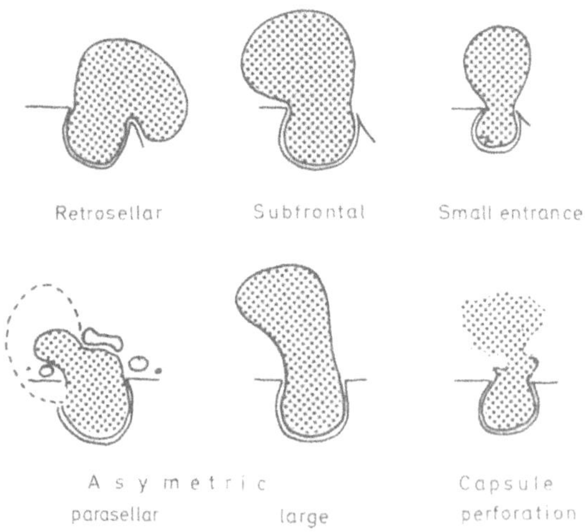

Fig. 3. Tumor forms and extension which make a transcranial (transfrontal or transfrontotemporal) approach necessary

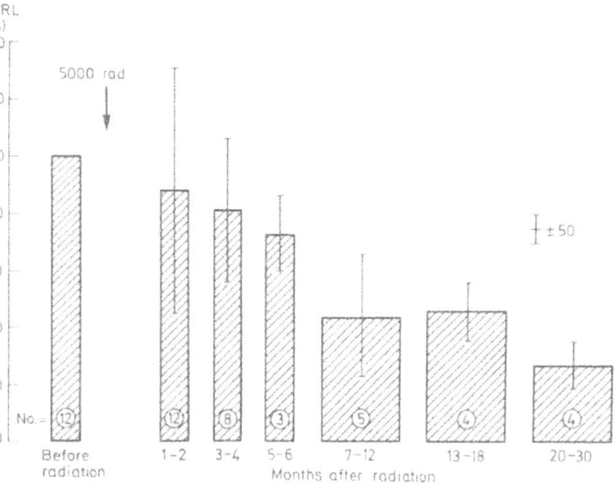

Fig. 4. Postoperative radiotherapy in 12 macroprolactinomas (29)

Operative Treatment of Cerebellopontine Angle Tumors with Special Consideration of the Facial and the Acoustic Nerve

M. SAMII

With all respect to the pioneer work of H. CUSHING (1), W.E. DANDY (2), H. OLIVECRONA (12), K.G. McKENZIE (11) and C.G. DRAKE (4,5), the decisive improvement in the surgical technique of cerebellopontine angle tumors occurred after the introduction of the operating microscope (6,7,8,9,15,16,17,18,19). Since 1968 we have applied the microsurgical technique to this field. The improved vision has helped us not only with the preservation of facial nerve function but also with reconstructive measures, such as end-to-end nerve suture or nerve graft, in the cerebellopontine angle.

We operate in the modified sitting position (lounging) recommended by JANNETTA (10). In this position the danger of air embolism is eliminated. The head of the patient is held anteflexed and turned 30° to the side with skull fixation (Fig. 1).

Figure 2 shows a relatively small neurinoma compressing the facial nerve and the acoustic nerve in a caudal direction. The nerves are visible immediately after the exposure of the cerebellopontine angle. After drilling away the posterior wall of the internal auditory canal, the tumor, originating from some fascicles of the vestibular nerve, was removed radically. The continuity of the facial and acoustic nerve is preserved (Fig. 3) and also the preoperative hearing.

In cases of large tumors, the facial nerve is neither visible at the brain stem nor at the internal auditory canal after exposure of the tumor. The gradual reduction in the tumor volume is performed through a 5 - 10 mm fenestration in the tumor capsule so that the capsule loses its tension. After further resection of the tumor capsule, the facial nerve can be identified at the brain stem.

Any direct manipulation of the facial nerve in the cerebellopontine angle will probably lead to a loss of function even if nerve trunk continuity is preserved macroscopically. The dissection of the facial nerve from the brain stem to the internal auditory canal has to be performed under the highest magnification. Using the microsurgical technique, the facial nerve may be preserved in its continuity in more than two-thirds of all cerebellopontine angle tumors. Often the acoustic nerve can also be preserved.

If one part of the facial nerve is damaged, the surgeon should not abandon his dissection. Accompanying the growth of the tumor, the facial nerve becomes lengthened. Thus, despite a loss of as much as 1 - 1,5 cm length during removal of the tumor, there is still the possibility of performing an end-to-end suture without tension, which gives the best results (Fig. 4a and b).

In the cases of larger defects, especially when the neurinoma grows into the internal auditory canal, the identification of the distal facial trunk may be impossible. Even electrostimulation is of no assistance here, for the stimulation of any distal stump in the internal auditory canal causes a contraction of the face muscles through spread of current into the facial nerve. Direct nerve grafting in the cerebellopontine angle is not to be recommended because of the criteria already mentioned.

To overcome these problems, DOTT (3) recommended anastomosing the central stump of the damaged facial nerve in the cerebellopontine angle to the extracranial part of the facial nerve in front of the stylomastoid foramen by means of a long nerve graft in two stages. It seems remarkable that after the good results obtained with this method, published by DOTT in 1958, only seven more cases - according to my knowledge - have been reported during the last 20 years. Most probably the reason for this is to be seen in the difficulty of dissecting the facial nerve at the brain stem without the aid of the operating microscope. Now that microsurgical operations have become common, one may expect that, in future, reconstruction of the facial nerve may become part of the surgical routine.

Instead of DOTT's surgical method, I have developed a technique that is performed in cooperation with otolaryngologic surgeons (WIGAND and DRAF). Figure 5 is an example of the exposure of a large acoustic neurinoma. The caudal nerves are compressed by the lower part of the tumor. The total removal of the tumor achieved by sacrificing the facial nerve preserving a 1.5 cm long nerve stump of the facial nerve at the brain stem is shown in Fig. 6.

After removal of a 5 cm long autologous nerve graft from the sural nerve, the graft was anastomosed to the central stump of the facial nerve at the brain stem (Fig. 7). The second end of the graft is to be placed as a loop into the internal auditory canal or dorsal to it between the labyrinth and the sigmoid sinus. Then the facial nerve is prepared by mastoidectomy in its mastoid and tympanic course. Subsequently, the internal auditory canal is approached by the translabyrinthine route, and the distal end of the graft is found. After cutting the facial nerve distal to the geniculate ganglion, the nerve stump can be displaced and anastomosed with the distal end of the graft (Fig. 8). In this manner, an intracranial-intratemporal anastomosis of the facial nerve can be performed by means of a 5 cm long graft. Figure 9a demonstrates the complete paralysis of the facial nerve after total removal of a large acoustic neurinoma and at the same time reconstruction of the facial nerve by intracranial-intratemporal anastomosis. The functional result 12 months after the operation is shown in Fig. 9b.

In summary, I should like to emphasize again the important contribution of microsurgical techniques to the management of cerebellopontine angle tumors. My experience indicates that there are great possibilities for preserving the function of the facial and acoustic nerves when the improved methods of dissection and the techniques of nerve suture and grafting are applied to the cerebellopontine angle.

References

1. CUSHING, H.: Tumors of nervus acusticus and syndrom of cerebellopontine angle. Philadelphia: Saunders 1971

2. DANDY, W.E.: An operation for the total removal of cerebellopontine (acoustic) tumors. Surg. Gynecol. Obstet. 41, 129-148 (1925)

3. DOTT, N.M.: Facial paralysis. Restitution by extrapetrous nerve graft. Proc. R. Soc. Med. 51, 900 (1958)

4. DRAKE, C.G.: Surgical treatment of acoustic neuroma with preservation or reconstruction of the facial nerve. J. Neurosurg. 26, 459-464 (1967)

5. DRAKE, C.G.: Total removal of large acoustic neurinomas. A modification of the McKenzie operation with special emphasis on saving the facial nerve. J. Neurosurg. 26, 554-561 (1967)

6. FISCH, U., WEBER, J.: Der diagnostische Wert der Pantopaque-Cisternographie. Méd. Hyg. 30, 1567-1568 (1972)

7. FISCH, U., YASARGIL, M.G.: Approach transtemporale, extradurale du conduit auditif interne. Pract. otorhinolaryngol. 30 (Basel), 377 (1968)

8. HOUSE, W.F.: Surgical exposure of the internal auditory canal and its contents through the middle cranial fossa. Laryngoscope 11, 1363-1385 (1961)

9. HOUSE, W.F.: Monograph transtemporal microsurgical removal of acoustic neuromas. Arch. Otolaryngol. 80, 597-756 (1964)

10. JANNETTA, P.J.: Bell's Palsy: A theory as to etiology. Observations in six patients. In: The laryngoscope. Vol. LXXXVIIII, No. 5, pp. 849-854, 1978

11. McKENZIE, K.G., ALEXANDER, E.: Acoustic neurinoma. Clin. Neurosurg. 2, 21-36 (1955)

12. OLIVECRONA, H.: Acoustic tumors. J. Neurol. Neurosurg. Psychiatry 3, 141-146 (1940)

13. OLIVECRONA, H.: Ablation des neurinomas acoustiques. J. Neurosurg. 26, 100-103 (1967)

14. OLIVECRONA, H.: The surgical treatment of intracranial tumors. 1) Meningiomas of posterior surface of the petrous bone, pp. 181-184. 2) The neurinomas, pp. 192-222. In: Handbuch der Neurochirurgie. OLIVECRONA, H., TÖNNIS, W. (eds.), Vol. 4, part 4. Berlin, Heidelberg, New York: Springer 1967

15. RAND, R.W.: Microneurosurgery for acoustic tumors. In: Microneurosurgery, pp. 126-155. St. Louis: Mosby 1969

16. RAND, R.W., KURZE, T.L.: Facial nerve preservation by posterior fossa transmeatal microdissection in total removal of acoustic tumors. J. Neurol. Neurosurg. Psychiatry 28, 311-316 (1965)

17. RHOTON, A.L.: Microsurgery of the internal acoustic meatus. Surg. Neurol. 2, 311-318 (1974)

18. SAMII, M.: Nerves of the head and neck. In: Management of peripheral nerve problems. Philadelphia: Saunders 1978

19. YASARGIL, M.G.: Mikrochirurgie der Kleinhirnbrückenwinkel-Tumoren. In: Kleinhirnbrückenwinkel-Tumoren, Diagnostik und Therapie, pp. 215-257. Berlin, Heidelberg, New York: Springer 1978

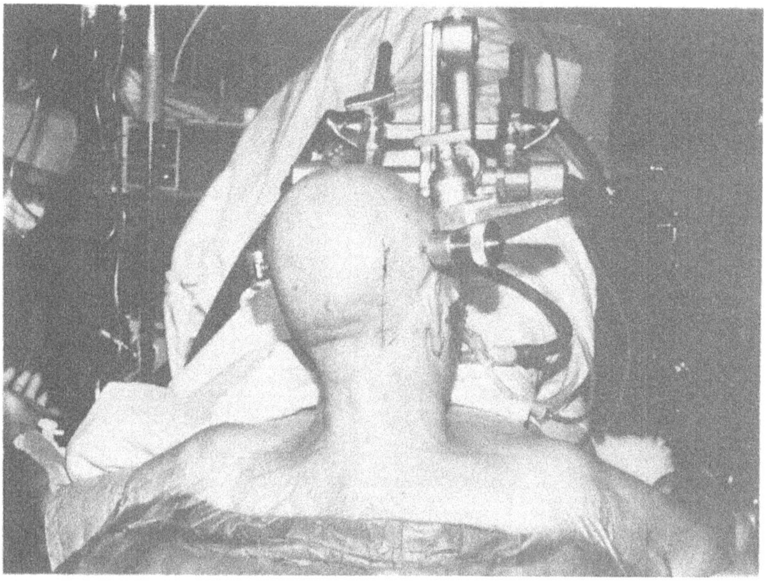

Fig. 1. Position of the patient during operation of an acoustic neurinoma. The head of the patient is held anteflexed and turned 30° to the side with skull fixation

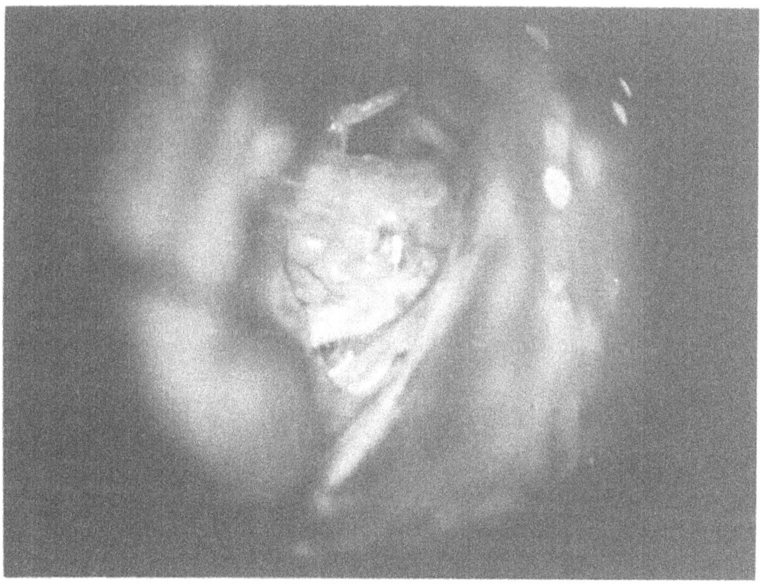

Fig. 2. Operative exposure of the cerebellopontine angle neurinoma. The facial and acoustic nerves are visible and are compressed in caudal direction

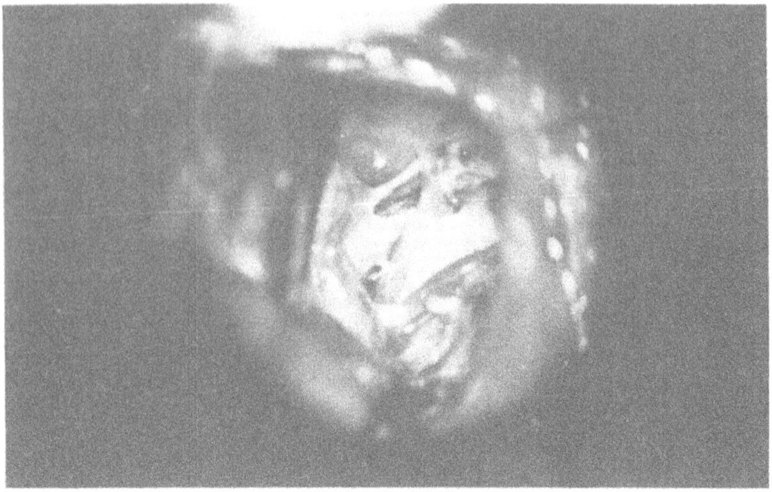

Fig. 3. Same case as Fig. 2. Condition after opening of the internal auditory canal and total removal of the tumor. The continuity of the facial and acoustic nerve is preserved

Fig. 4. See p. 143

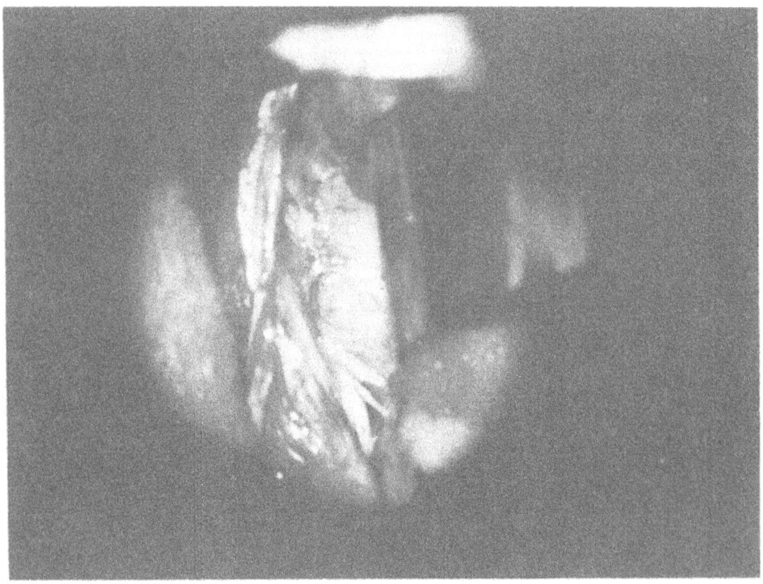

Fig. 5. Exposure of a very large acoustic neurinoma after the lateral suboccipital approach. The caudal nerves are compressed by the lower part of the tumor

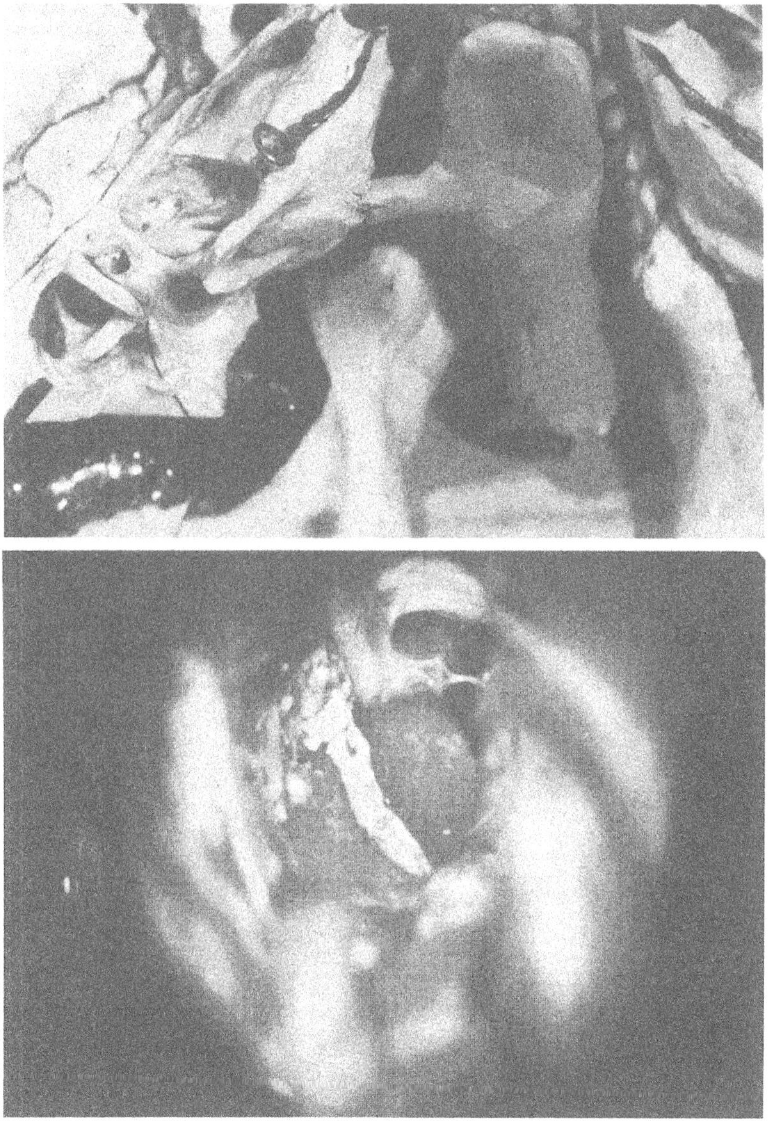

Fig. 4. a Model of the technique of an end-to-end suture of the facial nerve *(above)*. b End-to-end suture of the facial nerve after removal to the tumor *(below)*

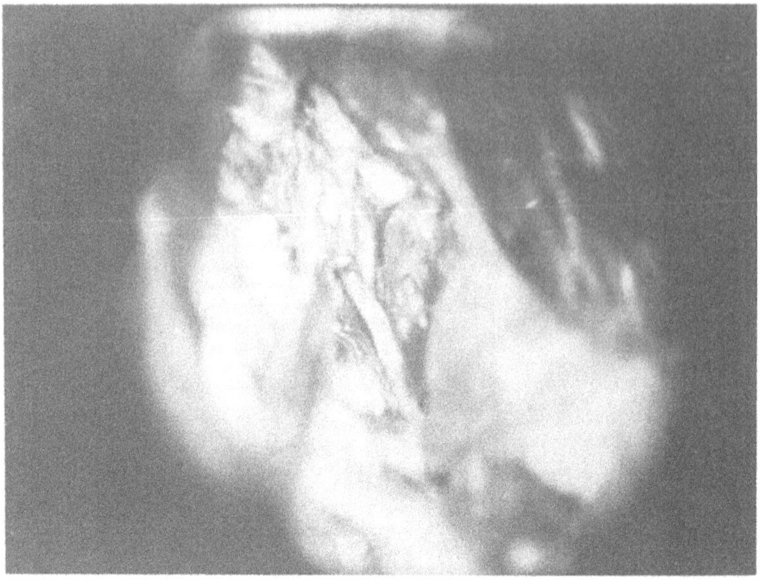

Fig. 6. Same case as Fig. 5. Total removal of the tumor and dissection of a 1.5 cm long nerve trunk of the facial nerve at the brain stem

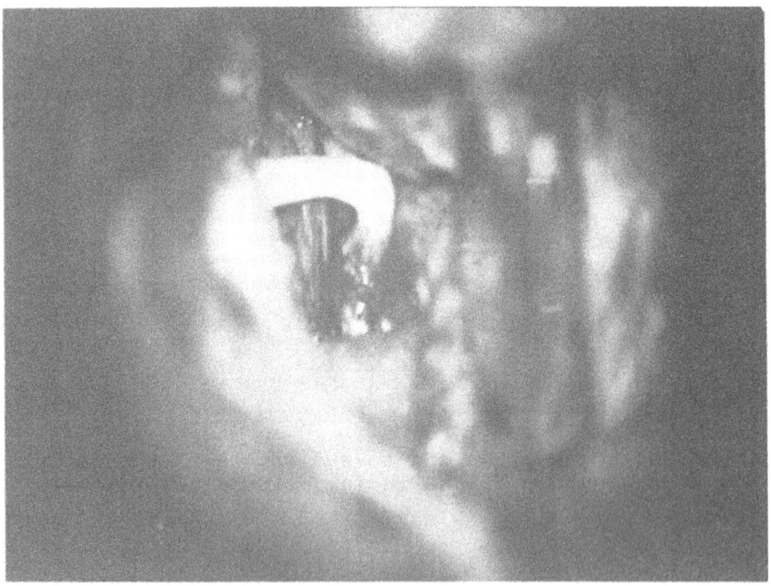

Fig. 7. Same case as Fig. 5. Anastomosis between the central stump of the facial nerve at the brain stem and a graft from the sural nerve

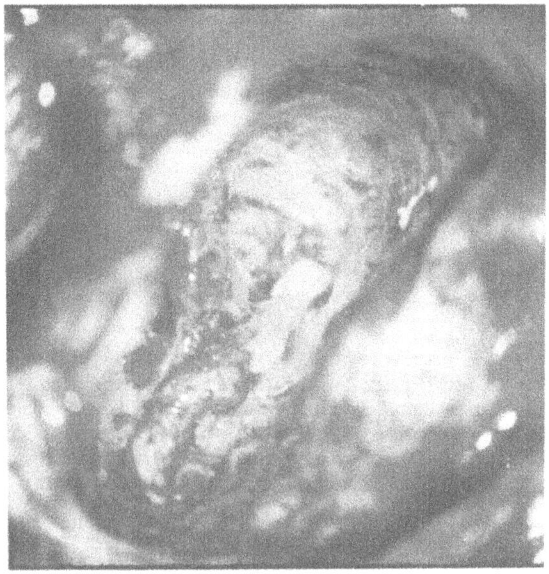

Fig. 8. Same case as Fig. 5. Transmastoidal exposure of the facial nerve in its mastoid and tympanic course and exposure of the distal end of the graft. After cutting of the facial nerve distal to the geniculate ganglion and displacement to ventral, the distal end of the graft is anastomosed with the facial nerve

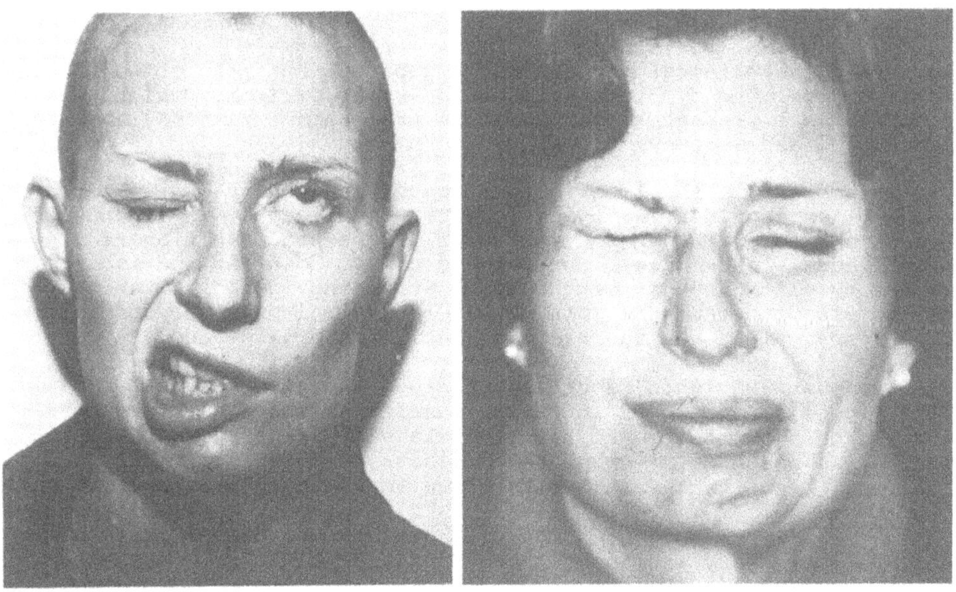

Fig. 9. a Same case as Fig. 5. Complete paralysis of the facial nerve on the left side after total removal of a large acoustic neurinoma with intracranial-intratemporal anastomosis simultaneous to a nerve graft *(left)*. b Same case as Fig. 5. Functional result 12 months after the operation *(right)*

Cervical Localized Spondylosis as Cause of Brachial Radicular Pain

J. CÁRDENAS, J. VERDURA, and S. RESNIKOFF

Cervical unilateral spondylosis is a well-defined pathologic condition that causes narrowing or stenosis of the diameter of the intervertebral foramina. This process produces compression of the corresponding root that comes from the spinal canal. This pathologic condition results in a specific syndrome that differs from the one caused when several unilateral foramina or bony bars extend posteriorly into the spinal canal. If long tract signs are present that are the result of medullar compression, the clinical picture may be interpreted as neuropathy, syringomyelia, multiple sclerosis, etc.

The purpose of this communication is to analyze the symptomatology and clinical neurological signs that are present in single localized unilateral cervical spondylitis. It is also important to review the radiologic findings. This report discusses the results of surgical treatment in 50 cases from our personal experience. Details of the surgical technique used to alleviate this condition are included.

Symptoms and Signs

In general, the clinical picture has a subacute but more often a chronic course. The symptoms produced by radicular compression when osteophytes are present in one foramina are: pain, weakness, numbness, hypoesthesia and atrophy.

Pain. It appears in the lower posterior cervical spine and radiates mostly to the shoulder, arm, and forearm. Occasionally it extends to the neck and occiput and as a rule down to the hand and fingers (thumb, index, and middle). The pain is almost constant and is aggravated by all movements of the head. Straining, coughing, and sneezing also increase the pain, by elevating the pressure and volume of the spinal fluid and the blood of the intraspinal veins.

Motor Symptoms. Patients report spontaneous muscular weakness, mostly in the biceps, triceps, or intrinsic muscles of the hand. In general, motor weakness is related to the time elapsed. Pain and weakness together cause patients to drop heavy objects, such as a pitcher or a thick book. Manual skilled work is often impaired by pain and fatigue.

Sensory Symptoms. Numbness and paresthesias in the distal parts of the fingers are very prominent.

Neurological Signs. The clinical neurological examination confirms the data obtained from a detailed patient history. Palpation and pressure in the supraclavicular space and along the nerve trunks produces tenderness or even real pain. Careful observation of the muscles can reveal atrophy. Diminished bicipital or tricipital osteotendinous reflexes are often found. Hypoesthesia with segmental distribution corresponding to C5, C6, or C7 are present. We must look for these signs, remembering the overlapping of the dermatomes.

Radiological Findings. Plain X-ray films of the cervical spine are very helpful. Lateral and oblique right and left are the most useful views to clearly see the osteophytes protruding into the intervertebral foramen. In the oblique position, we observe the diminution of the diameter of the space where the root makes its exit (Table 1).

Table 1. Radiologic findings

	No. of patients
Narrowing of intervertebral space with spondylotic changes	45
Flattening of the normal cervical curve	16
Foraminal osteophytes	3

Cervical myelography can confirm the diagnosis. We routinely use 9 cc of isophendylate (Pantopaque). This procedure can show a defect of the column of the corresponding space in which the root is compressed by the bony spurs or osteophytes.

Cases

The cases of 50 patients from the American-British Cowdray Hospital during the last 10 years are presented. The age range was 22-55 years, with 2 cases in the 2nd decade, 24 in the 3rd, 16 in the 4th, 8 in the 5th (Table 2).

Table 2. Sex and age distribution

Sex	No.
Male	30
Female	20
Age	
2nd decade	2
3rd decade	24
4th decade	16
5th decade	8

The duration of the symptoms varied from 1 month to 3 years (Table 3). The space between C6-C7 was affected in 32 cases and between C5-C6 in 18 cases. Only five patients had a history of trauma that could be considered the cause of the clinical picture. Of the patients, 50 complained of cervicobrachial pain, 46 had paresthesias in the thumb, index, and middle fingers, and 25 described spontaneously slight muscular weakness (Table 4). The neurological examination revealed muscular paresis in 45 patients, depressed triceps reflex in 25,

Table 3. Location and duration of symptoms

Space	No.
C6-C7	32
C5-C6	18
Duration of symptoms	
1-3 years	20
1-12 months	30

Table 4. Types of symptoms

	No. of patients	%
Cervicobrachial pain	50	100
Paresthesias (fingers)	46	90
Weakness	25	50

depressed biceps reflex in 15, hypoesthesia in 26, and atrophy in 16 (Table 5). Myelography showed a defect one side in the anteroposterior views, as had been previously seen in the transverse position in all 50 cases.

Table 5. Neurological signs

	No. of patients	%
Muscle weakness	45	90
Hypoactive or absent triceps reflex	25	50
Hypoactive or absent biceps reflex	15	30
Hypoesthesia	20	40
Atrophy	16	21

Surgical Technique

Under intratracheal general anesthesia, the patient is in a reclined position, and both legs are slightly elevated and bandaged with elastic antiembolic stockings. Both arms extend in the horizontal position parallel to the plane of the floor, which causes the roots to adopt a horizontal position as they emerge through the foramen and facilitates the removal of the osteophytes. An intravenous catheter in the arm introduced to the terminal portion of the superior cava vein and a Doppler are used to detect an air embolus. Basically, the operation consists of exposing the laminae of no more than three vertebrae. This is accomplished through an incision not longer than 6 or 7 cm. The muscles are well dissected from the midline of the affected side until the facets are well exposed. With the aid of a Syremovil unit (Siemens), the interspace is precisely located in the television screen. Using an air-driven spheric drill, a hole 1 cm in diameter is made between the two laminae, away from the midline. Afterwards, the opening is enlarged with fine Kerrison forceps. The root is exposed as the bony spurs, which are removed with fine curettes.

Very often the root is surrounded by fibrotic adhesions. The microscope is very useful for liberating the root from this abnormal tissue. The peridural veins are coagulated with the bipolar forceps.

Two complications must be avoided: injury to the vertebral artery and lesion to the root of the opening of the covering dura. A perfect hemostasis must be accomplished. The closure of the wound is performed in the usual manner. No drainage is left.

Using the described technique, we have operated on 50 patients with brachial radicular syndrome caused by unilateral and one single root compression. In all cases osteophytes were found. It is noteworthy that the bony spurs are more prominent in the lower part of the foramen. The root must be freed from adhesions as well. Careful handling of the root is very important. All of the patients were relieved from pain; those with a long history took longer but eventually the pain, motor symptoms and sensory symptoms disappeared. When atrophies were present, physiotherapy and rehabilitation were mandatory. Patients were followed for a period of 1 month to 10 years (Table 6).

Table 6. Follow-up

No. of patients	Years
23	5 - 10
27	1 - 5

There was no mortality or morbidity. Patients were allowed to walk the day after the operation; no collars were used.

Discussion

Unilateral cervical spondylosis localized at one level is a frequent cause of cervical brachial radiculopathy. EHNI (1) in 1945 mentioned that YOUNG had seen 84 patients with brachial pain, of which 62 had lesions of the cervical nerve roots and 55 had unique radicular lesions produced by spondylosis, herniated disk, or both.

EPSTEIN et al. (2) reported 20 cases with this syndrome and compression produced by bony spurs or disks, which were demonstrated both by X-rays and surgery. It is not uncommon that these patients suffer for years, during which time they are diagnosed variously as having rheumatism, bursitis, neuritis etc. The treatments are manifold: vitamins, psychiatric, hypnotism, steroids, analgesics, acupuncture, snake venom, X-ray therapy and so on.

Results

When a correct diagnosis is made and proper treatment initiated, the results are very gratifying. The etiology is uncertain. Some authors, such as MAYFIELD (3), believe that trauma plays an important role, although other reports (4) do not support this theory. In our series of 50 patients, only five had a history of trauma. The differential clinical diagnosis between a single chronic disk and localized spondylitis is difficult to establish.

Summary

Single nerve root compression caused by osteophytes narrowing a given cervical foramina constitutes a well-defined pathologic condition, which gives rise to a neurological syndrome that is characterized by neck and arm pain, muscle weakness, and reflex and sensation changes, limited to a very specific single nerve root distribution. The importance of X-ray examination is emphasized. The present report deals with a group of 50 patients suffering from the above-described syndrome whose neurological signs and symptoms were completely relieved by surgical decompression of the nerve root at the foramen, total facectomy, osteophyte removal, and lysis of root adhesions, all of which was performed through a single "keyhole" by the posterior approach.

References

1. EHNI, G.: Some observations on causes of cervicobrachial pain. Med. Rec. Ann. 44, 325-328 (1950)
2. EPSTEIN, I., LAVINE, L., ARONSON, J., EPSTEIN, B.: Cervical spondylotic radiculopathy. Clin. Orthop. 40, 113-123 (1965)
3. MAYFIELD, F.: Cervical spondylosis. A. Source of pain paresthesias, paralysis and plaintiffs. Is it traumatic. Bull. Am. Co. Surg. 51, 5-11 (1966)
4. GOTTEN, N.: Survey of 100 cases of whiplash, injury after settlement of ligation. J.A.M.A. 865, 192-195 (1956)

Atlanto-Axial Dislocation in Rheumatoid Arthritis with Cervical Cord Compression (Myelopathy)

K. SCHÜRMANN

Introduction

We have performed fusion operations on the cervical spine over a 10-year period since 1967 in more than 250 patients. In about 20 of these cases, vertebral body grafts after partial or total removal of the body were performed. In 27 cases, a dorsal suboccipitocervical fusion operation was indicated (Fig. 1). In this paper, the diagnosis, indication for surgery, the surgical technique, complications, and results in 16 cases of Primary Chronic Polyarthritis (PCP) in the atlantoaxial articulation are discussed (Table 1).

Table 1. Indication for 27 dorsal suboccipitocervical fusion operations

27		
Trauma	Tumor	PCP
6	5	16

Etiology and Diagnosis

In the nosology, we distinguish between *Juvenile Bechterev Disease* (JBD) and PCP (Table 2).

Table 2. Short summary of the clinical differential diagnosis between JBD and PCP

Nosology	
Juvenile Bechterev-disease	Primary chronic polyarthritis
JBD	PCP
Age: from 18-30 years	Age: from 50-70 years
Atlantoaxial dislocation = early (first) symptom	Atlantoaxial dislocation = late symptom
Bipolar manifestation: caudal pelvic lesion = ileosacral ankylosis cranial spine lesion = Atlas axis	Together with generalized PCP of all joint capsules, tendinous luxations, peripheral neuropathy etc.

Differential diagnosis is easy because the average age of patients with JBD is between 18 and 30 years, whereas the PCP patients have an average age of 50-70 years.

Moreover, it is to be emphasized that the atlantoaxial dislocation in JBD patients is an *early* symptom of the so-called bipolar manifestation of the disease, namely caudal pelvic lesion (ileosacral ankylosis) concomitant with the cranial spinal lesion (destruction of atlas-axis ligaments). On the other hand, in the elderly PCP patients there is a more or less long history of generalized PCP affecting all joint capsules with arthrodeformities, tendinous luxations, peripheral neuropathy with resulting muscular atrophy, etc. In PCP patients, the atlantoaxial dislocation is a *late* symptom in the long progress of this chronic disease. In general, the chronic proliferative inflammation of all synovial tissue leads to severe lesions of discs, bone, joint capsules, and ligaments. These lesions are more frequently found at the atlas-axis level (20%-34% in the literature) than is commonly known.

The destructive inflammatory process of the atlas-axis articulation affects mainly the transverse and the cruciform ligaments of the atlas, the alar ligaments of the axis (*ligamentum apicis dentis*), the anterior and posterior atlantooccipital membranes, and especially the "axe" of the axis (odontoid process) itself (Table 2, Fig. 2). As a result of this destruction, there is a *severe instability* of the atlas-axis articulation and a ventral dislocation of the atlas in certain cases (see Figs. 2 and 3).

Clinical Signs

The clinical signs are characterized in the early stage by dorsal neck pain, combined with rigidity of the neck and followed by a rigid torticollis caused by blocked rotation movements. These very early signs are already alarming symptoms and that is why one must urgently warn against "chiropraxis" or manipulation therapy. The subsequent symptoms are caused by incipient cord compression. Patients complain of dysesthesia in hands and fingers, sandpaperlike sensations, and/or sudden shooting pains into the legs caused by compression of the posterior fascicle of the cord by the anteriorly dislocated arch of the atlas. These alarm symptoms occasion urgent diagnostic measures. In a high percentage of cases, the diagnosis is not made before further myelopathic symptoms appear, generally in the following sequence: disturbed bladder function, urinary incontinence or urinary retention, then weakness in arms and legs with diminishing motor power in the four limbs, and finally quadrispasticity. We did not observe total quadriplegia.

Radiologic Signs

In most cases a rarefaction of the "axe" of the axis is to be seen. The ventral dislocation of the atlas varies from 4 to 20 mm. If the dislocation did not amount to more than 9 mm, then we did not find any neurologic deficits. On the other hand, if the dislocation amounts to more than 12 mm (up to 20 mm), then a more or less severe myelopathy is seen. In our series we found a narrowing of the high cervical channel to between 13 and 5 mm (the normal width is 22 mm). A tilt gliding of the atlas by more than 10° is not infrequent (Fig. 3). "Pseudobasilar invagination" (penetration of the axe into the foramen, magnum) is occasionally observed.

Surgical Treatment

The aims of the treatment are (1) decompression of the cervicobulbar cord, and (2) permanent stabilization of the unstable atlas-axis articulation (Figs. 4 and 5).

Surgical Technique

The patient lies in the abdominal position. Crutchfield tong traction is applied in order to achieve retroflexion of the cervical spine. A bone block is taken from the posterior iliac pelvis (Figs. 6 and 7). A midline skin incision is made into the dorsal neck, the arch of the atlas removed, and the foramen magnum enlarged. Then follows resection of the narrowed atlantooccipital cicatricial tissue ring. This is absolutely necessary, since without its removal, decompression of the dura is inadequate. The spinous process of C2 and C3 are removed. The posterior cortical wall of the arches of C2 and C3 are resected up to free spongiosa bone. Burr holes are applied bilaterally and suboccipitally. Steel wires are to be inserted through these as well as epidurally through the arches of C2 and C3. The two bone blocks are placed on the arches of C2 and C3 with the upper ends projecting into the burr holes on each side. They are then fixed by the previously inserted steel wires. The wound is now closed and a plaster of Paris diadem jacket is applied for 5 to 6 months. When this jacket has become hard (2-3 days), the Crutchfield tong is removed. The patient can then leave the bed and walk, provided that the neurologic status allows it (Figs. 8 and 9).

Complications

Of the total of 27 patients operated on, there was primary wound healing in 24 cases, and secondary wound healing in the cervical region in three cases. Two of the latter recovered completely with excellent spondylosyndesis. However, in one of them the bone graft had to be removed, and the neurologic signs of quadriparesis increased. There has still not yet been complete normalization of these symptoms. In two cases of osteomyelitis of the posterior iliac spine, both patients recovered well (see also Fig. 10).

Summary and Results

With the exception of one case, in which the bone grafts had to be removed because of infection, all cases operated on showed an excellent normalization of the quadrispastic symptoms. Moreover, they all showed a good stabilization of the suboccipital-cervical region.

In general, the best results in recovery of neurologic deficits were obtained in *PCP disease*, probably because the cord compression symptoms in these cases usually developed very slowly and therefore have a very good prognosis.

The recovery of neurologic deficits is slower and not so complete in *trauma* and in *tumor* cases.

References

1. BALL, J.: Pathology of the rheumatoid cervical spine. Ann. Rheum. Dis. 17, 121 (1958)
2. BALL, J., SHARP, J.: Rheumatoid arthritis of the cervical spine. In: Modern trends in rheumatology. HILL, A.G.S. (ed.), Vol. 117. London: Butterworths 1971
3. BÖHLER, J., SCHALLE, H.: Die angeborene Pseudoarthrose des Dens epistrophei (OS odontoideum) und ihre Behandlung. Z. Orthop. 93, (1960)
4. BRATTSTRÖM, H.: Operative Versteifung der Occipito-Cervikalregion bei CPC. ARO-Tagg. Lund, 13.-15.6.1977
5. DUNBAR, H.A., RAY, B.S.: Chronic atlanto-axial dislocations with late neurological manifestations. Surg. Gynecol. Obstet. 113, 757 (1961)
6. FRIED, L.C.: Atlanto-axial fracture-dislocations. J. Bone Joint Surg. 55-B, 490-496 (1973)
7. McGRAW, R.W., RUSCH, R.M.: Atlanto-axial arthrodesis. J. Bone Joint Surg. 55-B, 482-489 (1973)
8. MEYERS, K.A.E., van BEUSEKOM, G.Th., LUYENDIJK, W., DUYFJES, F.: Cervical dislocation in rheumatoid arthritis of the cervical spine. J. Bone Joint Surg. (1973)
9. NEWMAN, Ph., SWEETNAM, R.: Occipito-cervical fusion. J. Bone Joint Surg. 51-B, 423-428 (1969)
10. PATTERSON, F.P.: Instability of the upper cervical spine. J. Bone Joint Surg. 55-B, 456-457 (1973)
11. SCHILLING, F., HAAS, J.P., SCHACHERL, M.: Die spontane atlanto-axiale Dislokation (Ventralluxation des Atlas) bei chronischer Polyarthritis und Spondylitis ankylopoetica. Fortschr. Geb. Röntgenstr. Nuclearmed. 99, 518-538 (1963)
12. SHARP, J., PURSER, D.W.: Spontaneous atlanto-axial dislocation in ankylosing spondylitis and rheumatoid arthritis. Ann. Rheum. Dis. 20, 47 (1961)
13. SCHÜRMANN, K., REULEN, H.J., BUSCH, G.: Rekonstruktive und stabilisierende operative Maßnahmen bei Wirbelkörperverletzungen. 41. Jahrestagung D. Ges. f. Unfallheilkd. Berlin, 17.-19.11.1977, Kongreßbericht
14. SCHÜRMANN, K.: Rekonstruktive Chirurgie bei Wirbelkörperdestruktionen mit begleitenden Stabilisierungsmaßnahmen. Zbl. Neurochir. 37 (1976)

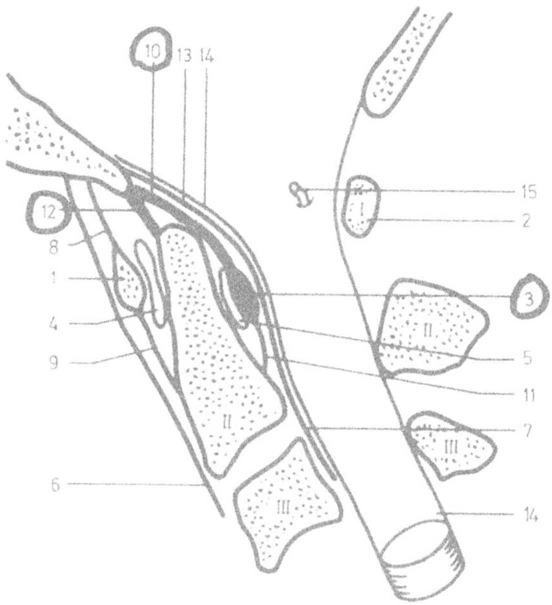

Fig. 1. Normal anatomy of the suboccipitocervical region (modified after SPALTEHOLZ, Lehrbuch für Anatomie), with distinguishings marks of the most important ligaments of the atlas-axis and axis-clivus:

3 Transverse ligament of the atlas
10 Cruciform ligament of the atlas
12 Apical ligament of the "axe" of the axis *(Ligamentum apicis dentis)*

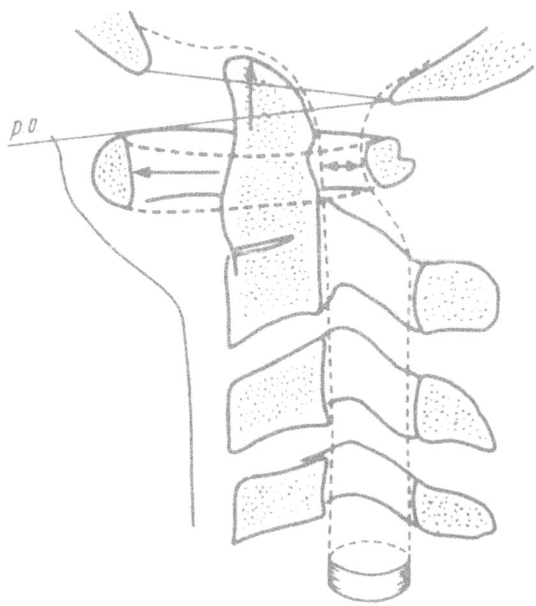

Fig. 2. Shows the severe instability of the atlas-axis articulation and a ventral dislocation of the atlas in JBD. If the dislocation amounts to more than 12 mm (up to 20 mm), then a more or less severe myelopathy is seen

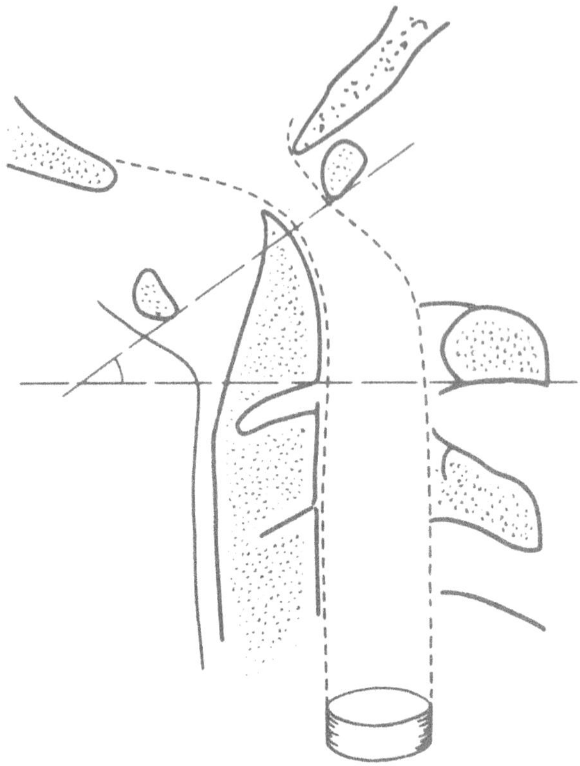

Fig. 3. Shows the often very severe instability of the atlas-axis articulation, combined with a not seldom extreme tilt gliding of the atlas in PCP patients. The narrowing of the high cervical channel is in our series to be found between 13 and 5 mm (the normal width is 22 mm). In the majority of PCP patients we saw also a remarkable rarefaction of the "axe" of the axis

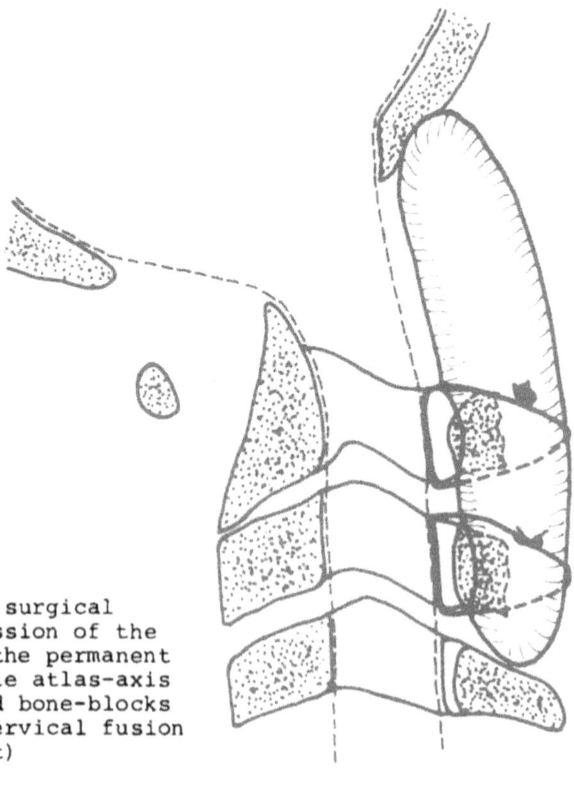

Fig. 4. Shows the result of surgical treatment: (1) the decompression of the cervicobulbar cord and (2) the permanent stabilization of the unstable atlas-axis articulation by the inserted bone-blocks for the dorsal suboccipitocervical fusion (surgical technique see text)

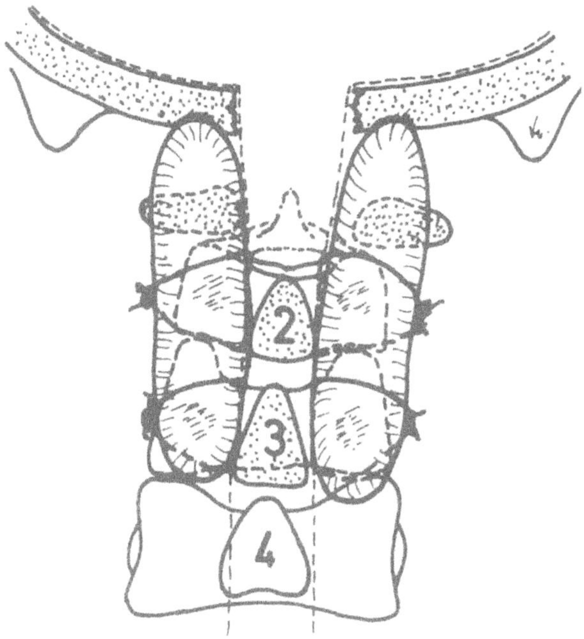

Fig. 5. The sketch shows the situation of Fig. 4 in the view from behind

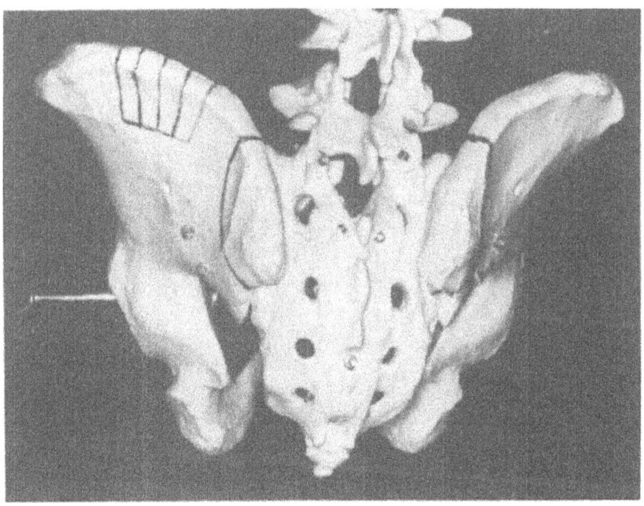

Fig. 6. The pelvis model shows the posterior iliac spine, from which the strong bone blocks are taken

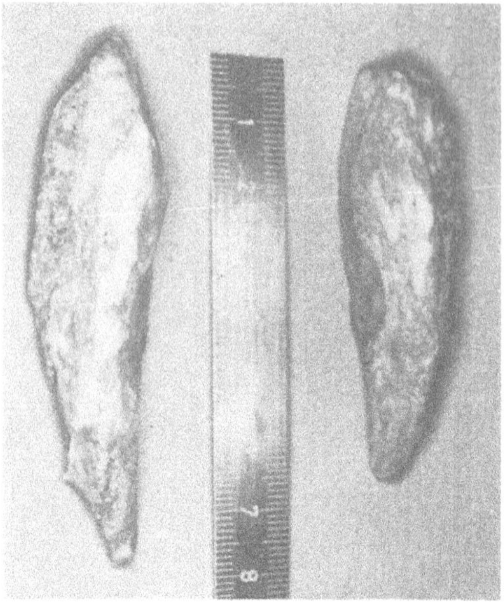

Fig. 7. The original bone blocks from the posterior iliac spine, applying the dorsal fusion. The length amounts to 70-80 mm

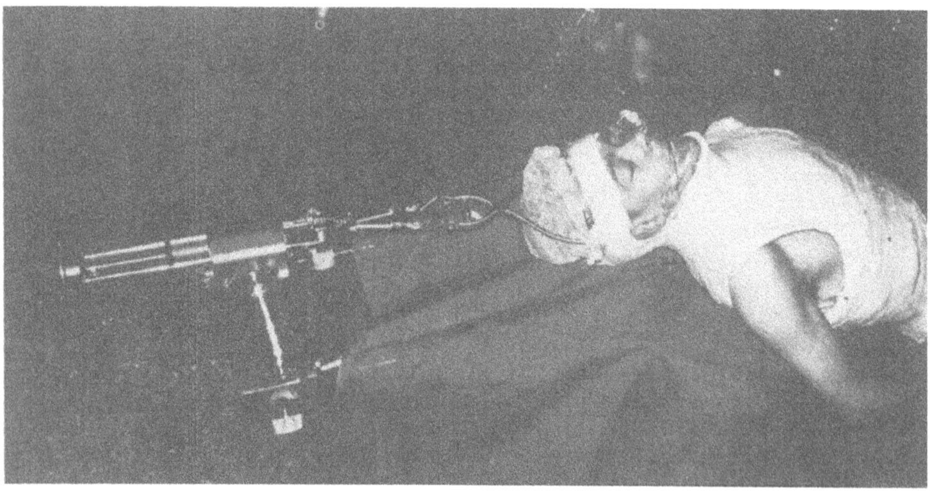

Fig. 8. Patient on the operating table after surgery, turned on his back for finishing the plaster of Paris diadem jacket. The Crutchfield-tong is connected with a mechanical winch (constructed by MAQUET AG, Kehler Straße 31, D-7550 Rastatt, FRG), which can increase the traction up to 30 kg and more. The winch is attached to the operating table with revolving arms, so that the traction can easily be changed in ante- or retroflexion position and the traction force can be changed as needed

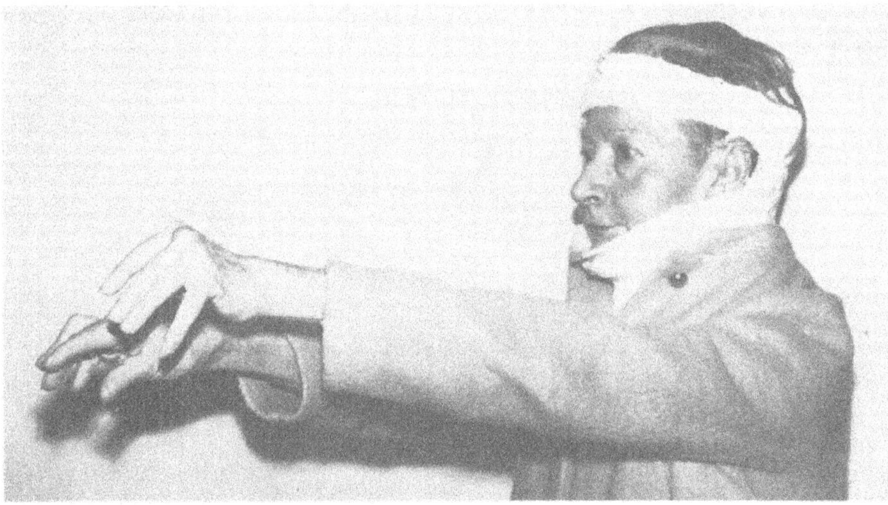

Fig. 9. A 62 year-old-lady with a severe PCP, ventral atlantoaxial dislocation and gliding, myelopathy (quadrispasticity), generalized arthrodeformities, tendinous luxations, peripheral polyneuropathy with consequent muscular atrophy, 6 days after surgery (see Figs. 3, 4 and 5)

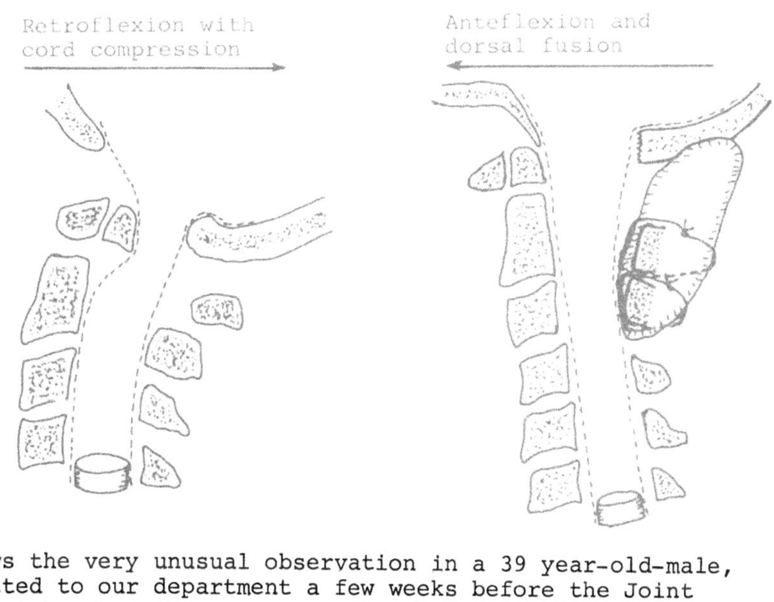

Fig. 10. Shows the very unusual observation in a 39 year-old-male, who was admitted to our department a few weeks before the Joint Meeting in Munich, when the paper was finished. In this case a *dorsal dislocation of the atlas* occurred and the "axe" of the axis was dislocated posteriorly and lies within the high cervical channel producing a cord compression and myelopathy (quadrispasticity). After surgery quadrispasticity improved in about 3 to 4 days so that the patient could walk with the plaster of Paris diadem jacket. Patient was operated upon on the 28th of September 1978 and left the hospital on the 5th October 1978, i.e., 7 days postoperatively, to celebrate the 80th birthday of his father

Necrosis of Vertebrae After Cloward's Operation of the Cervical Spine Using "Palacos" for Fixation

P. DISTELMAIER, I. VLAJIC, and J. WAPPENSCHMIDT

Introduction

Anterior cervical diskectomy in cervical disk lesions with vertebral body fusion using polymethyl methacrylate (Palacos) for fixation gives excellent results in most of our patients. We are now able to report on 618 patients operated on during the last 16 years. During the first few years we used a bone graft for fixation, but from 1968 on we preferred polymethyl methacrylate (Palacos). The results were very favorable, but we also observed a specific complication of these operations that may cause the patient pain and difficulties.

Materials and Methods

Between 1962 and 1977 we operated on 618 patients with cervical disk lesions according to Cloward's technique (2) with an anterolateral access. Since 1968, 405 of them were operated on using polymethyl methacrylate instead of a bone graft for fixation; 34% were women and 66% were men. Nine percent of the patients needed the operation because of a traumatic lesion. The distribution of the operations in regard to the localization of disk was: C2/3, 1; C3/4, 78; C4/5, 108; C5/6, 199; C6/7, 67; C7/TH1, 1; C2/C3 + C3/C4, 1; C3/4 + C4/5, 23; C4/5 + C5/6, 64; C5/C6 + C6/C7, 62; C3/C4 + C5/C6, 8; C4/C5 + C6/C7, 4.

Nearly all patients had a myelography or diskography before operation; all patients had X-rays before and immediately after the operation. In almost all patients, another X-ray was performed 6 months after the operation and in many 1 year after it. Most of them did not come back after this period, in general, simply because they were well. Some were followed up for 5-7 years, however.

Results

Of our patients operated on in this manner for cervical disk protrusions, 87% definitely improved. Naturally, our results vary according to the original neurological symptoms. From our experience, the results of the operations using *polymethyl methacrylate* for fixation have proved to be better than those of other techniques; we have less complications with these fusions than with bone graft. Nevertheless, we observed septic complications in 1% of our operations (Figs. 1 and 2). It is our intention to demonstrate another complication, which is not easy to distinguish from septic complications. This is the partial or complete aseptic necrosis of the vertebral body or the resorption, especially of the anterior part of the vertebral body after fusions using polymethyl methacrylate.

Clinical Symptoms

Aseptic necrosis of bone and resorption of bone as well as displacement by soft tissue or cicatrizing tissue is well known in surgery of the hip joint (Fig. 3). Comparable reactions may occur in the vertebrae as well. We observed similar reactions after 2% of our operations, most of them had had fusions of two levels. These patients never showed septic symptoms, fever, or alteration of blood tests. These patients never have difficulties in swallowing nor do they show severe neurological signs. Punctures of the prevertebral space near the fusion never led to the demonstration of bacteria. Typically, the initial neurological symptoms vanish immediately after the fusion, for example, brachialgia, and are replaced by completely uncharacteristic symptoms without radicular correlation. In general, the patients suffer from diffuse pain in the neck, sometimes increased by movements of the head or the arm. These pains are not too intense but impair the patient and may increase gradually. Psychic fixation of the patient on the pain is sometimes wrongly suspected. Nevertheless, patients are not content with the result of the operation as a rule.

Radiologic Symptoms

Initial symptoms do not occur within 1 month after the operation but can generally be observed 2-3 months later. In most cases, necrosis and resorption of parts of the vertebral body, especially of the anterior parts of the vertebra are the first symptoms (Fig. 4). A defect of the anterior part of the vertebral body may result without further deterioration. In about 50% of the patients with this reaction, the whole vertebral body is involved with collapse of the vertebral body with subsequent partial reconsolidation and osteosclerotic reactions of the bone (Fig. 5). Resorptive reactions may progress gradually and may lead to acute pain, especially in the anterior parts of the vertebra again. In Fig. 6 the resorptions are more impressive. In other cases osteophytic reactions may lead to a final osseous fusion and pain is vanishing (Fig. 5). The retropharyngeal space is not widened!

Discussion

In 2% of our patients with cervical disk protrusion operated on with a CLOWARD fusion but using polymethyl methacrylate for fixation, we observed a special reaction of the vertebral bone. Initially, there is a partial necrosis or a necrosis of the vertebral body followed by resorptive reactions and then in some cases osteosclerotic and even osteophytic reactions. The neighboring bone generally shows osteosclerosis. The resorption may progress for some years after the operation. Most of these patients had fusions at more than one level. In all cases no bacteria could be cultured. The origin of these pathologic changes is unknown to us. In our opinion there are four possible causes of these osseous reactions:

1) Necrosis of the bone by boiling of the bone because the exothermic reaction of the polimerization of the polymethyl methacrylate and perhaps secondary vascular lesions.
2) Vascular disturbance and ischemic necrosis of the bone due to lesions during the operation, especially when burring holes in the vertebrae to fix the polymethyl methacrylate.

3) Mechanical wear of the bone, perhaps because of a slight retraction of the polymethyl methacrylate after hardening and persistent low-grade motility with minimal but constant degeneration.
4) A specific reaction of the body against the polymethyl methacrylate as a hypersensitivity reaction or a foreign body reaction.

We cannot show histologic sections of these vertebrae since none of our patients had to be reoperated yet nor had the polymethyl methacrylate to be taken out. Histologic examination of material obtained at reoperations after implantation of artificial hip joints show extensive soft tissue with giant cells and cicatrizing tissue around the hip joint fixed with Palacos. As far as we know, the exact cause of these reactions and the resorptions has not been investigated yet. We think it is possibly of complex origin. Evidence of a second cause may be seen in the fact that these reactions are more frequently found after fusion at two levels. It may also be evidence for the first cause. The third cause may be that resorptions may occur more frequently in areas under excessive mechanical stress after the implantation of polymethyl methacrylate. Evidence for the fourth cause may be the histologic findings after hip joint surgery with the detection of giant cells.

In the literature about cervical diskectomy with interbody fusion by implantation of polymethyl methacrylate we found this complication mentioned in only one publication (7). They estimate it to be a form of transformation of the bone following these operations, which finally leads to an osseous fusion and is of no major importance. In agreement with them, we think that these reactions of the bone are no indication for reoperation as a rule. On the other hand, most of our patients had no osseous fusion of the intervertebral segment and some have slowly progressing resorption of the bone even some years after the operation, which may force us to reoperate in the future. In any case, patients suffer from diffuse uncharacteristic pain unless final osseous fusion is attained. These patients are not content with the result of the fusion, although in most cases they are distinctly better than before the operation. In the future, we intend to observe these pathologic changes closely. Ten years of experience with this form of the operation, i.e., with polymethyl methacrylate in the cervical spine, are perhaps not yet sufficient to judge the final results in cases of these complications. On the other hand, our results with these operations are very good and better than those of fusion with bone graft (4/5), and we think also better than those without interbody fusion (1/8), which is why we still recommend these operations and think that the described complications are tolerable.

Conclusion

In 2% of our patients treated with anterior cervical diskectomy with interbody fusion by polymethyl methacrylate, we observed necrosis and resorptions in the neighboring vertebral bodies, especially when fusion in two levels was performed. These alterations should be distinguished from septic complications, which is possible by observing clinical symptoms and radiologic mainly because of the lack of widening of the retropharyngeal space. In general, they are of minor importance, but can impair the patient by constant diffuse pain. Radiologically, the osseous alterations are characterized by resorptions, especially of the anterior part of the vertebral body and sometimes collapse of the vertebrae. The adjacent bones show osteosclerosis. These reactions of the bone are generally not an indication for reoperation, but further observations are necessary. In the literature, we found only one similar observation (7), but we think that in many cases these alterations are not observed either because they are not correctly interpreted or because patients could not be followed up. In our mind the value of these operations is not seriously impaired by these complications, which we regard as tolerable. Further observations and investigations to find the cause of these complications are necessary. The indication for operation of two disks ought to be deliberated thoroughly because these complications are generally seen in such cases.

Summary

We treated 618 patients with cervical disk lesions by anterior cervical diskectomy. Of them 405 were operated on by using polymethyl methacrylate for fixation. These patients were followed up. Two percent showed necrosis of the vertebrae, especially of the anterior part. The special clinical and radiologic features of the affection are described, and reasons for the necrosis of the bone are discussed.

References

1. BEECHER-SCOVILLE, WILLIAM, DOHRMANN, G.J., CORKILL, G.: Late results of cervical disc surgery. J. Neurosurg. 45, 203-209 (1976)
2. CLOWARD, R.B.: The anterior approach for removal of ruptured cervical discs. J. Neurosurg. 15, 602-617 (1958)
3. DEREYMAEKER, A., MULIER, J.: Nouvelle cure chirurgicale des discopathies cervicales. Neurochirurgie 2, 233-236 (1956)
4. GROTE, W., RÖTTGEN, P.: Die ventrale Fusion bei der zervikalen Osteochondrose und ihre Behandlungsergebnisse. Acta Neurochir. 16, 218-240 (1967)
5. GROTE, W., BETTAG, W., WÜLLENWEBER, R.: Indikation, Technik und Ergebnisse zervikaler Fusionen. Acta Neurochir. (Wien) 22, 1-27 (1970)
6. RILEY, L.H., ROBINSON, R.A., JOHNSON, K.A., WALKER, E.W.: The results of anterior interbody fusion of the cervical spine. J. Neurosurg. 30, 127-133 (1969)
7. ROOSEN, K., GROTE, W., BETTAG, W.: Komplikationen zervikaler ventraler Fusionsoperationen. Neurochirurgia (Stuttg.) 18, 1-11 (1975)
8. WILSON, D.H., CAMPBELL, D.: Anterior discectomy without bone graft. J. Neurosurg. 47, 551-555 (1977)

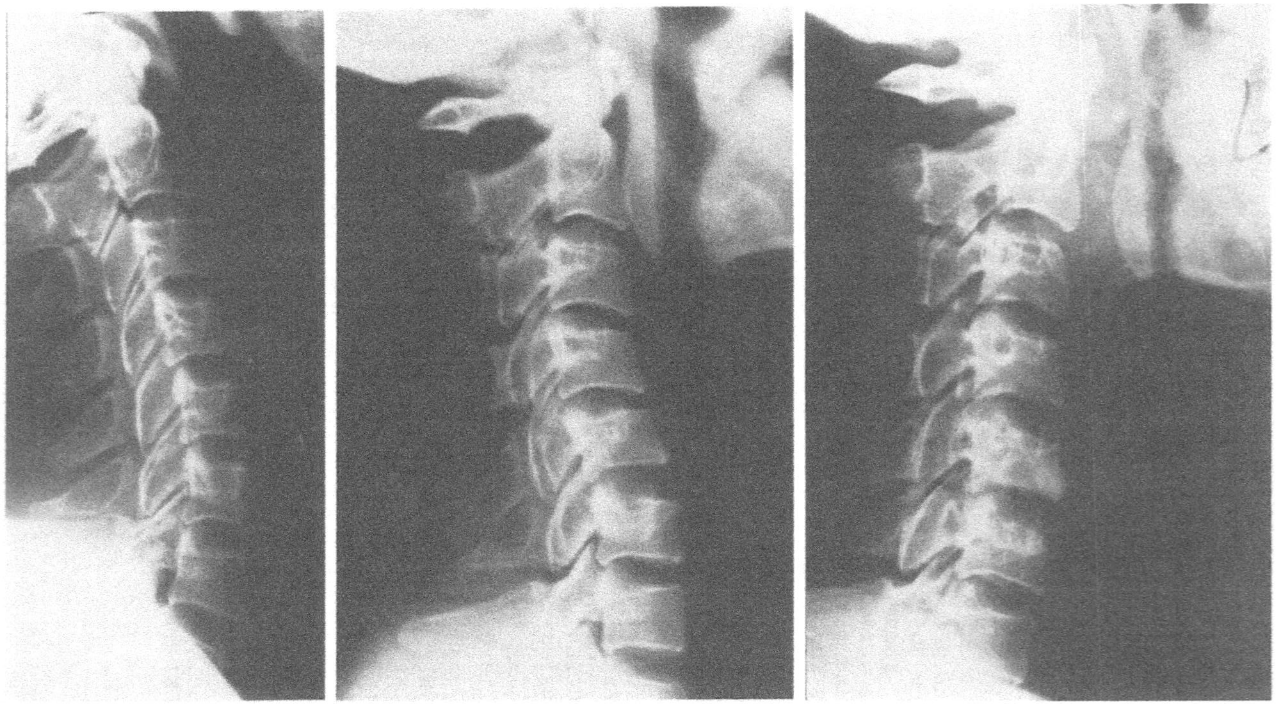

Fig. 1. A 31-year-old man with diskopathy C5/C6. *Left:* before operation; *middle:* immediately after diskectomy with interbody fusion by polymethyl ethacrylate; *right:* osteomyelitis, widening of the retropharyngeal space 1 month later

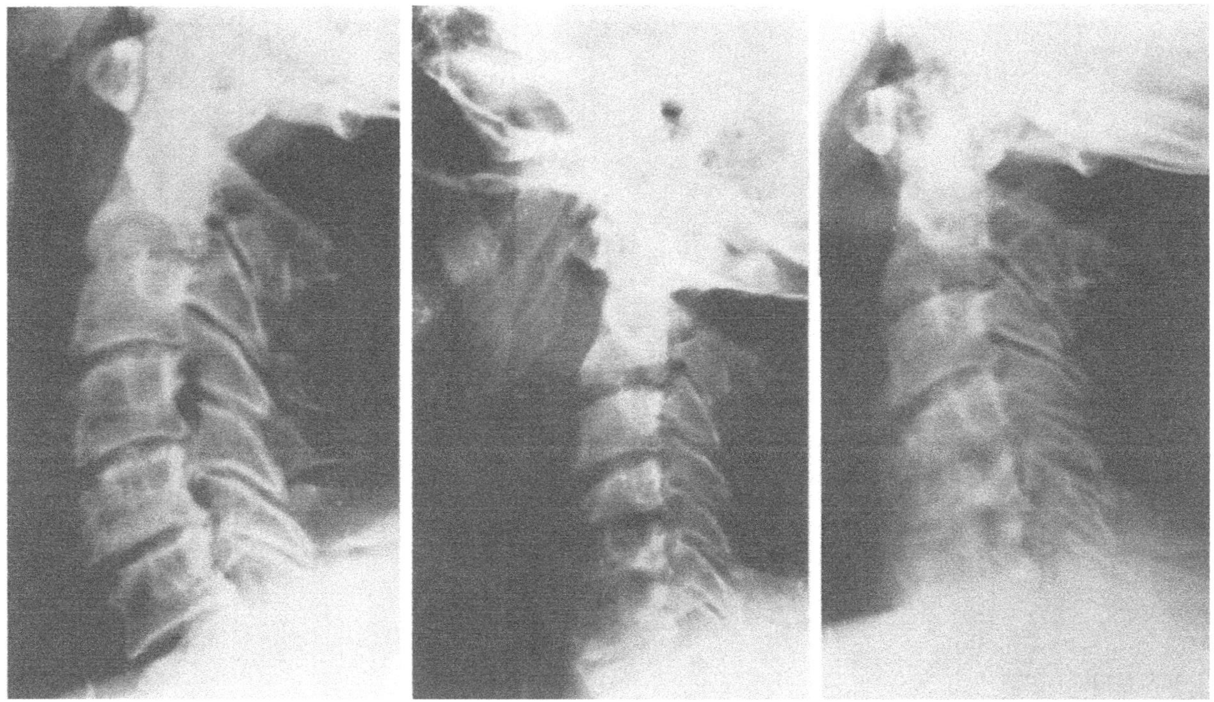

Fig. 2. A 56-year-old man with diskopathy C4/C5, C5/C6. *Left:* before operation; *middle:* 4 weeks after operation, osteomyelitis with partial destruction of the vertebrae, Crutchfield extension; *right:* 2 months later after removal of the polymethyl methacrylate consolidation

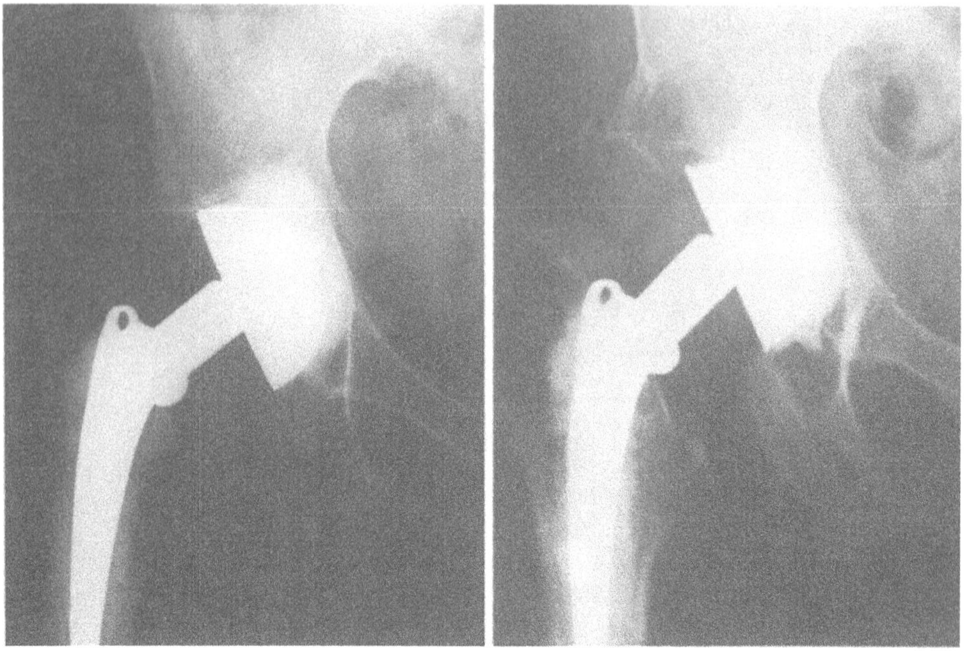

Fig. 3. A 68-year-old woman with artificial hip joint. *Left:* immediately after implantation, fixation by polymethyl methacrylate; *right:* 7 years later, extensive resorption of the surrounding bone, pain

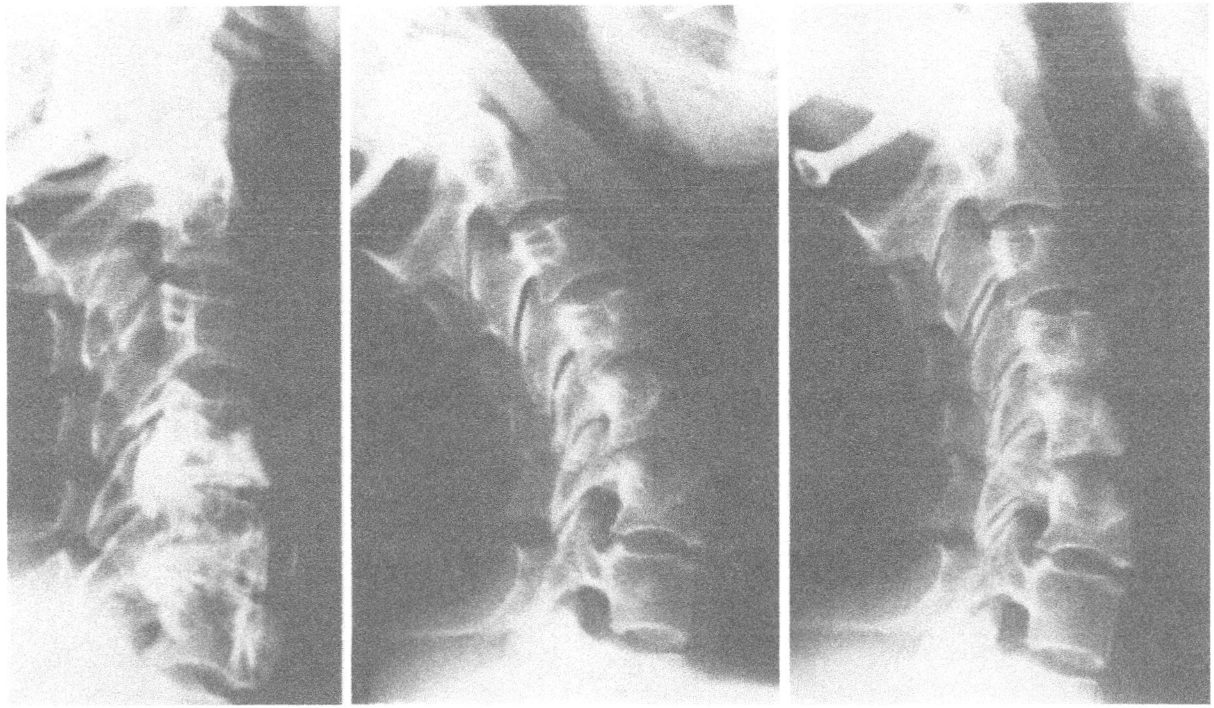

Fig. 4. A 47-year-old woman with diskopathy C4/C5, C5/C6. *Left:* diskography before the operation; *middle:* immediately after fusion; *right:* 3 months later, partial *necrosis* and resorption of the anterior parts of the vertebral bodies, no osteomyelitis

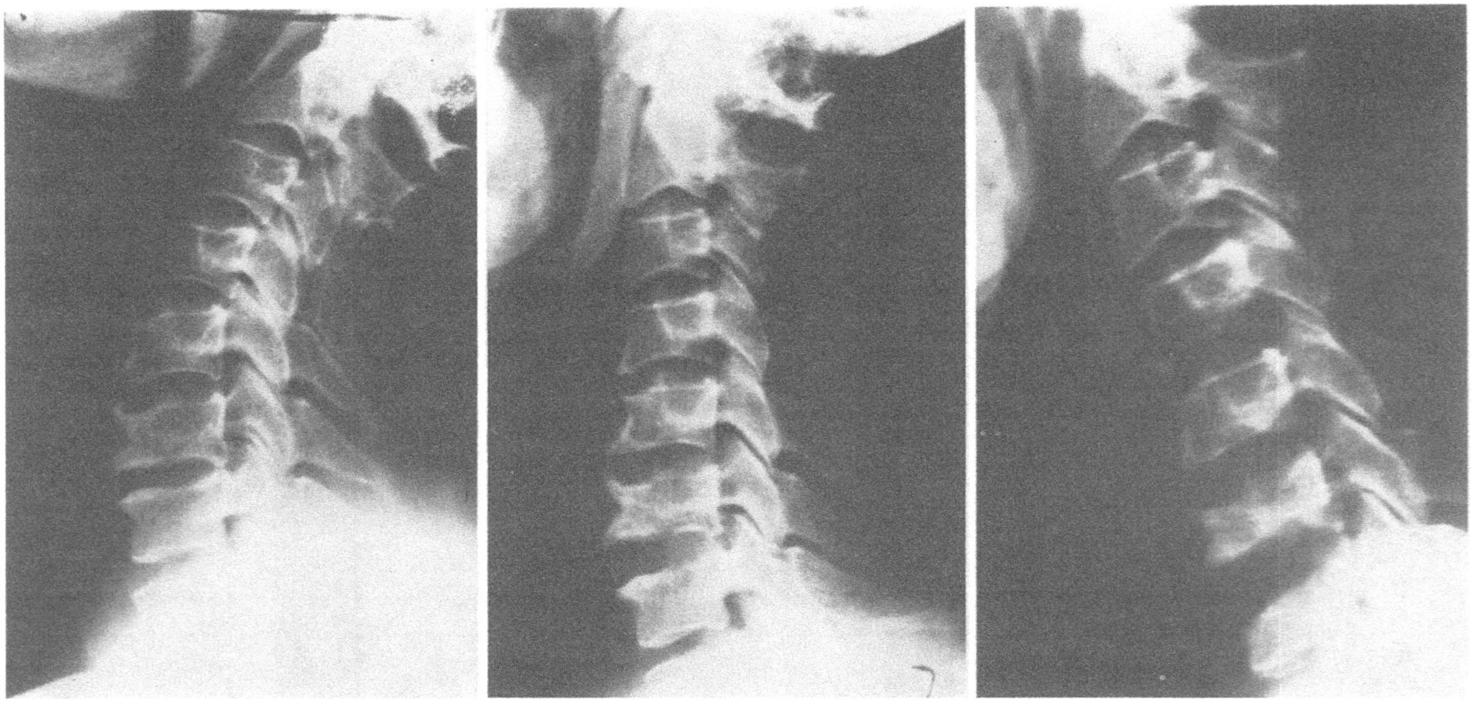

Fig. 5. A 55-year-old woman with diskopathy C5/C6, C6/C7. *Left:* before operation; *middle:* immediately after operation; *right:* 3 months after operation, collapse of the vertebral body, resorption, osteosclerosis

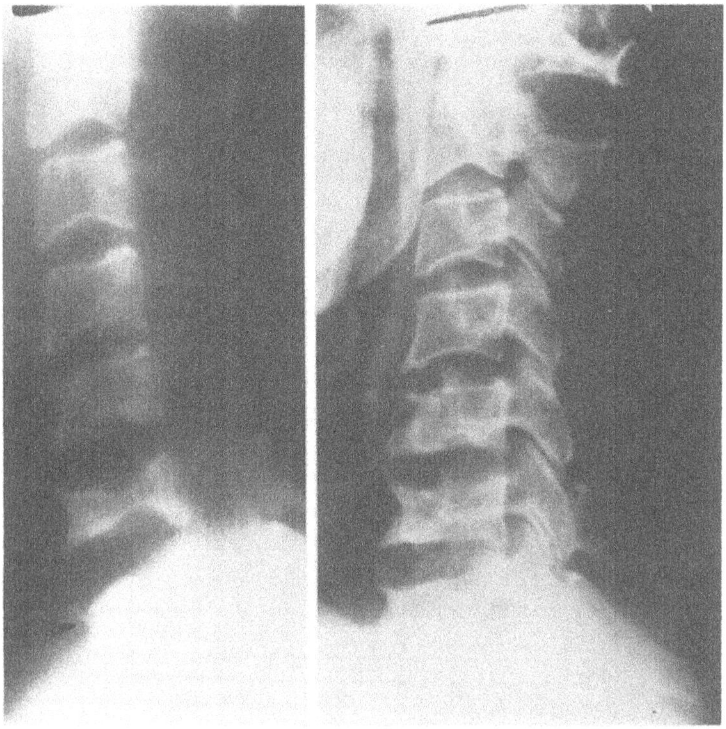

Fig. 5 *(continued)*. *Left:* corresponding tomography, no widening of the retropharyngeal space; *right:* 1 year later, beginning consolidation by osteophytic reactions, osteosclerosis

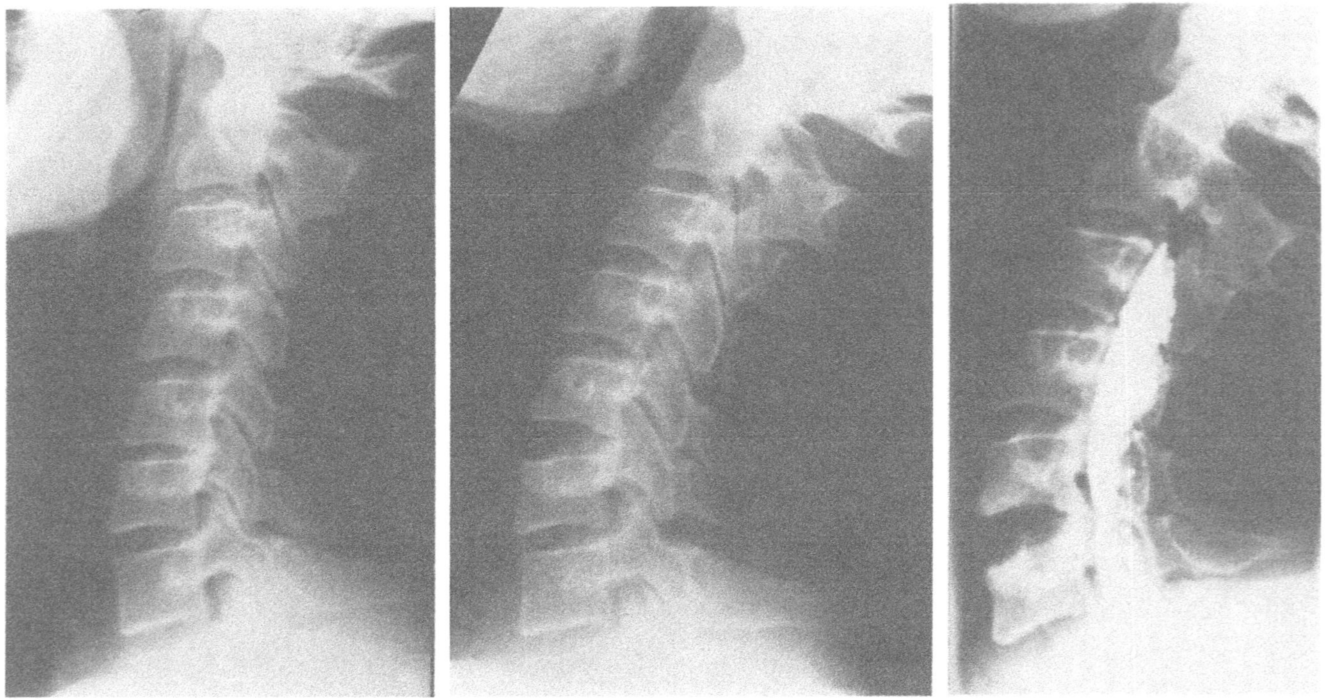

Fig. 6. A 53-year-old man with diskopathy C5/C6, C6/C7. *Left:* before operation; *middle:* immediately after operation; *right:* 1 month after operation, normal retropharyngeal space slight osteosclerosis in the fourth and fifth vertebrae

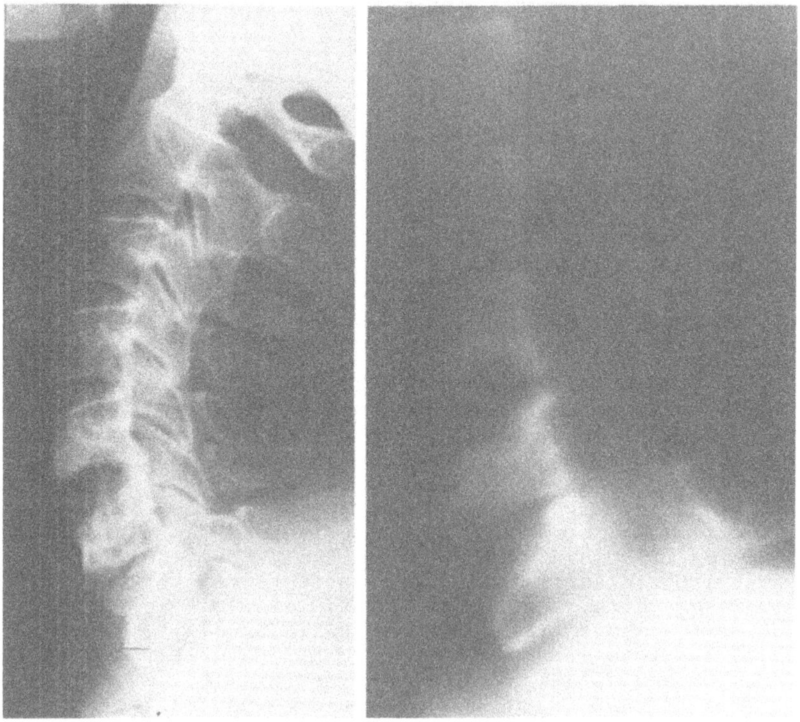

Fig. 6 *(continued)*. *Left:* 4 months later, diffuse pains in the neck, myelography without greater indentation of the spinal canal increasing osteosclerosis and resorption of the bones; *right:* 2.5 years later, collapse of the fifth vertebral body, resorption of anterior parts of the vertebrae nearby, no consolidation by osteophytes

Pain Relief by Chronic Mediothalamic Stimulation in Man

G. DIECKMANN and J. U. KRAINICK

Introduction

As long as stereotactic neurosurgery has existed, intraoperative stimulation procedures have been used to corroborate exact electrode positioning. However, only the method of chronic spinal cord stimulation with implantable systems (16) induced permanent deep brain stimulation for therapeutic purposes in chronic pain states. The appropriate target points were found by animal experiments inducing analgesia by electric stimulation (2,10,11,12) as well as the intraoperative observation in man that acute electric stimulations of certain structures, the destruction of which cause pain relief, were followed by a replacing of pain for a short time (MARK and ERVIN in (17)). Clinical application of these findings was carried out by MAZARS et al. (13,14), ADAMS et al. (1), FIELDS and ADAMS (5), HOSOBUCHI et al. (6), and RICHARDSON and AKIL (15). RICHARDSON and AKIL stimulated the periaqueductal and periventricular grey matter, MAZARS et al. (l.c.) the thalamic VPL nucleus, FIELDS and ADAMS (l.c.) the internal capsule, and ADAMS et al. (l.c.) as well as HOSOBUCHI et al. (l.c.) both the internal capsule and the sensory thalamic relay nuclei. Based on our own intraoperative observations, we have choosen the thalamic parafascicular-center median complex for chronic deep brain stimulation for pain control (4).

Surgical Technique

A flexible, four-polar deep brain electrode (Medtronic) was stereotactically implanted into the parafascicular-center median complex (Fig.1). Target coordinates used in this series were: 0-3 mm rostral Cp, 2-3 mm below ac-cp line, and 2 mm lateral of the wall of the posterior third ventricle. The exact electrode position was verified by acute electric stimulation and the electrode was then fixed in the burr hole by acrylic cement and attached to a percutaneous extension. During the postoperative trial period of about 14 days, stimulation was performed using a direct output pulse generator. Effective poles were determined, mostly pole 1 to 3 estimated lying within the parafascicular-center median complex, and appropriate stimulation parameters were evaluated. After having proved the clinical efficacy of the stimulation, the percutaneous extent was removed under general anesthesia, and a chronic extension with a radiofrequency receiver was attached to the electrode. The receiver was implanted in a subclavian pocket. Chronic stimulation was then performed by the patient himself with a radiofrequency transmitter giving the current by an antenna through the skin to the receiver by way of induction. Best stimulating parameters have been proved to be 50 cycles/s, pulse width of 0.8-1.0 ms. The strength varied in relation to pole combination and distance between receiver and antenna, normally 3 - 9 V transmitter output. Stimulation time had to be 10-20 min several times daily. After intervention disulfiram or amitriptyline were given daily to avoid development of tolerance to analgesia.

Subjects

The population evaluated consists of 22 patients with implanted deep brain stimulating electrodes. Taken into consideration here are only 19 patients with chronic unbearable pain states; the three others suffered from other diseases. Each patient of the pain group had proved to be not responding to a long period of medical treatment. Fifteen of them had previously undergone peripheral surgery. The ineffectiveness of these peripheral surgical interventions served as an important selection criterion. Since spinal cord stimulation in pain syndromes after traumatic cervical root avulsion had been proved ineffective, we primarily implant deep brain electrodes at present.

The psychological status of the patients was assessed by psychological tests and standardized psychological interviews by psychiatrists to avoid treating drug-addicted patients. The age of the patients ranged from 32-74 years. The time since surgery ranged from 1-22 months, with a mean of 12 months. More than 50% of the patients suffered from pain for more than 20 years, exactly 7-37 years. The stimulation effect was evaluated according to the self-estimated pain relief of the patients, in correlation with a reduced analgetic drug intake.

Indications

Principally, intermittent brain stimulation by chronically implanted stimulating systems is indicated in the management of chronic intractable pain after failure of peripheral invasive and ablative procedures. These indications are shown in Table 1.

Table 1. Indications for deep brain stimulation in cases of chronic intractable pain

1. Of central origin
2. Facial anesthesia dolorosa
3. Posttraumatic pain syndromes (spinal cord and peripheral nerves, especially after cervical root avulsion)
4. After failed spinal cord stimulation

Results

Table 2 shows sex, age, diagnosis, previous operative procedures, target point of the active surface of the electrode, internalization, complications, follow-up, results, and special remarks on all 22 patients in whom deep brain stimulation electrodes have been implanted.

Of the 19 patients with chronic pain, 16 (84%) demonstrated good pain relief by the stimulation during the postoperative trial period. Of the other three patients who failed to receive good relief, two belonged to those with phantom limb pain. They failed because of a dislodgment of the electrodes due to a hydrocephalic enlargement of the brain ventricles (Table 3). The third patient was paraplegic in whom

Table 2. Patients with implanted deep brain stimulation electrodes

No.	Sex	Age	Diagnosis	Previous op. proc.[a]	Target points[b]	Internalization	Complications related to implantation	Follow-up (months)	Result[c]	Remarks
1	M	74	Upper phantom limb pain		CGM, NPCMC	+	Dizziness	22	3	
2	M	44	Cerv. root avulsion	SCS: no pain relief	CGM, NPCMC	+		21	3	
3	M	37	Torticollis		H_1,V.o.i.	- no effect				
4	M	64	Lower phantom limb pain	SCS: insuff.1 pain relief	CGM - N. para.-CM-complex	+	Revision of the connector after 6 months	16	3	
5	F	56	Facial an-esth. dolorosa	Operation of Dandy	CGM, NPCMC	+		15	0 (during test period: 3)	Reimpl. in specific thalam. nucl.
6	M	32	Cerv. root avulsion	SCS: no pain relief	CGM, NPCMC	+		13	2	
7	M	45	Lower phantom limb pain	SCS: no pain relief SCS revis: no pain relief	CGM, NPCMC	-	Dislodgment			
8	F	62	Facial an-esth. dolorosa	Operation of Dandy	CGM, NPCMC	+		12	4	
9	M	66	Paraplegia (incompl.)	SCS: insuff.	CGM, NPCMC	+		12	3	
10	M	38	Cerv. root avulsion	SCS: insuff.	CGM, NPCMC	+		11	2	
11	F	41	Psychiatric disease		Rostral thalam.	+		11	good	

12	F	56	Torticollis		H_1, V.o.i.	- no effect				
13	M	46	Cerv. root avulsion		CGM, NPCMC	+		10	4	
14	F	56	Paraplegia complete	SCS: negative	CGM, NPCMC	- no pain relief				
15	M	43	Cerv. root avulsion		CGM, NPMC	+		7	4	
16	M	42	Cerv. root avulsion	SCS: insuff.	CGM, NPCMC	+		6	3	Stimulation addict
17	M	48	Facial anesth. dolorosa	Operation of Dandy	CGM, NPCMC	+		6	4	
18	M	66	Lower phantom limb pain	SCS: negative	CGM, NPCMC	-	Dislodgment			
19	M	45	Paraplegia (complete)	SCS:negative	CGM, NPCMC	+		4	0	
20	M	39	Cerv. root avulsion	SCS:insuff.	CGM, NPCMC	+		4	2	
21	M	69	Facial anesth. dolorosa	Thermorhizotomy 4 times	CGM, NPCMC	In test period				
22	M	41	Cerv. root avulsion		CGM, NPCMC	In test period				

a SCS, spinal cord stimulation. b CGM, central grey matter; NPCMC, parafascicularis-center median complex; H_1, V.o.i.
c 0, no pain relief; 1, up to 25% pain relief; 2, up to 50% pain relief; 3, up to 75% pain relief; 4, up to 100% pain relief.

Table 3. Test and final implantation of deep brain stimulation electrodes

Diagnosis	No. of test implantation	No. of final implantation	Remarks
Cervical root avulsion	8	7	1 patient in test period
Facial anesthesia dolorosa	4	3	1 patient in test period
Phantom limb	4	2	Electrode dislodgment in 2 patients
Paraplegia	3	2	
Torticollis	2	No effect	
Other	1	1	
Total	22	15	

the cause of the failure is unknown. A chronic extension was not internalized in these patients. In two other patients, the internalization has not yet been performed because they are still in the trial period. Therefore, from the 19 patients in whom electrodes were inserted for purposes of pain relief, only 14 were internalized.

Of these 14 patients, 9 (64%) presently show good pain relief of 75%-100% (Table 4). Three patients experienced relief of about 50%, and in two others the benefit did not continue. The relief of pain is estimated by the patients themselves and noted according to the classification of the Minneapolis Pain Seminar in 1973.

Table 4. Results of final implantation of deep brain stimulation electrodes

Diagnosis	No. of patients	Pain relief 0	up to 25%	50%	75%	100%	Follow-up (months)
Cervical root avulsion	7	-	-	3	2	2	4-21
Facial anesthesia dolorosa	3	1	-	-	-	2	6-15
Phantom limb	2	-	-	-	2	-	16-22
Paraplegia	2	1	-	-	1	-	4-12
Total (pain)	14	2	-	3	5	4	4-22
Other	1		good result				11
Total	15						4-22

The follow-up ranges from 1-22 months. The longest *successful* stimulation period in our patients is 22 months. Most of the patients mentioned here have a stimulation time of about 1 year.

Complications

As mentioned above, an electrode dislodgment occurred in two patients. Both patients had an enlarged ventricular system due to brain atrophy. Because of the vicinity of the target point to the wall of the posterior third ventricle, one may assume that the tip of the electrode invaded the ventricular system.

One patient reported dizziness during 50/s stimulation of the center median, which disappeared after changing the frequency to 30/s and resulted in good pain relief. One other patient seems to be addicted to the stimulation itself. Presently, he tries to stimulate himself several hours per day and demands a second stimulator for use. A revision of the connector was necessary in one patient because of an isolation defect.

Discussion

Significant pain relief was observed in the eight patients with pain after cervical root avulsions verified by myelography. All of them could be internalized except one who is still in the trial period. They represent the majority of our patients because other surgical procedures have been proved ineffective in this indication.

In contrast, phantom limb pain can be relieved with good results by percutaneous spinal cord stimulation, thus avoiding the necessity of deep brain stimulation. Therefore, the number of those patients is small in our series. The failure in two of four patients was due to technical reasons and does not reflect the efficacy of the procedure.

It is a striking finding that chronic parafascicular-center median stimulation in patients with phantom limb pain and facial anesthesia dolorosa resulted in the same good pain relief as stimulation of somatosensory systems since stimulation of the latter is considered to be the main indication of so-called deafferentation pain "lack of proprioceptive stimuli" (7,14). The reason is yet unknown.

Stimulation of parafascicular-center median complex probably activates the same pain-inhibiting system in the medial brain stem as stimulation of periventricular grey matter (15). Today one assumes (3,9) that electric stimulation of this system releases endogenous, morphine-like substances, endorphines, which directly act at the opiate receptor sites of the pain-inhibiting system. Therefore, it is understandable why the administration of disulfiram or amitriptyline may impede development of tolerance to analgesia since both substances are ingredients for the preparation of these opioid peptides the releasing of which is introduced or enhanced by the electric stimulation. Furthermore, it is understandable that inhibition of pain could be prevented by injection of the opiate antagonist naloxone (8,15).

During the acute intraoperative and chronic unilateral stimulation of parafascicular-center median complex, it was always observed that tingling and temperature sensations only occurred in those contralateral body areas that were affected by the pain, not in other pain-free areas. The tingling and temperature sensations then masked the pain. The pain might be localized in the arm, leg, or in the face; the electric stimulation of the same cerebral site always causes masking paresthesias only in that area of the body affected by the pain if one uses threshold stimuli. The mechanism of this restricted, local specific answer by stimulating a target point belonging to the nonspecific thalamic activating system is not yet known.

Summary

Chronically implanted electrodes in thalamic parafascicular-center median complex allowed repeated self-stimulation by means of an induction-receiving system and external stimulator. Good results were obtained in seven patients with cervical root avulsions, in two patients with anesthesia dolorosa, and in two patients with phantom limb pain. Patients with paraplegic pain did not to respond well. The surgical procedure is described, and the mechanism of thalamic stimulation in the relief of pain is discussed.

References

1. ADAMS, J.E., HOSOBUCHI, M.S.Y., FIELDS, H.L.: Stimulation of internal capsule for relief of chronic pain. J. Neurosurg. 41, 740-744 (1974)
2. AKIL, H., MAYER, D.J.: Antagonism of stimulation-produced analgesia by p-CPA, a serotonin synthesis inhibitor. Brain Res. 44, 692-697 (1972)
3. AKIL, H., MAYER, D.J., LIEBESKIND, J.C.: Antagonism of stimulation-produced analgesia by naloxone, a narcotic antagonist. Science 191, 961-962 (1976)
4. DIECKMANN, G., KRAINICK, J.-U., THODEN, U.: Pain-modulation by electrical stimulation of nonspecific thalamic nuclei. 3rd Meeting of the European Society of Stereotactic and Functional Neurosurgery. Freiburg 1977
5. FIELDS, H.L., ADAMS, J.E.: Pain after cortical injury relieved by electrical stimulation of the internal capsule. Brain 97, 169-178 (1974)
6. HOSOBUCHI, Y., ADAMS, J.E., FIELDS, H.L.: Chronic thalamic and internal capsular stimulation for the control of facial anesthesia dolorosa and dysesthesia of thalamic syndrome. Adv. Neurol. 4, 783-787 (1874)
7. HOSOBUCHI, Y., ADAMS, J.E., RUTKIN, B.: Chronic thalamic and internal capsule stimulation for the control of central pain. Surg. Neurol. 4, 91-92 (1975)
8. HOSOBUCHI, Y., ADAMS, J.E., LINCHITZ, R.: Pain relief by electrical stimulation of the central gray matter in humans and its reversal by naloxone. Science 197, 183-186 (1977)
9. LIEBESKIND, J.C.: Pain modulation by central nervous system stimulation. In: Advances in pain research and therapy. BONICA, J.J., ALBE-FESSARD, D. (eds.), Vol. 1, pp. 445-453. New York: Raven Press 1976
10. LIEBESKIND, J.C., GUILBAUD, G., BESSON, J.H.: Analgesia from electrical stimulation of the periaqueductal gray matter in the cat: behavioral observations and inhibitory effects on spinal cord interneurons. Brain Res. 50, 441-446 (1973)
11. MAYER, J., WOLFE, T.L., AKIL, H., CARDER, B., LIEBESKIND, C.J.: Analgesia from electrical stimulation in the brainstem of the rat. Science 174, 1351-1354 (1971)
12. MAZARS, G., ROGÉ, R., MAZARS, Y.: Résultats de la stimulation du faisceau spinothalamique et leur incidence sur la physiopathologie de la douleur. Revue Neurol. (Paris) 103, 136-138 (1960)

13. MAZARS, G., MERIENNE, L., CIOLOCCA, C.: Stimulations thalamiques intermittentes antaligiques. Note preliminaire. Rev. Neurol. (Paris) 128, 273-279 (1973)

14. MAZARS, G., MERIENNE, L., CIOLOCCA, C.: Traitement de certains types de douleurs par des stimulateurs thalamiques implantables. Neurochirurgie 20, 117-124 (1974)

15. RICHARDSON, D.E., AKIL, H.: Pain reduction by electrical brain stimulation in man. Part 2: Chronic self-administration in the periventricular gray matter. J. Neurosurg. 47, 184-194 (1977)

16. SHEALY, C.N., MORTIMER, J.T., RESWICK, J.B.: Electrical inhibition of pain by stimulation of the dorsal columns: Preliminary clinical report. Anesth. Analg. (Cleve) 46, 489-491 (1967)

17. WHITE, J.E., SWEET, W.H.: Pain and the neurosurgeon: a 40-year experience. Springfield, Ill: Thomas 1969

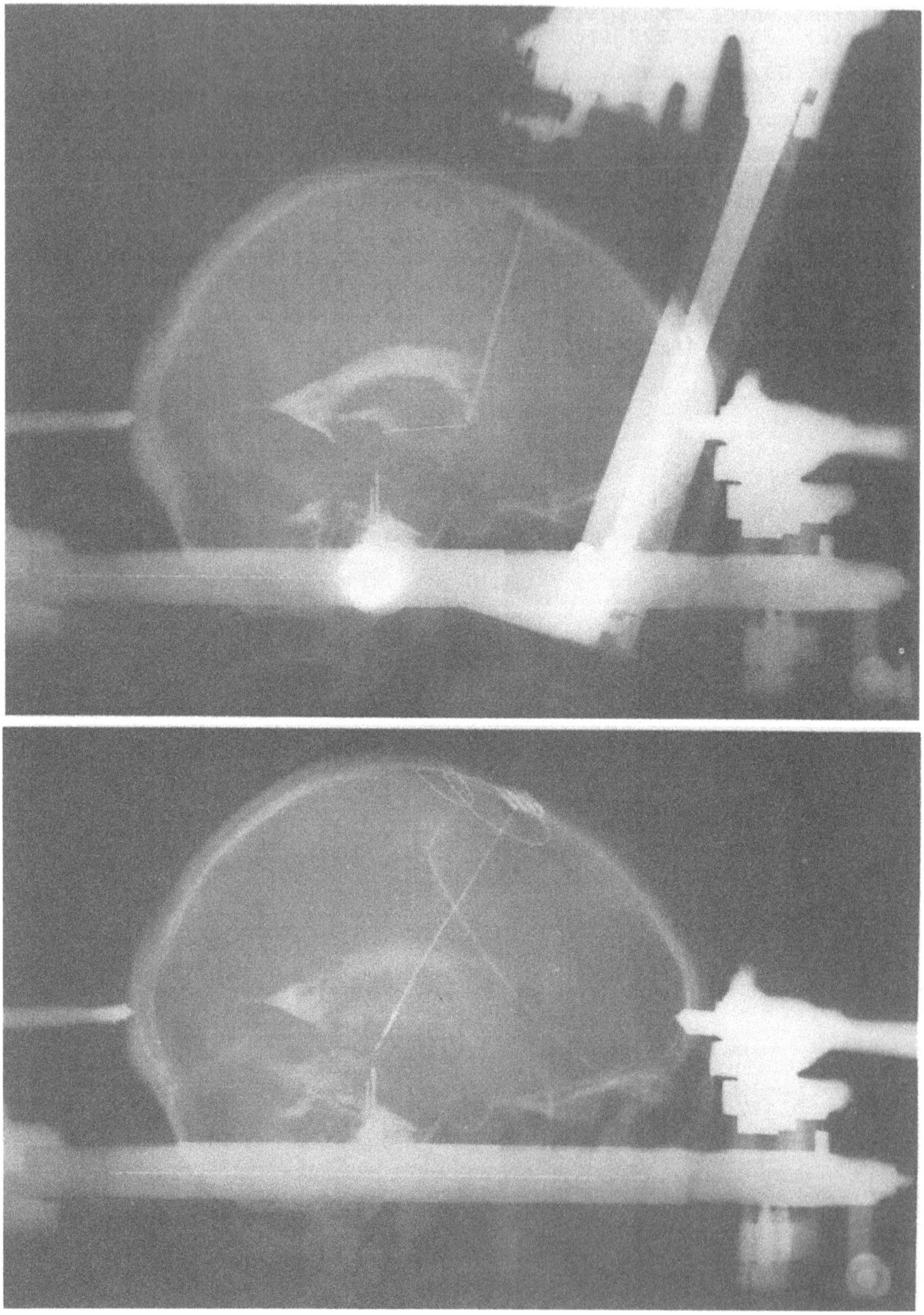

Fig. 1. Lateral ventriculogram showing deep brain electrode in situ. The active surface of the electrode is situated in the parafascicular-center median complex. Rostrally one sees the cannula for contrast medium injection

Radiofrequency Percutaneous Gasserian Ganglion Surgery

B. M. ONOFRIO

Trigeminal neuralgia in its pure form consists of severe paroxysmal pain localized to the sensory domain of the trigeminal nerve uniformly induced by stimuli to the sensory endings of the trigeminal nerve. The pain begins abruptly, lasts seconds to minutes, and ends as suddenly as it began having varying pain-free intervals between paroxysms. There are several avenues of approach for amelioration of this pain. Firstly, a history and neurological examination are done to rule out the possibility of a mass lesion as the cause of trigeminal neuralgia. Sensation in the distribution of the fifth cranial nerve should be tested. The pin is appreciated in this patient as sharp on the right and over the third division on the left. The pin not only is appreciated as sharp in the left second and first divisions but also provokes typical paroxysms of the patient's pain. Touch similarly causes pain. Fifth cranial motor function, including temporalis and pterygoid, is tested. The presence of numbness or motor weakness should alert the physician to the likely presence of a mass involving the posterior root or the gasserian ganglion. Corneal sensation is checked. Some of the maneuvers that precipitate pain are demonstrated. Skull X-rays with stereo base views are taken to rule out bony pathology along the course of Meckel's cave or the three exiting foramina of the respective three divisions of the fifth cranial nerve. A general examination and routine laboratory studies are also done.

The first step in the treatment of trigeminal neuralgia is institution of either diphenylhydantoin (Dilantin, United States) or Carbamazepine (Tegretol, United States), in increasing doses until the pain is controlled. If the patient has pain that is refractory to this medical management or if toxic levels are needed to produce pain relief, the next step may be considered, namely, stereotaxic coagulation of the gasserian ganglion or posterior sensory root. A full discussion of the procedure, its possible complications, and the method of the operation are entered into in detail.

Knowledge of the anatomy of the base of the skull and Meckel's cave are essential to the success of the procedure. With the naked skull in the position used to accomplish the operation, 30° hyperextension and 15° rotation to the opposite side, the needle is seen to be inserted in the most medial portion of the foramen ovale. As the needle is inserted in the yellow clay facsimile of the gasserian ganglion, it can be seen piercing the third division and gasserian ganglion coming to rest at approximately the depth of the petroclinoid ligament and in good position for coagulation to produce second division analgesia. Next the needle is introduced at a steeper trajectory with reference to the posterior clinoid to lie in a position for accomplishing first division analgesia. A facial view of the needle insertion demonstrates the relationship of the foramen ovale.

This same area with intact soft tissues is viewed from the facial aspect. With the needle in place in the foramen ovale, one can see the relationships of the following structures: (1) middle meningeal, (2) foramen ovale with the third division, (3) foramen rotundum and second division, (4) pterygoid fossa with the attachments of the pterygoid muscles, (5) carotid canal, (6) sphenoid sinus, and (7) superior orbital fissure.

As the specimen is rotated, the following intracranial structures are dipicted: (1) foramen spinosum, (2) foramen ovale, (3) foramen rotundum, (4) superior orbital fissure, (5) anterior clinoid, and (6) the posterior clinoid with petroclinoid ligament running from the posterior clinoid to the petrous ridge. The petroclinoid ligament marks the boundary of posterior aspects of Meckel's cave. The posterior root and the gasserian ganglion are reflected anteriorly revealing the most medial portion of Meckel's cave. The fifth cranial motor root is seen lying on the most medial portion of the gasserian ganglion running in a superior to inferior direction to exit from the foramen ovale. The first division exits from the superior orbital fissure. The opening of Meckel's cave appears underneath the petroclinoid ligament. The lateral boundary of the cavernous sinus, namely, the gasserian ganglion, has been stripped away, showing the carotid artery, the third cranial nerve superiorly and the sixth nerve running in the cavernous sinus on the lateral side of the carotid artery. The needle trajectory here is positioned for accomplishing first and second division analgesia.

On the day of surgery, the patient is taken to the fluoroscopy room and placed on the X-ray table. An IV is in place in the arm for later administration of sodium methohexital (Brevital, United States) during the actual coagulation of the ganglion. The area of pain is outlined. The face is prepped with colorless aqueous thimerosal (Merthiolate, United States) over the cheek on the involved side and the opposite forehead. The opposite forehead is infiltrated with lidocaine (Xylocaine, United States) and an 18 gauge indifferent spinal needle is introduced so it lies in the subgaleal space. On the painful side of the face, a point 2.5 cm lateral to the angle of the mouth is infiltrated with lidocaine. This point is directly lateral to the angle of the mouth when third division analgesia is desired and more in the caudal direction from this point to accomplish second or first division analgesia.

The thermistor needle used for making the lesion is a thin-walled 20 gauge spinal needle 11 cm in total length: the hub and needle are entirely coated with three coats of epoxylite except for the small side arm extending from the hub and the 5 mm exposed needle tip. There is a stylet, which is kept in place in the needle until the needle has achieved optimal final positioning, and the thermistor-dipped stylet, which is then placed for measuring the needle tip temperature at the time of coagulation. The exposed needle tip measures 5 mm. The stereotaxic needle is then introduced with a gloved palpating finger lying against the buccal mucosa to assure against entering the oral cavity; by free hand trajectory the needle can be felt passing between the ramus of the manible and the buccal mucosa. The needle is inserted about half its entire length and directed so that if extended it would be in planes bisecting the middle of the pupil and 3 mm anterior to the external auditory meatus.

The fluoroscopy is then used to correct the needle position to the desired part of the foramen ovale along the most medial border for accomplishing first and/or second division numbness or into the middle of the foramen for third division numbness. The needle now is anterior and medial to the foramen ovale. The needle is repositioned.

When fluoroscopy shows good position in this plane, a permanent film is taken in this projection. A lateral permanent X-ray is taken. The permanent oblique film shows the needle optimally placed for achieving first and second division analgesia. The foramen ovale and the needle in its superior medial quadrant lie above the ramus of the mandible in this projection. When preliminary X-rays indicate a proper needle trajectory, the needle is ready for insertion into the cranial vault.

The insertion of the thermistor needle with gentle pressure through the foramen ovale causes pain at this point, and the patient is forewarned of this. A small pop is felt as the dura propria is penetrated. The lateral film is essential for measuring the desired angle and depth of the needle. Here the needle on X-ray is in optimal position for accomplishing third division analgesia and is relatively shallow in the middle fossa. The outline shows the sella, the dotted line is the petroclinoid ligament, and the solid line anterior to it is the bony landmark of the clivus. The posterior root, darker gasserian ganglion, and three divisions of the fifth cranial nerve are depicted on the X-ray. The course of the motor root is shown here in red going from superior to inferior along the most medial portion of the posterior root and gasserian ganglion. The needle is inserted deeper and is now in its optimal final position for accomplishing first and second division analgesia. At this point the stylet is removed, the spinal fluid is seen eminating from Meckel's cave, and the thermistor bead-tipped stylet is introduced into the needle. The active electrode is placed on the hub of the needle. The temperature monitoring probe is connected to the radionics generator as well as connecting the indifferent electrode in the opposite forehead. Stimulating voltage varies between 0.1-1.0 V and is used to verify the position of the exposed needle tip in the ganglion. The radionics machine can be regulated with a timer to accomplish the desired 30- to 60- to 90-s burn of the gasserian ganglion and posterior root, and the temperature during the burn is monitored with the thermistor probe at 80°. Next the patient is cautioned of impending face pain as ganglion stimulation is carried out. She complains that the stimulus reproduces her first and second division pain. This adds another element of positioning accuracy of the exposed needle tip. Each time the patient is stimulated she is warned of precipitation of sharp pain. Usually patients will tolerate this maneuver reasonably well. Next, the patient is given 3-6 cc of sodium methohexital depending on age and body habitus. As the lesion is made, a dense erythema is almost always seen over the surface of the face in which analgesia is developing. Here erythema of the left upper vermilion border and cheek is marked. As the patient begins to awaken from the short-acting sodium methohexital, a stimulus in the suspected areas of sensory deprivation accomplishes a reasonable index of what the patient will display when she is awake as far as sensory loss is concerned and is judged by grimace. As the patient awakens, the dense erythema in the second division can still be seen and lasts for a considerable period of time. After an appropriate period has been allowed to elapse for the patient to regain full consciousness, she is asked to evaluate the areas of numbness in her face, and formal testing outlines areas that are analgesic or hypalgesic. The conjunctiva is markedly red on the operated side indicating that there has also been erythema and vasodilation in the area supplied by the first division. Here stimulus of the first and second division shows absence of pain appreciation on the left. Sensation is, of course, intact on the right. There is also a modest hypalgesia of the left third divison.

The erythema is still persistent, especially on the vermilion border of the upper lip and over the malar eminence. The presence of the erythema is a good indicator of a durable lesion and here can be seen readily to be present on the left and absent on the right. After completion of a good lesion, the needles are removed and the needle sites washed. Sensory testing again shows dense analgesia of the first and second divisions on the left as well as part of the third division. Here the corneal sensation is seen to be absent on the left and present on the right, and this patient will require a welder's shield on the left side of her glasses to help prevent corneal ulceration. The patient, after she is dismissed the following morning, is again checked for the areas of analgesia, possible motor weakness, and the possible need for wearing a shield if first division analgesia is accomplished. Should conjunctival redness or blurred vision occur on the side of the analgesia, she should see her ophthalmologist immediately for the prevention or treatment of corneal ulceration. Here the patient shows that she is analgesic to cotton in the first and second divisions on the left. The pin is appreciated as sharp on the right, sharp in the third division on the left, and dull in the second and first division. There is good pterygoid and good masseter function. The extraocular nerves are investigated and shown to be all intact. Maneuvers that preoperatively caused her pain are unable to provoke discomfort postoperatively. We have found that this procedure carried low morbidity and is tolerated well by even the most debiliated patients.

Discussion

Using the technique described, our results in 359 patients having undergone radiofrequency procedures are as follows. The divisional distribution of pain in these patients is depicted in Table 1.

Table 1. Divisions involved by trigeminal neuralgia (359 patients)

V_1	V_2	V_3	No. patients
X			6
	X		66
		X	62
X	X		78
	X	X	122
X	X	X	25

Of the 359 patients, 300 achieved a pain-free state in the series. The postoperative follow-up has been from 8 years to 6 months. Table 2 shows that 40 patients required repeat procedures to obtain relief.

Fifty-nine patients were considered to be failures of this form of treatment. Table 3 shows that 46 patients resorted to some other method of pain control after one procedure. Most of these were disuaded from further radiofrequency attempts either due to poor quality analgesia obtained after a concerted first attempt or prompt recurrence of their pain within 3-6 months. The patient's considered failures after multiple radiofrequency procedures usually chose a more definitive open procedure, either via the subtemporal or posterior fossa approach. The method of affording relief in these 59 patients is depicted in Table 4.

Table 2. Radiofrequency treatment for trigeminal neuralgia in successful cases: No. of procedures

Lasting relief	No. patient
After 1 RF procedure	260
After 2 RF procedure	33
After 3 RF procedure	7
After 4 RF procedure	0
Total	300

Table 3. Radiofrequency treatment for trigeminal neuralgia in cases considered failures: No. of procedures

Failure	No. patients
After 1 procedure	46
After 2 procedure	8
After 3 procedure	4
After 4 procedure	1
Total	59

Table 4. Radiofrequency treatment for trigeminal neuralgia failures among 359 patients

	No. patients
Residual pain but no further treatment	16
Further treatment	43
Repeat alcohol block	9
Resumption carbamazepine	9
Craniectomy: subtemporal	14
posterior fossa	4
Peripheral neurectomy	1
For anesthesia dolorosa: fluphenazine hydrochloride and amitriptyline	6
Total	59

The complications of the radiofrequency procedures in these patients are described in Table 5. There were no intra- or extracranial vascular injuries and no mortality.

The unwanted first division analgesia, a problem earlier in our series, has become less frequent. As SHURMAN and others have shown, this can for the most part be avoided by using neuraleptic analgesia instead of sodium methohexital alone so that sensory testing may be done as the lesion is being made. In Table 6, the ten patients having facial pain or other than trigeminal neuralgia experienced poor palliation of pain.

Table 5. Radiofrequency treatment for trigeminal neuralgia complications among 359 patients

	No. patients
Anesthesia dolorosa	6
Unwanted 1st division numbness	34
Corneal ulceration	8
Cleared without loss of vision	6
Associated with some loss of vision	2
Transient 6th nerve palsy	1
Transient aseptic meningitis	1
Total	50

Table 6. Radiofrequency treatment for pain other than trigeminal neuralgia

Kind of pain	Relief	No relief
Craniofacial malignancy	0	3
Traumatic neuritis (secondary to ENT procedures)	0	3
Anesthesia dolorosa	0	2
Atypical face pain	1	2[a]

a Anesthesia dolorosa developed in 1.

As the length of follow-up of these patients increases, there will be a higher percent of failures, but the procedure, because of ease of technique and low morbidity, remains an excellent form of treatment in patients suffering from trigeminal neuralgia.

Changes in Current Threshold During Controlled Thermocoagulation for Treatment of Trigeminal Neuralgia: a New Parameter for Judging the Result of Loss of Pain

R. MÜKE and H. SCHMIDT

The substantial advantage of controlled thermocoagulation is the possibility of selective destruction of pain fibers, preserving all or most of the touch sensation. Until now, analgesia was thought to be necessary for a good result (3,5). When we performed our first controlled thermolesion, a few patients who achieved complete pain relief experienced no sensory loss. First we found it strange and thought they would turn out as poor results, but then we heard the reports from Stockholm (1). In 1957 LEKSELL performed stereotactic irradiation of the trigeminal root and ganglion on some patients with typical trigeminal neuralgia. In two patients a follow-up examination could be made 18 years later. They had been completely free from pain without any sensory loss. In 1975 this occurrence led to a further trial. This time 23 patients were treated with the gamma unit. Most of them experienced improvement or complete pain relief after a latency of 1 day to 4-5 weeks. There was a mean follow-up of 12 months. In no case were there any significant sensory disturbances or dysesthesia or other inadvertent effects.

With this information it appeared possible to obtain a similar effect with thermolesion. The problem was how to test this effect. Since we wanted no sensory loss, we checked the sensitivity threshold for 100 Hz current as indicated by changes in voltage and for temperature before and after each lesion. We found that the threshold for 100 Hz current measured before the first lesion had to be raised in the average four to five times and for temperature by 50% before obtaining any loss of sensitivity. Table 1 gives some examples of threshold changes during controlles thermolesions. Fig. 1 demonstrates graphically the relation between the extension of the thermolesion and the threshold for a 100-Hz current and for temperature in one patient. The lesion was increased stepwise by 5° starting with 55°. Prior to the first lesion, the threshold for 100 Hz current was 0.1 V for a temperature of 45°. Before reaching hypalgesia, the 100-Hz threshold had to be elevated five times, and before reaching analgesia eight times. There are individual differences.

One could argue that threshold changes for a 100-Hz current are relevant only for judging the function of A α and β fibers but not the function of A γ and C fibers, the threshold of which is much higher. We know from investigations by LETCHER and GOLDRING (2) on the saphenous nerve of the cat that when conduction in both the A γ and C fibers was interrupted by heating, the A α and β fibers amplitude was also reduced to 10% - 20%. In addition, we observed that the threshold for a 100-Hz current is elevated at least four to five times in cases where analgesia is combined with normesthesia. It is also well-known from percutaneous cordotomies that one can produce different forms of paresthesias before eliciting pain sensation secondary to stimulating the spinothalamic tract with a 100 Hz current.

Table 1. Threshold changes for 100-Hz current and temperature during thermolesion (nine patients)

Threshold prior to the first lesion		First lesion		Threshold after the first lesion		Second lesion		Treshold after the second lesion	
100 Hz	Temp.			100 Hz	Temp.			100 Hz	Temp.
0.1 V	45°	70°	60 s	0.3 V	50°	75°	60 s	0.48 V	68°
0.15 V	51°	70°	60 s	0.6 V	55°	75°	60 s	0.8 V	75°
0.12 V	48°	75°	60 s	0.4 V	60°	80°	60 s	0.6 V	70°
0.1 V	48°	75°	60 s	0.4 V	64°	80°	60 s	0.6 V	73°
0.1 V	50°	65°	60 s	0.3 V	59°	68°	60 s	0.5 V	68°
0.1 V	49°	65°	60 s	0.4 V	58°	70°	60 s	0.65 V	62°
0.12 V	50°	65°	60 s	0.4 V	65°				
0.08 V	46°	70°	60 s	0.5 V	55°				
0.11 V	45°	65°	60 s	0.2 V	50°	70°	60 s	0.3 V	50°
						75°	60 s	0.68 V	55°

Table 2. Patients after thermolesion without pain, sensory loss, or recurrences

Patient	Date of operation	History of attacks before operation (years)	Threshold prior to lesion (100 Hz)	Threshold after lesion (100 Hz)	Temp. (°)
1	26 Apr 1977	14	0.12 V	0.7 V	70
2	5 May 1977	8	0.15 V	0.5 V	65
3	14 June 1977	15	0.12 V	0.6 V	70
4	28 Oct 1977	2	0.15 V	0.4 V	65
5	4 Aug 1977	11	0.15 V	0.6 V	65
6	25 Aug 1977	6	0.1 V	0.6 V	73
7	29 Sept 1977	2 1/2	0.1 V	0.5 V	68
8	24 Nov 1977	4	0.12 V	0.65 V	62
9	6 Dec 19771	7	0.12 V	0.4 V	60

Since we knew these correlations between threshold, sensitivity, and pain relief, we tried to free the patients from pain by elevating the 100 Hz threshold only three to five times to preserve as much sensory perception as possible. This could not be achieved in all cases. Sometimes an unintended hypalgesia or hypesthesia developed. Nervetheless, the number and degree of hypesthesia were definitely decreased. Table 2 shows the data of nine patients all of whom are free from pain since the thermolesion and have no or only very small sensory loss. All of these patients had complained of heavy attacks over a long period of time prior to surgery and had reacted insufficiency to carbamazepin (Tegretal, Germany). Prior to thermolesion, the threshold for a 100-Hz current was never higher than 0.15 V. The threshold for temperature before thermolesion was about 45°-50° C. All of these patients are free from pain until now, without any sign of dysesthesia. Some of them had a delayed improvement with continued attacks from 2-14 days postoperatively.

We have had experience in thermolesions with 86 patients. It is possible that the recurrence rate in cases without sensory disturbances will be higher than in those with analgesia. However, experience with stereotactic irradiation in Stockholm and our own follow-up studies for more than 1 year let us hope that it will be tolerable. Additionally, the controlled thermolesion can easily be repeated involving no more difficulties than the original procedure.

We think that the most serious problems disturbing patients postoperatively are paresthesias (4). We know that paresthesias are less frequent in thermocoagulations but cannot always be avoided, as SWEET reported 3 years ago in Heidelberg (6). To reduce these paresthesias, he discontinued the thermolesion with hypalgesia in some cases. Therefore, we think our procedure is justified. Besides, we have the impression that it is easier and more exact to determine the threshold than to examine the sensory function of patients at the time of operation. This is underlined by the fact that most patients with trigeminal neuralgia are elderly patients who often have difficulty in distinguishing between different sensory qualities, especially after anesthesia (even after a very short one).

Summary

To avoid troublesome paresthesia, it is necessary to keep the lesion small. We found it possible to stop trigeminal paroxysms by lesion causing no sensory disturbance - by elevating the 100-Hz current threshold only three to five times. We, therefore, recommend threshold measurements to control the effects of thermolesion.

References

1. HAKONSON, S., LEKSELL, L.: Stereotactic radiosurgery in trigeminal neuralgia. Unpublished information
2. LETCHER, F.S., GOLDRING, S.: The effect of radiofrequency current and heat on peripher nerve action potential in the cat. J. Neurosurg. 29, 42-47 (1968)
3. ONOFRIO, B.M.: Radiofrequency percutaneous gasserian ganglion lesions. J. Neurosurg. 42, 132-139 (1975)
4. SCHÜRMANN, K., BUTZ, M., BROCK, M.: Temporal retrogasserian resection of trigeminal root versus controlled elective percutaneous electrocoagulation of the ganglion of Gasser in the treatment of trigeminal neuralgia. Report on a series of 531 cases. Acta Neurochir. (Wien) 26, 33-53 (1972)
5. SIEGFRIED, I.: Results of percutaneous controlled thermocoagulation of the gasserian ganglion in 300 cases of trigeminal pain. Advances in Neurosurgery. Vol. 3, pp. 287-296. Berlin, Heidelberg, New York: Springer 1975
6. SWEET, W.H.: Percutaneous differential thermal trigeminal rhizotomy for the management of facial pain. Advances in Neurosurgery. Vol 3, pp. 274-286. Berlin, Heidelberg, New York: Springer 1975

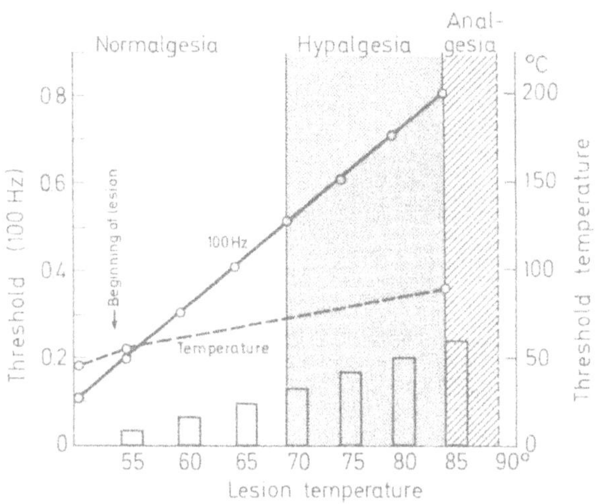

Fig. 1. Changes in threshold during thermolesion

Chronic Cerebellar Stimulation in Cerebral Palsy

W. WINKELMÜLLER, B. U. SEIDEL, and G. GRAUBNER

Introduction

Spasticity, athetosis, and ataxia are the most frequent symptoms of persisting pyramidal and extrapyramidal lesions in cerebral palsy. The hypertonic movement disorders may be lessened by early physiotherapy or orthopedic interventions. In the majority of patients, motor ability worsens during puberty so that, in severe cases, no alternative but neurosurgical treatment exists.

Since the introduction of chronic cerebellar stimulation by COOPER in 1973 (1), new trails have been followed in the treatment of complex motor disorders in cerebral palsy. In contrast to the traditional open and stereotactic lesions within the pyramidal afferents, this nondestructive method utilizes physiologic cerebellar control functions on unbalanced motor performance. It is supposed that electric stimulation of the anterior lobe leads to inhibition of neocerebellar circuits via dentatothalamocortical pathways and, on the other hand, reduces the spinal activity, especially of the γ-motoneurons by way of reticulospinal projections (Fig. 1).

Material and Methods

At the Medical School of Hannover 13 patients suffering from cerebral palsy have undergone implantation of a bilateral cerebellar stimulator. All children had a quadriplegia and were subdivided into four different groups according to the clinical manifestation of spastic and dyskinetic symptoms (Table 1). The age of the surgically treated patients ranged from 9 to 35 years. The operation is performed under general anesthesia.

Table 1. Groups according to clinical manifestation of symptoms

Diagnosis	No.	Age/years
CP and quadriplegia	13	$\bar{x}$ = 14,38
Spasticity	3	9, 14, 18
Spasticity > Athetosis	6	10, 10, 11 13, 13, 14
Athetosis > Spasticity	2	10, 13
Athetosis	2	17, 35

The electronic implant is composed of a platinum electrode, which is connected to a receiver. The electrodes are placed bilaterally on the anterior lobe of the cerebellum (Fig. 1), and the leads emerge through small craniectomies and are passed subcutaneously down to the neck to the radio receiver implant on the anterior chest wall. Radiofrequency pulses are sent form a transmitter box via an antenna applied to the skin over the receiver.

For evaluation of the therapeutic benefits, we used the following pre- and postoperative testing combining clinical estimation and apparative methods, which permit quantitating clinical signs.

A standardized questionnaire is directed to parents, physiotherapists, occupational therapists, and teachers.

Neurological symptoms are graduated semiquantitatively.

In addition, a test chart of motor ability is performed.

Muscular resistance is recorded by repeated myotonography.

The electromyogram (EMG) is recorded with special preference to the silent period.

Results

The beneficial effect of stimulation as revealed by clinical examination covers various symptoms of cerebral palsy. Apart from the reduction of muscular hypertonia, of muscle tone variations, of hyperkinetic movements, and of salivation, progressive improvement of statomotor functions and skillful movements are observed (Table 2).

Table 2. Number of improved patients by cerebellar stimulation (clinical results)

	Tonus	Skilled movement	Stato-motor control	Hyper-kinesia	Salivation
Spasticity No. = 3	3	3	2		1
Spasticity > Athetosis No. = 6	3	5	2	1	
Athetosis > Spasticity No. = 2	1	2	1	1	2
Athetosis No. = 2	2	2	1	2	1

For quantifying muscle tone we developed myotonography. This is the recording of muscular resistance to passive flexion and extension of an extremity by means of a special device. Electric activity of agonistic and antagonistic muscle groups is recorded simultaneously during motion.

In Figures 2 and 3, the curve and statistical evaluation in the case of a 10-year-old boy who suffers from a mixed spastic-athetoid-tetraplegia is demonstrated. On the left side the increased unstable muscular resistance is recorded during extension and flexion of the arm from 80 to 180°. Cerebellar surface stimulation with 30 cps leads to a stabilization of the curve, which approaches normal values. In correspondence with the reduced muscle tone, the EMG shows decreased amplitudes in the agonistic and antagonistic muscle groups. In the same case, the mean values of tonus maxima as well as the standard deviation are significantly lower during cerebellar stimulation.

Special interest was given to the pre- and postoperative recording of the silent period in the EMG. This is the cessation of electric activity induced by the electric stimulus of the tibial nerve during maximal voluntary innervation. In five of seven cases investigated, a significant prolongation of the silent period is apparent after stimulation. A single record of silent period with and without stimulation is shown in Fig. 4.

The mean value of 81 recordings in the same patient who experienced a marked muscular relaxation induced by stimulation shows an increase of the silent period from 90.8-125 ms as compared to preoperative values (Fig. 5). It is supposed that one of the factors generating the silent period is the cessation of afferent muscle spindle impulses. Thus, the prolonged silent period after cerebellar stimulation in cases with predominant spasticity may be interpreted as a suppression of muscle spindle excitability.

Summary

The date obtained by myotonography and silent period recordings correspond with our clinical impression that the stimulation-induced decrease of muscle tone mainly affects palsied patients with predominant spastic symptoms (Table 3).

Table 3. Number of improved patients by cerebellar stimulation (myotonography and EMG)

	Tonus No. = 13	Tonusvariation No. = 13	Silent period No. = 7
Spasticity No. = 3	3 (3)[a]	1 (3)	1 (1)
Spasticity Athetosis No. = 6	6 (6)	5 (6)	3 (4)
Athetosis Spasticity No. = 2	1 (2)	2 (2)	1 (1)
Athetosis No. = 2	1 (2)	2 (2)	(1)

a Numbers in brackets indicate patients investigated.

The beneficial effect on athetosis consists in a stabilization of varying muscle tone and suppression of hyperkinetic movements. In spite of the small number of patients, we believe that chronic cerebellar stimulation is a valid method for treating spasticity and dyskinesia in cerebral palsy. Even if the changes are not dramatic, improved control of posture and of purposeful movements means a facilitated performance of daily activities in the restrained patients.

References

1. COOPER, J.S., CRIGHEL, E., AMIN, I.: Clinical and physiological effects of stimulation of the paleocerebellum in humans. J. Am. Geriatr. Soc. 21, 40-43 (1973)
2. COOPER, J.S., RIKLAN, M., SNIDER, R.S.: The cerebellum, epilepsy and behavior. New York: Plenum Press 1974
3. COOPER, J.S., RIKLAN, M., AMIN, I., WALTZ, J.M., CULLINAN, T.: Chronic cerebellar stimulation in cerebral palsy. Neurology (Minneap.) 26, 744-753 (1976)
4. COOPER, J.S.: Cerebellar stimulation in man. New York: Raven press 1978

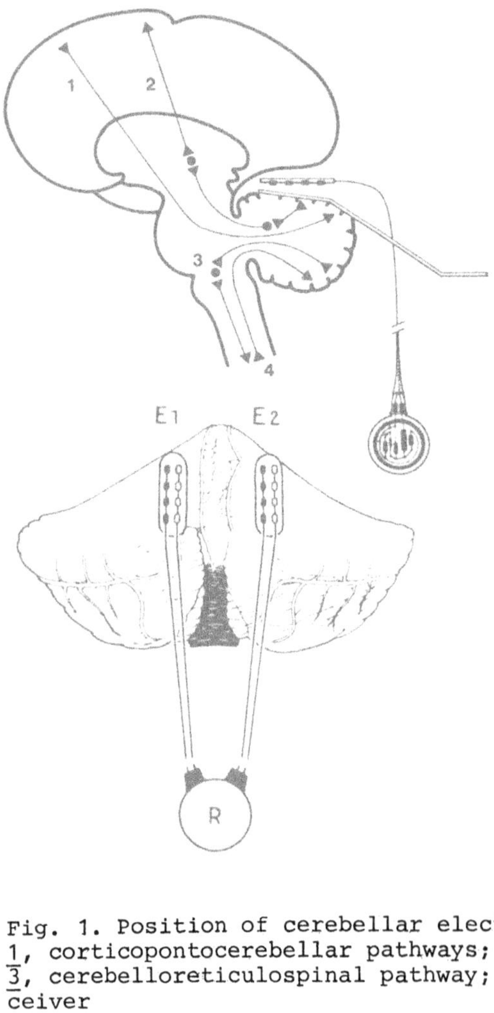

Fig. 1. Position of cerebellar electrodes
1, corticopontocerebellar pathways; 2, dentatothalamocortical pathway; 3, cerebelloreticulospinal pathway; 4, spinocerebellar pathway; R receiver

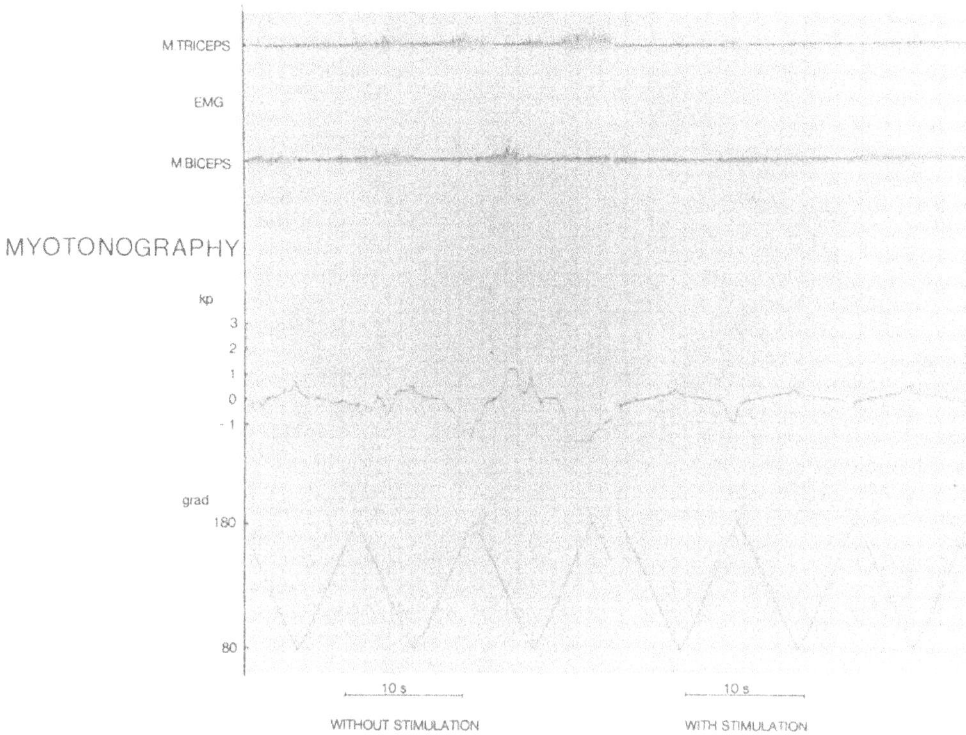

Fig. 2. Myotonogram prior to *(left side)* and after *(right side)* stimulation. Both *upper tracings* show the EMG. *Middle tracing*, muscular resistance to distension in kilopond times centimeters (torque). *Lower tracing*, course of passive distension and flexion in the elbow

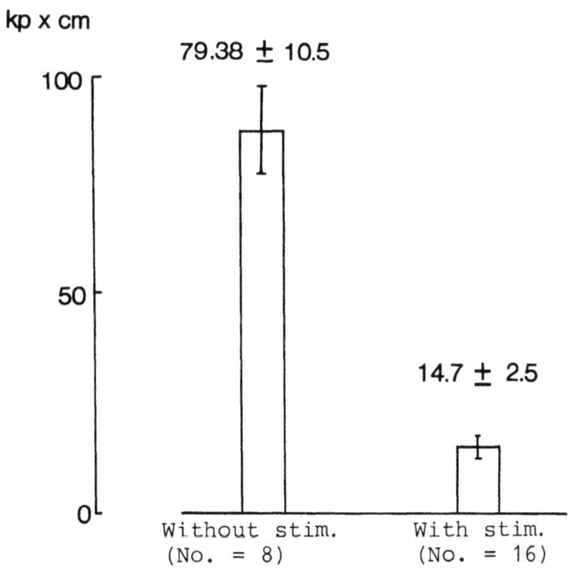

Fig. 3. Myotonography with and without stimulation (C.K. 291 167).
No. = number of recordings

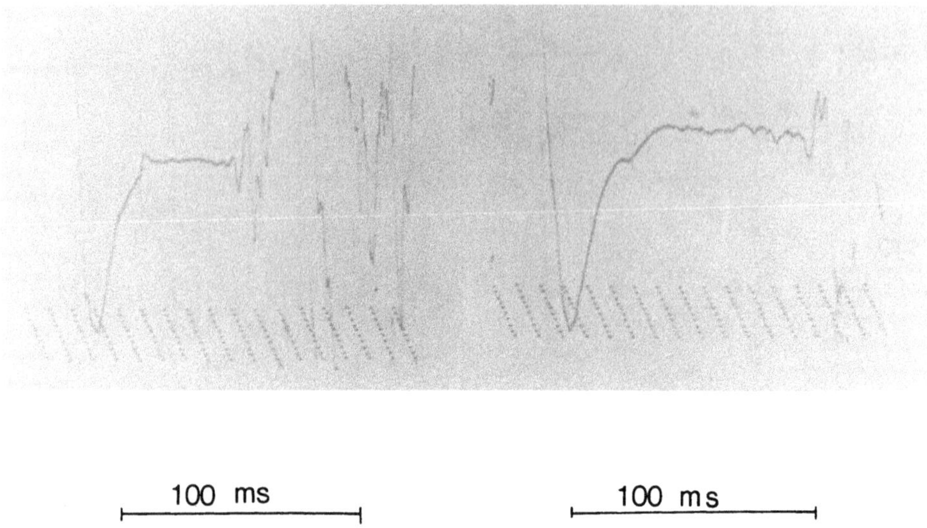

Fig. 4. Single shock to n. tibialis during maximal innervation. Recording with surface electrodes over m. gastrocnemius. Silent period. *Left:* without stimulation; *right:* with stimulation

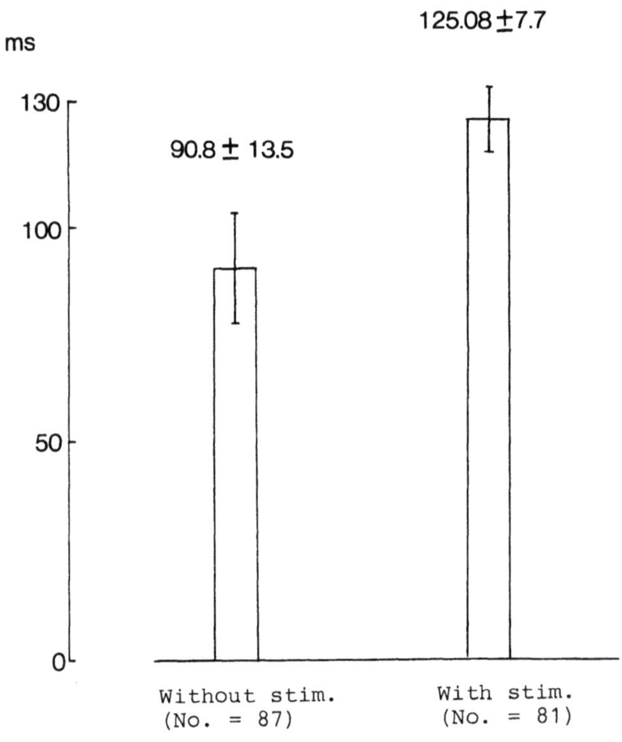

Fig. 5. Silent period with and without stimulation (C.K. 291 167). No. = number of recordings

Quantitative Measurement of Parkinsonian Tremor Before and After Stereotactic Operation

F. BRANDT and F. OPPEL

The quantification of tremor parameters is of considerable importance for the evaluation of the therapeutic effects of stereotactic operations. A new method of data processing is presented here together with the results of its application on parkinsonian tremor.

Materials and Methods

The finger tremor of five Parkinsonian patients was recorded before and immediately after stereotactic operation. All the patients had a marked resting and postural tremor, which resisted pharmalogic treatment. The operations were performed at the Neurosurgical Clinic of the Klinikum Steglitz, Berlin. In all cases the zona incerta was reached by stereotactic technique and electrically coagulated. The same method of recording the tremor was tested on 17 other patients who had been operated on 1-9 years before. Five other patients, who had previously been operated on were medicated with BUDIPIN[1], a presumptive dopamine liberator. Figure 1 illustrates the process of recording and data processing. The tremor was recorded by a piezoelectric transducer, which was positioned between the thumb and index fingers of the patients. The tremor signals were amplified by an EEG amplifier and then recorded on magnetic tape. For the evaluation of the frequencies of the tremor signals, we used the EEG interval spectrum analysis device (EISA). This instrument digitizes the intervals of oscillations and plots them oscillographically at corresponding points on the abscissas. The measured frequencies ranged from 1-30 cps. The total measuring time of 100 s was drawn on the ordinates. A pattern of calibrated lines was laid over the photographed EISA-grams, and thus the denset accumulation of points within a certain frequency range could easily be determined. For the amplitude analysis, a cumulative distribution curve was constructed by an analogue digital computer with a signal averager. As special modules, we used a pulse-height analyzer and a histogram-signal shaper. The amplitude range of 1-1800 mV corresponds to a mechanical amplitude range of 0.5-10 mm. The ordinate values represent the cumulative frequencies of the amplitudes. They have been evaluated at two fixed points on the abscissas: first at 400 mV, which was representative for the low-amplitude range and second at 1600 mV for the high-amplitude range. The proportion of high tremor amplitudes relative to low amplitudes was expressed by $\frac{\underline{N}_{1600}}{\underline{N}_{400}} - 1$. $\underline{N}$ are the cumulative frequencies of 400 and 1600 mV amplitudes. A flat ascent between 400 and 1600 mV together with a high 400-mV value was an indication of a clinical tremor improvement. In healthy persons this quotient converges to 0.

---

1 1-tert-butyl-4,4-di-phenyl-piperidine-hydrochloride, Byk-Gulden, Konstanz.

Results

As a result of stereotactic operation, the proportion of low tremor frequencies decreased, and the peak of the spectrum and the mean shifted to a higher value. Figures 2 and 3 illustrate this effect with the original record of a single exemplary case above the corresponding diagrams of the absolute number of counted points within a distance of 5 mm below. The tremor frequency of the patients examined before stereotactic operation had a distinct maximum of density at 6-7 cps, which changed postoperatively into a 8-13 cps band. The postoperative increase in tremor rate is also clearly reflected in the average tremor rates in Table 1. The 17 patients examined 1-9 years postoperatively again showed low-frequency tremor and had worsened in their clinical symptoms in ten cases.

Table 1. Influence of stereotaxic operation and Budipin medication on mean and peak values of tremor rate

Frequency Time	Maximum	Average
Before operation	6 - 7 cps	8 cps
Immediately after operation	8 -13 cps	15 cps
1 - 9 years after operation		12 cps
Under medication of Budipin + stereotaxic operation		
Before medication		8.7 cps
After medication (1-3 x 10 mg/day)		9.9 cps

The comparison of immediate and long-term postoperative results shows a reduction of the therapeutic effects with time. With the administration of Budipin, a moderate acceleration of tremor rate was obtained (see Table 1). The parameter, which expresses most directly the clinical state, is naturally the tremor amplitude. The sometimes drastic postoperative clinical improvement is reflected by a marked decrease of the high amplitude proportion of the amplitude distribution (Fig. 5). It is also illustrated by the shape of the cumulative amplitude frequency distribution in Fig. 4, which postoperatively - like a normal physiologic tremor - forms a plateau at a relatively low amplitude. The tendency to normalization is also expressed by a numeric value, a quotient, which relates the proportions of high and low amplitudes of the distribution. It was reduced from 1.6 before the operation to 0.27 immediately afterward. After 1-9 years the mean quotient was 0.66. The reduction of high-tremor amplitudes pharmacologically was documented by the depression of the quotient from 0.8 to 0.4.

Discussion

The method of tremor frequency analysis by means of the EISA device was first presented by OPPEL and UMBACH in 1977. The management of this apparatus is fairly easy, and we also found the EISA (TÖNNIES 1969) a useful technical instrument for quick clinical orientation and documentation of the operative effect. Our results demonstrate that after stereotactic subthalamotomy a marked increase in the rate of parkinsonian tremor together with a significant diminution of tremor amplitudes as correlates of clinical improvement can be observed. The long-term deterioration of the good immediate postoperative results may reflect the progressive nature of the underlying degenerative process. Our data are compatible with the two component hypotheses of parkinsonian tremor as proposed by LANCE in 1970, who postulates that parkinsonian tremor is constituted by a low-frequency resting tremor and a high-frequency action tremor component. The latter type of tremor, which can be seen in about 60% of all parkinsonian patients, represents exaggerated physiologic tremor (LANCE 1963). Stereotactic subthalamotomy would thus predominantly affect the low-frequency/high-amplitude resting tremor component. According to DIETZ et al. (1976), the observed decrease of tremor amplitude is a mere consequence of the increased tremor rate. These authors have convincingly shown that tremor is the envelope of the periodic contractions of single motor units with the lowest discharge rates.

Summary

A new way of recording Parkinsonian tremor under practicable clinical conditions has been developed. The tremor movements were recorded by a piezoelectric transducer and then analyzed as regards their frequency and amplitude. For the frequency-analysis the EEG-interval-spectrum-analyser (EISA)-device was used. For the amplitude-analysis an analogue-digital-cumputer with a signal averager constructed cumulative distribution curves by means of a histogram-shaping module. The new method was successfully applied for measurements before and after stereotaxic operations and for postoperative follow-up studies. The aid of additional pharmacological therapy has been examined.

References

1. DIETZ, V., FREUND, H.J., ALLUM, J.H.J.: Parkinsonian tremor during rest and voluntary contraction and its correlation with single motor unit activity. In: Advances in Parkinsonism. BIRKMAYER, W., HORNYKIEWICZ, O. (eds.). Basel: Editiones Roche 1976

2. LANCE, J.W.: A physiological approach to neurological disease. London: Butterworths 1970

3. LANCE, J.W., SCHWAB, R.S., PETERSON, E.A.: Action tremor and the cogwheel phenomenon in Parkinson's disease. Brain 86, 95-110 (1963)

4. OPPEL, F., UMBACH, W.U.: A quantitative measurement of tremor. Elekctroencephalogr. Clin. Neurophysiol. 43, 885-888 (1977)

5. TÖNNIES, J.F.: Automatische EEG-Intervall-Spectrumanalyse (EISA) zur Langzeitdarstellung der Schlafperiodik und Narkose. Arch. Psychiatr. Nervenkr. 212, 423-445 (1969)

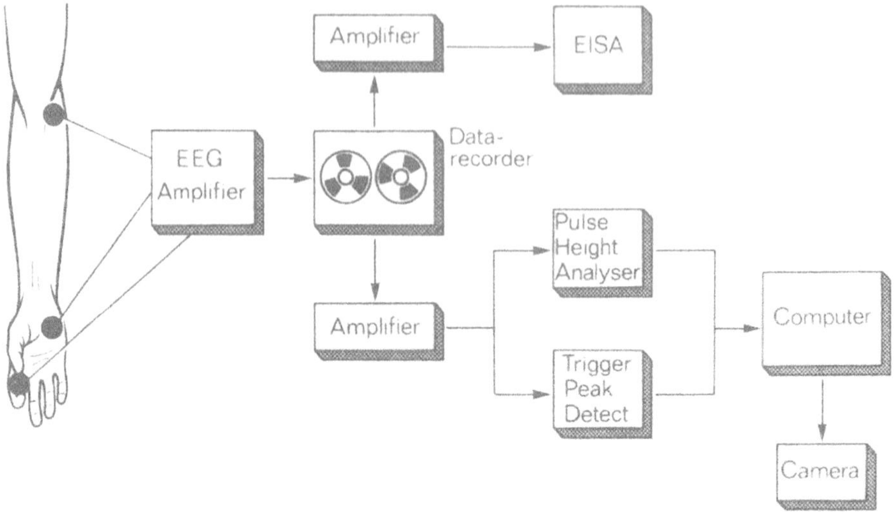

Fig. 1. Recording and data processing system

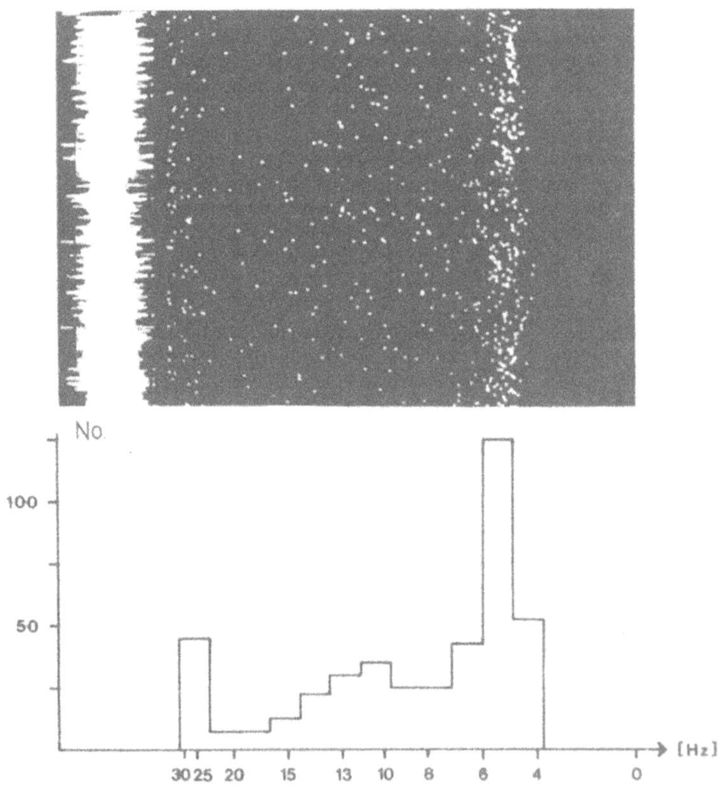

Fig. 2. Frequency distribution of parkinsonian tremor before subthalamotomy. *Upper half*, original records of EISA spectograms; *abscissa*, tremor frequency increasing from right to left; ordinate, recording time. Each *dot* represents the frequency component of a tremor beat recorded at the corresponding time. *Lower half*, frequency spectrum of the absolute number of counted dots within a distance of 5 mm

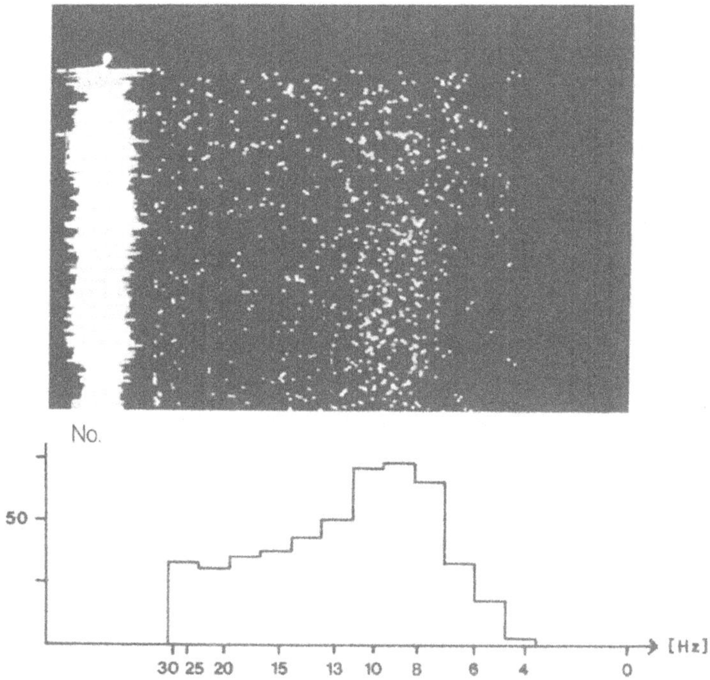

Fig. 3. Postoperative control. The area of highest dot concentration has shifted into a higher frequency range

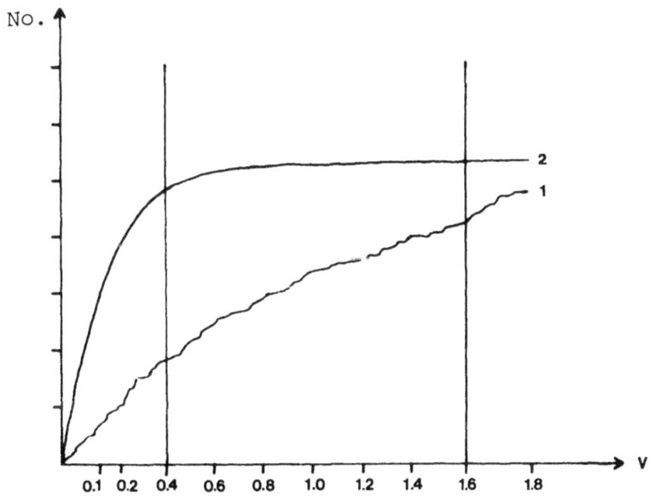

Fig. 4. Cumulative frequency distribution of parkinsonian tremor amplitude before (1) and after (2) stereotactic operation. As with normal physiologic tremor, plateau is reached at a low amplitude after operation

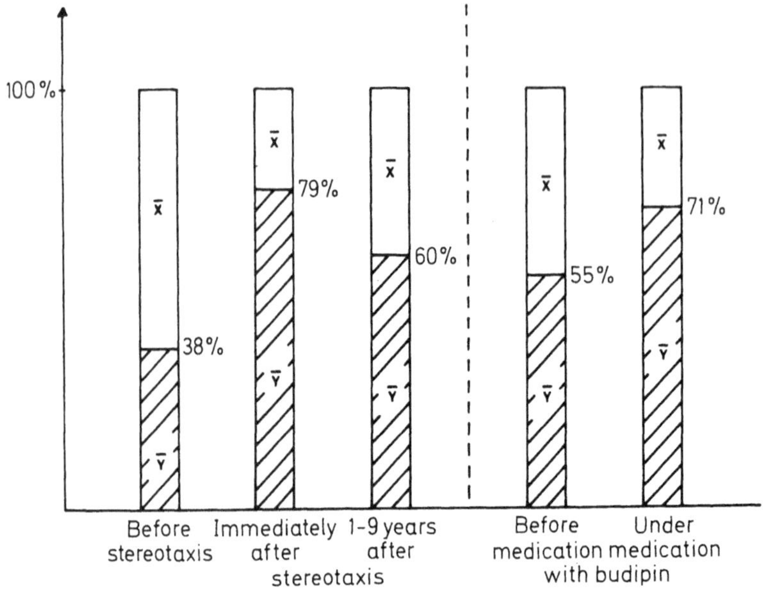

Fig. 5. Proportion of low ($\bar{x}$) and high ($\bar{y}$) amplitudes of parkinsonian tremor

Motor Control Analysis During Stereoencephalotomy [1]

A. STRUPPLER, F. ERBEL, H. ALTMANN, C. H. LÜCKING, and F. VELHO

Stereotactic interventions for the treatment of hyperkinesias give us to opportunity to investigate motor control in awake human subjects (STRUPPLER et al. 1977). In contrast to clinical lesions, such as stroke or head injury, the localization of the lesion can be precisely determined. Furthermore, we gain information by recording from, as well as by stimulating at, the target point prior to the destruction.

Table 1. Clinical findings following thalamotomy (VL) and subthalamotomy

Rigor		↓
Tremor	Resting	
	Postural	↓
	Intentional	
Tonic stretch reflexes		↓
Postural tone		↓
Load compensation		↓
Phasic stretch reflexes		=
Maximal force		=

The clinical findings following subthalamic and thalamic lesions for the treatment of different kinds of tremor are seen in Table 1. Abolition of tremor seems to be correlated to hypotonia. One can speculate that there may be a common mechanism underlying the clinical symptoms, tremor, and muscle tone. Therefore, we investigated the changes in motor control following the lesions in patients suffering from hemiparkinsonism during various motor performances. The motor tasks, such as holding or moving, were modified by proprioceptive stimuli or command. The goal was to analyze and distinguish between more reflex-evoked automatic motor effects and supraspinal or transcortical (long latency) responses. Two torque motors, electrically coupled in series, were used to deliver constant torques between 0.5 and 6 Nm (Newton meter) to both forearms in either flexion or extension. An additional torque disturbance could be added in either direction, providing stretching or unloading. An electromyogram (EMG) was recorded from the brachialis and triceps muscles on both sides using wire electrodes; the potentials were rectified and averaged. Angular displacement (mechanogram) in the elbow joints were registered simultaneously (Fig. 1).

1 Supported by Deutsche Forschungsgemeinschaft (SFB 50 Kybernetik).

During load compensation of an external force in normal subjects, three early EMG components can be distinguished (1,2). The first two peaks appear after a latency of 30 ms, which is comparable to the latency of the phasic muscle stretch reflex. It is followed by a second peak at approximately 60 ms. This latency is definitely briefer than the minimal reaction time to kinesthetic stimuli (about 85 ms). A third peak appears at about 90-110 ms. This latency lies partially within the time period for the shortest reaction (Fig. 2).

Following lesions there is a remarkable switching from reflex-compensated motor responses to more governed responses (Fig. 3).

Since muscle tone is dependent upon the sensitivity of muscle spindles, which are innervated by γ-motoneurons, we investigated the α-γ-coactivation by microneurographic recordings as described by VALLBO and HAGBARTH (4).

Figure 4 shows the discharge characteristics of a muscle spindle afferent in the median nerve. The phasic discharge during passive increase of muscle length (Fig. 4d) is typical for primary muscle spindle afferents in contrast to secondary muscle spindle afferents. The discharge during the relaxation phase following twitch contraction permits discrimination of this afferent fiber from Ib afferents, originating from Golgi tendon organs.

Figure 5 gives an example of how muscle spindles can be activated by subthreshold repetitive stimulation at the target point. During thalamic stimulation with a frequency of 30/s (Fig. 5b), the spindle discharges either twice of three times following the twitch contraction in contrast to the control in Fig. 5a.

The sensitivity of the muscle spindle was increased by intracerebral stimulation at the very point where stimulation enhanced tremor and destruction abolished it. The role of the gamma system needs to be further studied. The following conclusion may be drawn: stereotactic lesions change motor control; external disturbances are compensated mainly by volition and less by reflex.

References

1. HAMMOND, P.H.: The influence of prior instruction to the subject as an apparently involuntary neuro-muscular response. J. Physiol. (Lond.) 132, 17-18 (1956)

2. MARSDEN, C.H., MERTEN, P.A., MORTON, H.B.: Servo action in human voluntary movements. Nature 238, 140-143 (1972)

3. STRUPPLER, A., GERILOWSKY, L., VELHO, F., ERBEL, F., ALTMANN, H.: Mode of innervation following stereoencephalotomy. (In press)

4. VALLBO, A.B., HAGBARTH, K.E.: Impulses recorded with microelectrodes in human muscle nerves during stimulation of mechanoreceptors and voluntary contractions. Electroencephalogr. Clin. Neurophysiol. 23, 392 (1967)

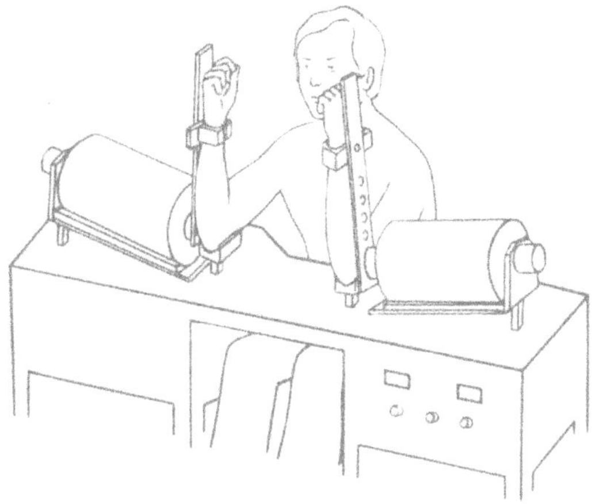

Fig. 1. Torque motors applying extension or flexion at both elbow joints simultaneously. Initial torque: 2-6 Nm; Disturbance torque: 4-14 Nm; EMG: brachial m. + triceps m; Muscle spindle afferents recording in musculocutaneous nerve; Mechanogram of the elbow joint

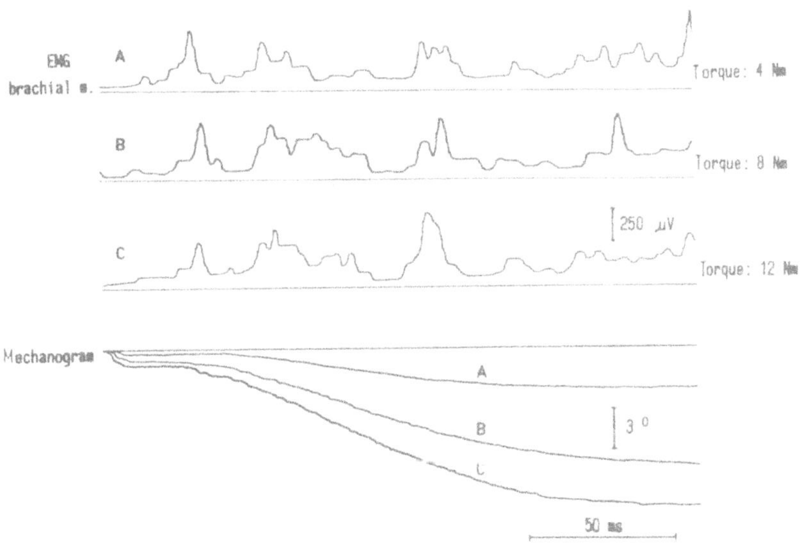

Fig. 2A-C. Load compensation of a torque-induced disturbance in an isometrically contracted muscle of a normal subject. Rectified and averaged EMG activity (No. = 16) during three different disturbance torques (identical initial torque of 4 Nm; A, B, and C). Corresponding mechanograms are superimposed *below*

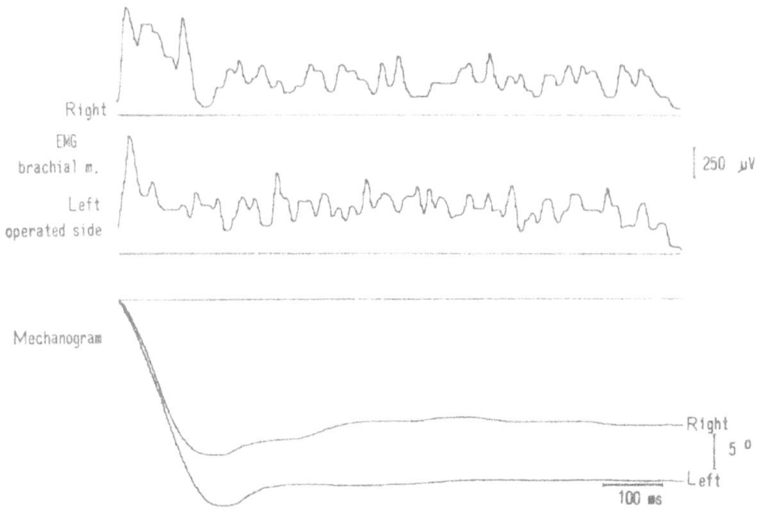

Fig. 3. Load compensation of a torque-induced disturbance in an isometrically contracted muscle. Patient with hemiparkinsonism, following stereoencephalotomy. Disturbance torque applied bilaterally simultaneously (8 Nm, initial torque 4 Nm) (see Fig. 2)

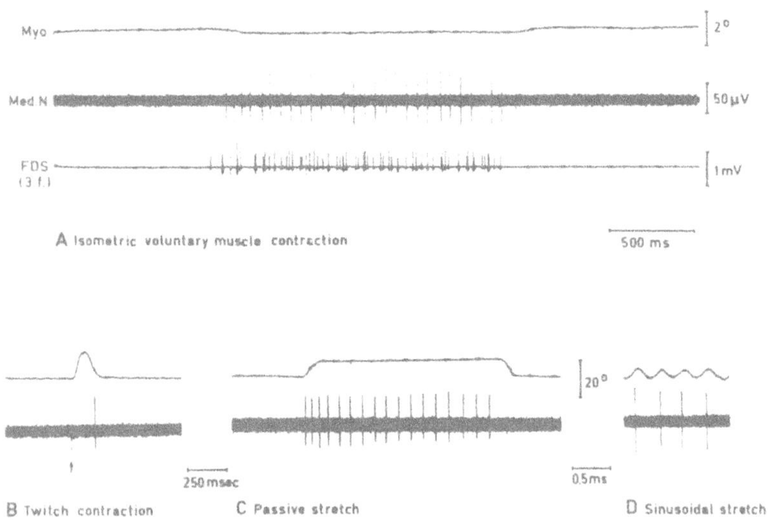

Fig. 4 A-D. Muscle spindle afferent identification scheme. A During voluntary contraction of the flexor digitorum superficialis, showing α-γ-coactivation; B in the relaxation phase of a twitch contraction (*arrow* indicates stimulus artifact); C during passive stretch; D during sinasoidal stretch of the same muscle

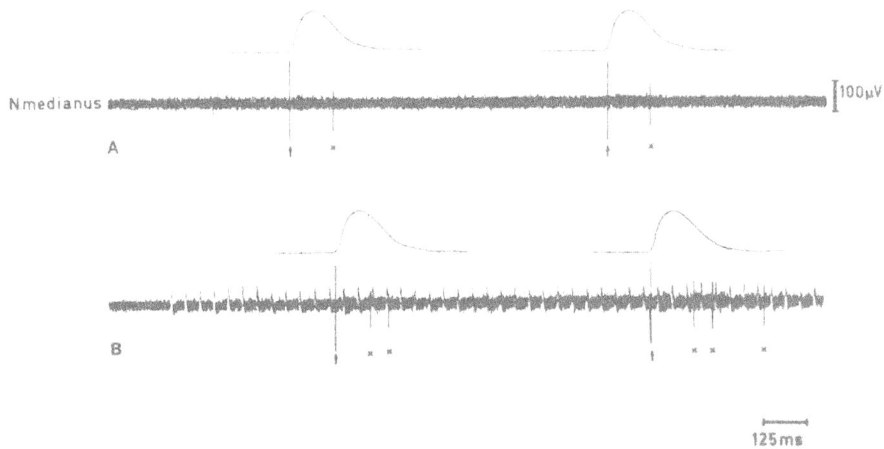

Fig. 5 A,B. Effect of thalamic stimulation (B) on muscle spindle discharge elicited by twitch contraction. A Mechanical muscle twitch; B primary muscle spindle afferent in the contralateral median nerve (*arrows* indicate nerve stimulus artifacts, *crosses* spindle discharges)

Chronic Hyperpathia: an Experimental Animal Model

B. S. NASHOLD, JR., D. ALBE-FESSARD, and M. CH. LOMBARD

After traumatic root avulsion of the brachial plexus, a patient may suffer from intractable hyperpathia in the deafferentated limb. The neurophysiologic basis of this type of chronic central pain has been explained as due to a lack of inhibition of central synapses caused by the deafferentation or the development of hypersensitization of central synapses forming a quasi-epileptic focus. To duplicate the pain syndrome of brachial plexus avulsion in an animal, we have performed unilateral dorsal root avulsions and surgical sections of mulitple cervical dorsal roots in a group of rats and studied the evolution of their abnormal behavior related to the deafferentation (Fig. 1).

The exact details of the experimental techniques have already been reported, and only the experimental results are emphasized here (1,4). The animals were observed for periods up to 1 year, and in one group of deafferentated rats microrecordings were made in the thalamus after they had developed the abnormal behavior resulting from deafferentation (5). Sham surgical operations were carried out in a control group of animals for comparison.

Results

Most of the animals with multiple dorsal cervical root lesions (avulsion or surgical section) developed hypersensitivity in the area of skin closely adjacent to the zone of the deafferentation. In some rats, the area of hypersensitive skin extended across the body into the contralateral intact upper limb; the hypersensitive zone was designated as the "mirror" dermatomes in contrast to the denervated dermatomes. The hyperalgesic reaction appeared between 3 and 10 days postoperatively, which is comparable in time to the appearance of the pain after a brachial plexus avulsion in man. The lightest touching of the animal's skin in the hypersensitive area elicited vocalization and a withdrawal response lasting many months after surgery. The animals with five cervical roots sectioned or avulsed exhibited the most intense hypersensitivity to cutaneous stimulation as compared to those animals with only four cervical roots sectioned. The onset of the syndrome appeared earlier after root sections than after an avulsion injury. When the hypersensitive skin reaction appeared, the animals began scratching the skin both ipsilaterally and contralaterally to the injury (Fig. 2). After a delay of many days, the scratching behavior caused skin wounds, usually on the ipsilateral side and occasionally on the contralateral side, which healed spontaneously only to reappear. At a later time, the animals mutilated their limb, but the area of mutilation was confined to the area of total denervation (digit of the upper limb) (Fig. 2).

The thalamic recordings were made in rats exhibiting skin hypersensitivity, scratching, and biting behavior from 27-493 days postoperatively (5). Rats with four cervicodorsal roots sectioned showed only normal thalamic electric activity, while those animals with five roots sectioned exhibited abnormal spiking thalamic activity at a rate of 10 Hz, which originated from the sensory thalamus (VP) 6 months postoperatively (Fig. 3). The abnormal thalamic activity consisted of bursts of spikes followed by a positive slow wave with a 10-ms period of silence before the next 10-Hz burst (Fig. 4). Bursting thalamic activities were recorded from the ipsilateral and contralateral thalamus. No thalamic bursting activity was ever seen in the control group of animals.

Conclusions

Our observations in chronic rats are similar to those of other authors who have produced the hyperalgesic syndrome with bilateral nerve root sections. Our report is the first where a clinical syndrome as observed in man with traumatic avulsion of the brachial plexus was reproduced in animals resulting in a hyperalgesic syndrome. BLACK noticed cutaneous hypersensitivity with skin scratching in the zone of the fifth nerve of the cat after producing an experimental epileptic focus in the brain stem (2). LOESER and WARD have recorded abnormal electric activity from the spinal cord of man and in cats after spinal cord trauma and dorsal root section (3,6). The discovery of the spontaneous thalamic spiking in the thalamus of the denervated rats is a new observation, and its relationship to the hyperalgesic syndrome needs further study. Chronic hypersensitivity can result in animals after unilateral deafferentation and may mimic the pain syndrome seen in similar circumstances in man. Neurophysiologists are now developing experimental models that can be studied in detail and may give us clues as to the origins of central pain in man and hopes for therapeutic relief.

References

1. ALBE-FESSARD, D., NASHOLD, B.S., Jr., LOMBARD, M.C., YAMAGUCHI, Y., BOREAU, F.: Rat after dorsal rhizotomy. A possible animal model for chronic pain (in press)
2. BLACK, R.G.: Trigeminal pain. In: Pain and suffering. CRUE, B.L. (ed.), pp. 119-137. Springfield, Ill.: Thomas 1970
3. LOESER, J.D., WARD, A.A., Jr.: Some effects of deafferentation on neurons of the cat spinal cord. Arch. Neurol. 17, 629-636 (1967)
4. LOMBARD, M.C., NASHOLD, B.S., Jr., ALBE-FESSARD, D.: Deafferentation hypersensitivity in the rat after dorsal root rhizotomy: A possible animal model of chronic pain (in press)
5. LOMBARD, M.C., NASHOLD, B.S., Jr., PELLISIER, T.: Thalamic recordings in rats with hyperalgesia (in press)
6. WARD, A.A., Jr.: Mechanisms of neuronal hyperexcitability. EEG, Suppl. 3 (1972)

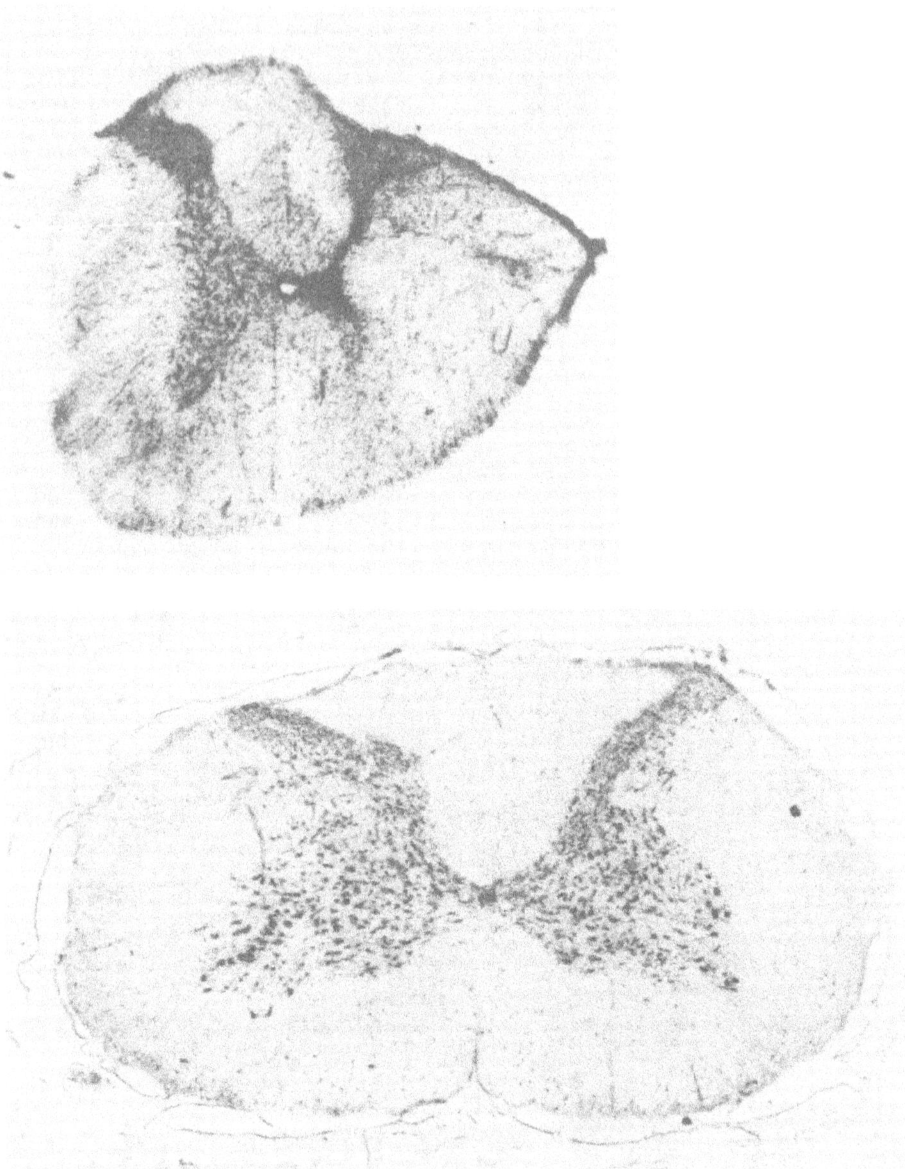

Fig. 1. Cross section of rat spinal cord. Effects of avulsion of dorsal rootlets *(above)* and postdorsal root section *(below)*

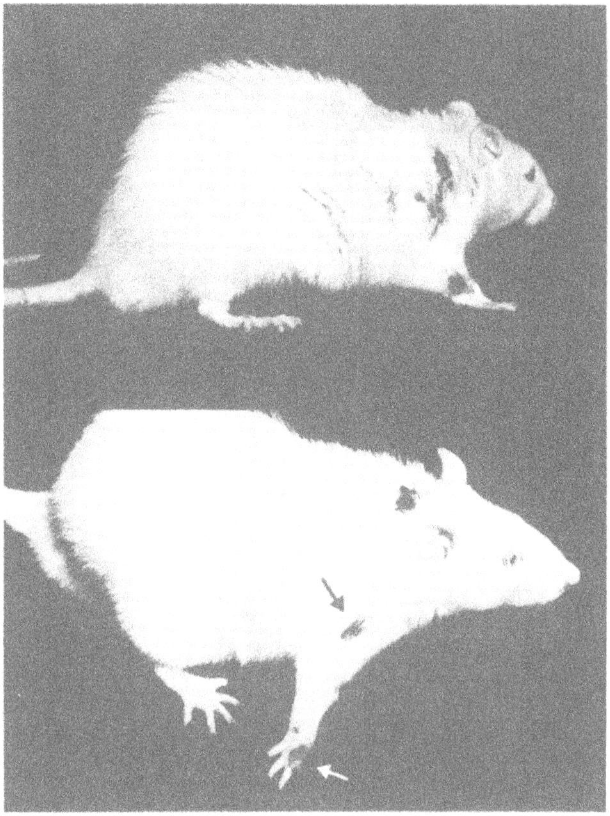

Fig. 2. Skin lesions following deafferentation

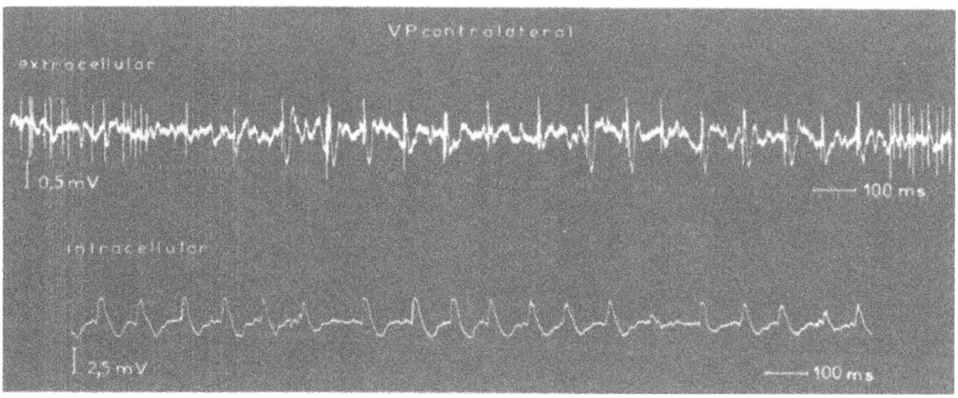

Fig. 3. Abnormal thalamic spiking following deafferentation. VP, sensory thalamus

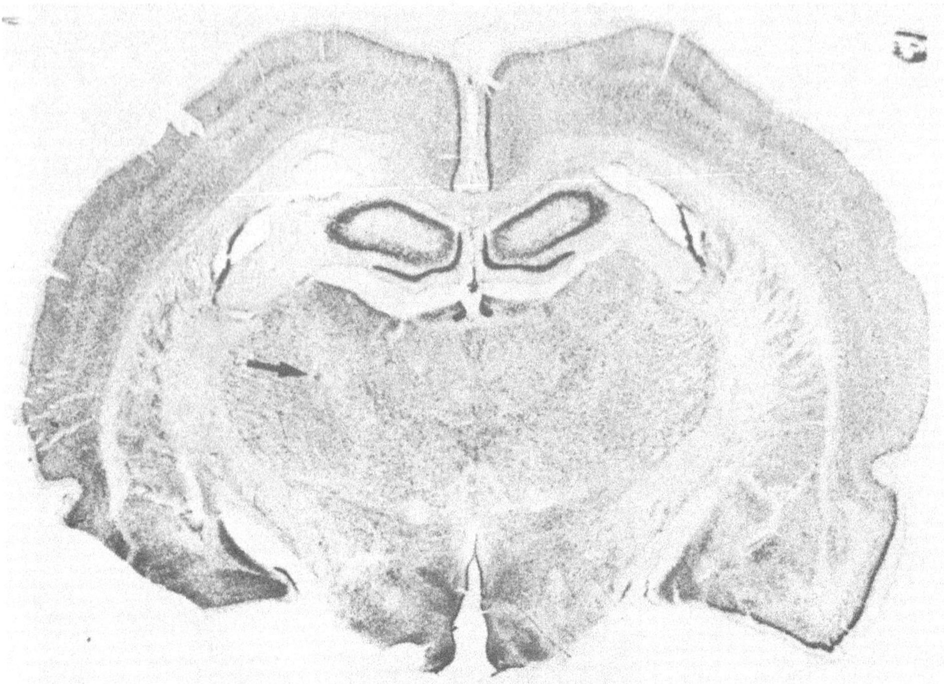

Fig. 4. Cross section of thalamus. *Arrow* indicates region in VP where abnormal spiking neurons were recorded

Electric Stimulation of the Brain: a Search for Safe Stimulus Protocols

R. H. PUDENZ, W. F. AGNEW, T. G. H. YUEN, L. A. BULLARA, S. JACQUES, and C. H. SHELDEN

Introduction

In 1968 BRINDLEY and LEWIN reported their implantation of an 80-electrode array activated by radiofrequency transmission on the visual cortex of a blind nurse (3). The pattern of phosphenes seen by this patient when the electrodes were stimulated suggested that technical refinements of this technique might enable blind persons to not only move about in their environments but even to read.

This exciting report led the National Institute of Neurological and Communicative Disorders and Stroke to initiate a series of investigations on the feasibility of developing a visual prosthesis. Investigators at many university and independent research centers were recruited to participate in these studies. Subsequently, these investigations were broadened to include investigations of functional electric stimulation of the cerebellum, spinal cord, spinal nerve roots, and peripheral nerves.

In 1970 our neurosciences research laboratories in Pasadena became involved in this program. The goal of our studies has been to find techniques for chronic stimulation of the brain that would not injure neurons or other tissue elements underlying the electrodes.

Material and Approach

Up to the present time we have carried out approximately 600 acute and chronic stimulations of the cerebral cortex of cats. In these studies we have evaluated electrode materials in various sizes, shapes, and configurations and have designed numerous electrode arrays and a large number of stimulus protocols. In these latter protocols, we have varied current amplitude, wave form, pulse duration, frequency and polarity, as well as the charge per phase, charge density, current density, and total charge. Histologic changes at the stimulated and control electrode sites have been observed with both light and electron microscopy. Preliminary pH measurements have been made in acute experiments. Observations of circulatory changes at stimulated electrode sites have been made both with the surgical microscope and with specialized apparatus available in the microcirculation laboratories of the California Institute of Technology. Observations in many of these studies have been published previously (1,7). In this report we wish to present briefly some of the highlights.

Results

Electrodes. Platinum and rhodium have proved to be the most satisfactory metallic electrode materials. Histologic changes have been similar beneath the stimulated and control electrodes fabricated from these metals. Capacitor electrodes fabricated from tantalum pentoxide show considerable promise but require further refinement and study. These electrodes are allegedly self-cleansing and do not pass electrons or cause oxidation-reduction reactions.

Blood-Brain Barrier (BBB) Effects. The effects of electric stimulation on the BBB have been evaluated in both acute and chronic experiments using Evans blue as the intravital dye marker (6). We agree with MORTIMER and his associates (5) that extravasation of the dye into the neuropil during stimulation is an index of impending neural damage. This observation, however, is valid only in the acute stimulations because it has been shown that the BBB will be restored in 1 month even in the presence of extensive neural damage.

Electrode Arrays. It has been observed that silicone rubber sheeting on which electrodes are mounted may migrate into the underlying brain and actually become embedded. We have solved this problem by using Dacron mesh, which causes only minimal cortical compression and tends to maintain its position even though it has been implanted for weeks and months.

Current Wave form. It is essential that the charges in each half wave of the stimulating pulse be balanced as completely as possible if neural damage is to be minimized or avoided. It is problematic whether this can be easily achieved with either symmetric biphasic wave forms or with capacitively coupled monophasic wave forms. Direct-coupled monophasic wave forms are extremely destructive of neural tissue and blood vessels and should never be used.

Effect of Charge. In our search for safe stimulus protocols, we have varied the charge per phase, charge, and current density and the total charge delivered. We have also evaluated continuous and intermittent stimulation and varying pulse durations and train lengths.

In our neural damage model studies reported in 1975, we stated that the charge per phase should not exceed 0.45 μC if continuous stimulation is used. Studies in progress in our laboratories suggest that total charge density might be a better criterion in designing a stimulus protocol.

BROWN and his colleagues at the University of California at Los Angeles have reported that stimulation of the monkey cerebellum for 205 h with a charge of 0.5 μC/ph and an estimated charge density of 7.4 $\mu C/cm^2$/ph will not damage the cerebellar structures (4). This charge per phase is about five times threshold for evocation of cerebellar efferent activity.

Histopathology

Light Microscopy. Cortical lesions resulting from electric stimulation tend to have the shape of an inverted cone with the greatest damage in the superficial grey layers. In the most severe lesions, damage may extend beyond the edge of the electrode, and hemorrhage may occur in the underlying neuropil. Both light and electron microscopy have demonstrated that neurons and astrocytes are the most vulnerable cells, whereas oligodendrocytes and endothelial cells are least affected.

Neuronal damage is characterized in the early stages by vacuolization of the cytoplasm, which can extend to chromatolysis and disappearance of these cells in the more severe lesions. In the early stages of neural damage, astrocytes proliferate particularly in the molecular grey layer. However, in the presence of extensive injury, clasmatodendrosis and disappearance of these cells from the neuropil will be noted (Figs. 1 and 2).

The PAS stain for glycogen is particularly valuable in determining the site and extent of cortical injury. Under normal conditions, glycogen is essentially undetectable in the adult mammalian brain except in certain paraventricular structures, e.g., the area postrema. In damaged cortical areas, there is extensive deposition of glycogen granules in the neuropil. In the most severely damaged areas, free glycogen disappears creating the so-called PAS-negative zone.

Electron Microscopy. Changes observed in our ultrastructural studies include gliosis, mitochondrial swelling, lipid inclusions, degenerating cells, neuronal loss, and phagocytic activity (Fig. 3). A finding of particular interest to us has been the presence of dense crystalline inclusions preferentially located in the mitochondria of several cell types and in postsynaptic dendrites. These dense bodies have been identified as calcium hydroxyapatite by electron diffraction and energy dispersive X-ray analysis. A possible explanation of the mechanism of this calcium deposition is that increased cyclic AMP levels, which are known to occur with electric stimulation, cause increased plasmalemmal permeability (2).

Discussion

We are living in an era of neuroaugmentative surgery. Electronic devices activated by radiofrequency transmission are being implanted in various areas of the central and peripheral nervous systems to treat convulsive seizures, dyskinesias, pain, behavioral problems, the neurogenic bladder, and selected musculoskeletal disorders. Our knowledge of the physiologic and pathologic effects of stimulation as well as the optimum stimulation parameters is markedly deficient. It is obvious that much additional study is required before many of the residual problems will be solved.

References

1. AGNEW, W.F., YUEN, T.G.H., PUDENZ, R.H., BULLARA, L.A.: Electrical stimulation of the brain. IV. Ultrastructural studies. Surg. Neurol. 4, 438-448 (1975)
2. AGNEW, W.F., YUEN, T.G.H., BULLARA, L.A., JACQUES, D., PUDENZ, R.H.: Intracellular calcium deposition in brain following electrical stimulation. Neurol. Res. (in press)
3. BRINDLEY, G.S., LEWIN, W.S.: The sensation produced by electrical stimulation of the visual cortex. J. Physiol. 196, 479-493 (1968)
4. BROWN, W.F., BABB, T.L., SOPER, H.V., LIEB, J.P., OTTINO, C.A., CRANDALL, P.D.: Tissue reactions to long-term electrical stimulation of the cerebellum in monkeys. J. Neurosurg. 47, 366-379 (1977)

5. MORTIMER, J.T., SHEALY, C.N., WHEELER, C.: Experimental nondestructive stimulation of the brain and spinal cord. J. Neurosurg. 32, 553-559 (1970)

6. PUDENZ, R.H., BULLARA, L.A., DRU, D., TALLALA, A.: Electrical stimulation of the brain. II. Effects on the blood-brain barrier. Surg. Neurol. 4, 265-270 (1975)

7. PUDENZ, R.H., BULLARA, L.A., JACQUES, S., HAMBRECHT, F.T.: Electrical stimulation of the brain. III. The Neural Damage Model. Surg. Neurol. 4, 389-400 (1975)

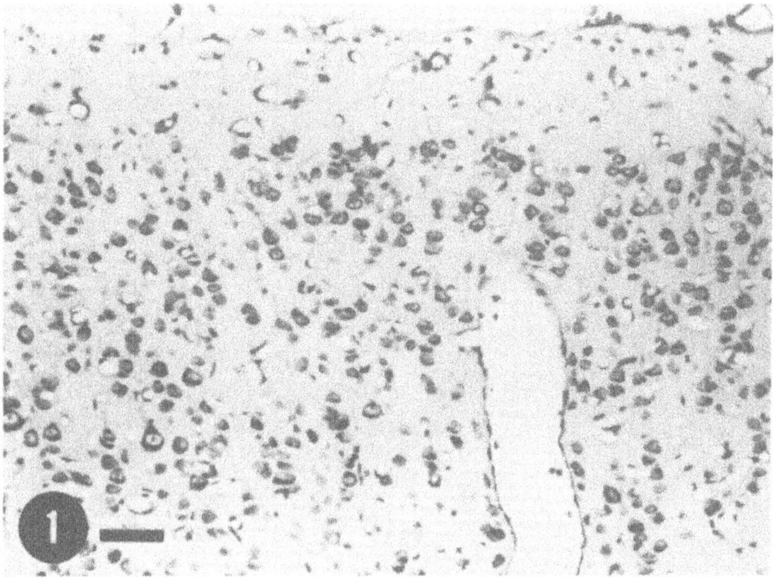

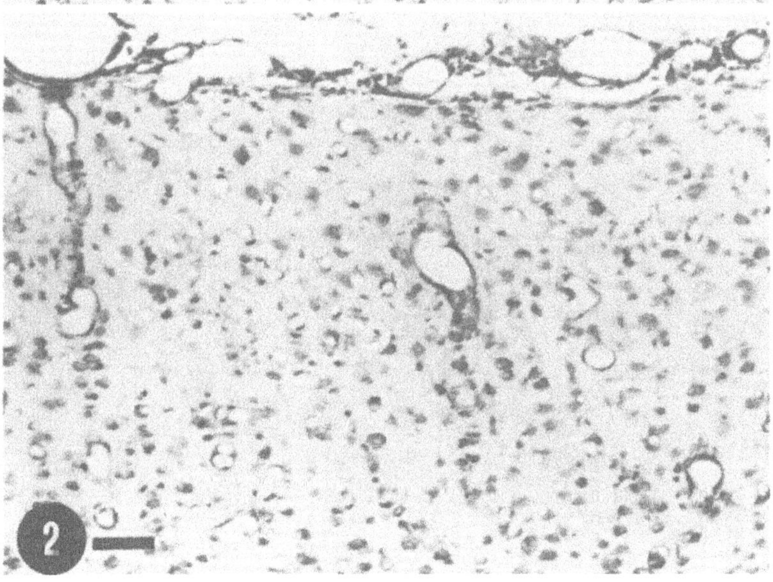

Fig. 1 *(above)*. Control cat parietal cortex immediately beneath an unstimulated 1.1-mm diameter platinum electrode showing normal molecular layer and cellular disposition. Nissl stain. *Bar* represents 50 μm

Fig. 2 *(below)*. Tissue beneath active alectrode of same animal as Fig. 1. Platinum electrode was stimulated continuously for 20 h using a charge density of 100 $\mu C/cm^2$/ph. Note extensive gliosis and loss of neurons in the superficial grey cortex. Nissl. stain. *Bar* represents 50 μm

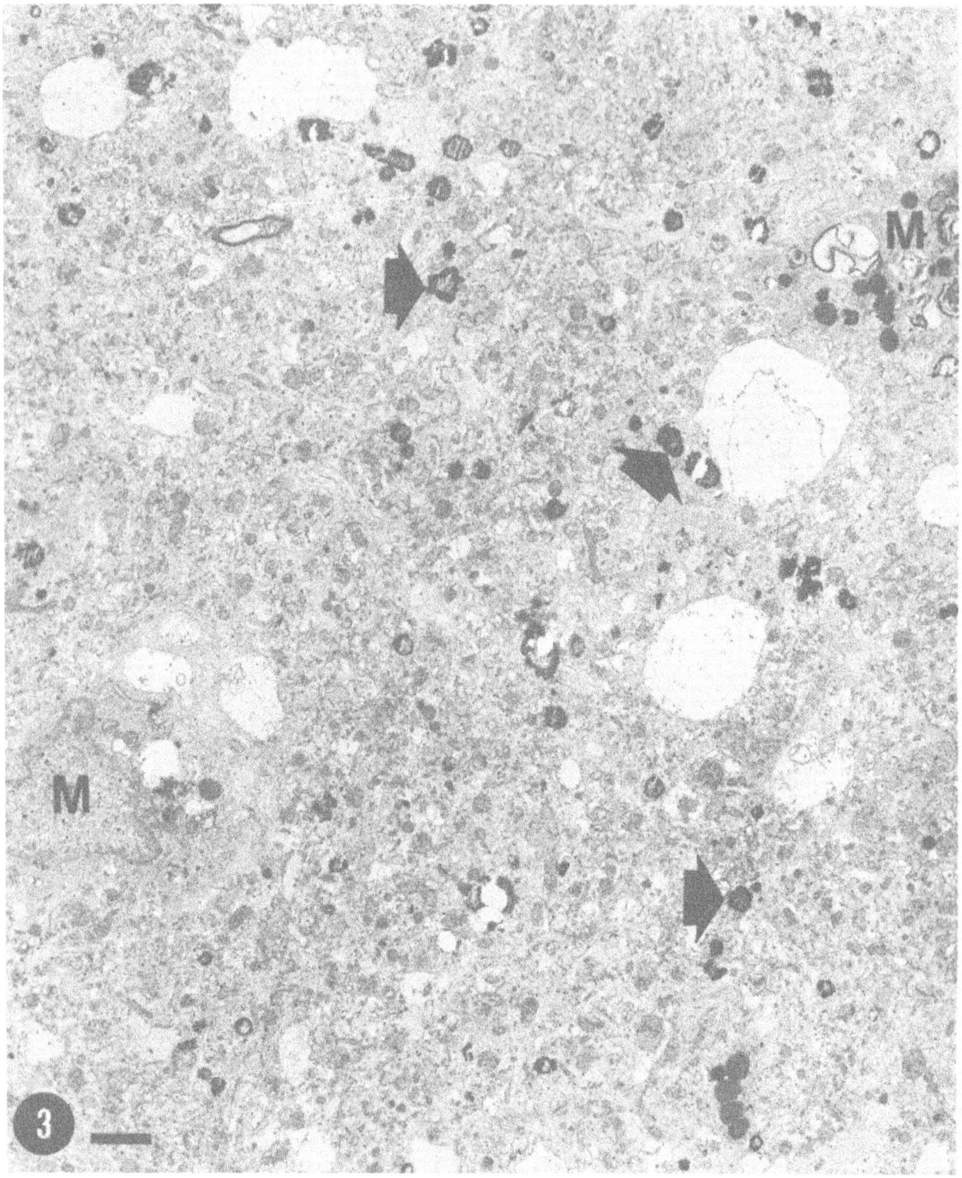

Fig. 3. Electron micrograph of the superficial cortex beneath a 1.1-mm diameter platinum electrode stimulated with a charge density of 100 μC/ cm^2/ph for 9 h/day for 4 days. Note numerous large vacuoles, abundant dense calcium hydroxyapatite crystals *(arrows)*, and debris-filled macrophages *(M)*. *Bar* represents 2 μm

"Otfrid Foerster Lecture"
Stimulation of the Posterior Columns of the Spinal Cord for the Suppression of Chronic Pain

W. H. SWEET

The gracious invitation to give the OTFRID FOERSTER lecture to this gathering gives me the opportunity to acknowledge a peculiarly significant personal debt to Professer FOERSTER. As a medical student in the early 1930s, I was aware of the decisive stimulus to WILDER PENFIELD of 6 months association with FOERSTER in 1928, which led PENFIELD to devote so much professional effort to epilepsy. I was impressed not only by this specific fact but also by the generalization that the medical world in the 1930s still turned for comprehensive documentation on any subject to the great German HANDBÜCHER. As a student at Oxford from 1932 to 1934 I was able to use about half of each year to work at the medical school in Würzburg, taking the German government examination in internal medicine at the close of that time. The experience led me to save enough money to buy the new edition of the giant 19 volume BUMKE-FOERSTER *Handbuch der Neurologie*, which appeared from 1935-1937. Many of the thousands of pages in the 18 principal volumes and the four supplementary volumes were written by FOERSTER himself. It remains for me a valuable storehouse of clinical observations.

However, my greatest debt to OTFRIED FOERSTER is directly related to the subject of this lecture. PATRICK WALL and I noted in 1966 that the threshold sensation on electric stimulation via needle electrodes into our own infra-orbital nerves was a tolerable tingling or buzzing sensation in the distribution of the nerve. During stimulation and for a brief interval thereafter, this same area was analgesic or hypalgesic to pinprick (47). Such an observation gave only meager support to the notion of electric stimulation for the suppression of pain. However, on the basis of his work in cats, PAT WALL thought that stimulation of large diameter afferent fibers might reduce pain (30). His studies showed that such stimuli caused a presynaptic depolarization reducing the excitatory effectiveness of afferent impulses on cells in the dorsal horn (46).

However, the impetus for me to pursue this approach lay in the clinical observations and most decisively the precisely recorded surgical experience of FOERSTER (43). In 1927 he drew attention to his own and other's observations that an isolated lesion of the posterior column of the cord often produced a severe hyperpathia of the skin or hairs - this while the nerve roots and all other parts of the grey and white matter of the cord were intact (15). Two of his own cases were the most convincing. In the first, his operation on an intramedullary tumor in the cervical and thoracic cord led him to sacrifice the posterior columns on both sides in the thoracic cord. There followed an intensive hyperpathia of the legs and abdomen on both sides. A second operation in this patient extended, in the right posterior column only, up to the C2 level. New hyperpathia ensued, now confined to the right side and extending up into the occipital hair, light stroking of which caused frightful paroxysms of pain. In his second patient with an intramedullary cyst, incision was made at C3-4 into the right funiculus gracilis of Goll. There resulted pronounced spontaneous unpleasant feelings and at times severe pain in the right leg and lower torso again corresponding well with the anatomic distribution of the severed pathway. Confirming these two dramatic surgical results by other clinical observations, FOERSTER concluded in 1936 (17):

The posterior column system exerts a moderating influence on the posterior horn - anterolateral column system. A stimulus to the body activates both systems in such fashion that in the rostral centers of the afferent systems excitation in the posterior horn and opposite anterolateral column is depressed by waves in the ipsilateral posterior column. The posterior column keeps the anterolateral column system in check, preventing both inordinately severe sensations of pain and any pain from non-noxious stimuli.

There it is in black and white in 1936, a superb example of prescient analysis of two surgical misadventures and the courage to record them to guide others, including me.

On another score, the documentation of recent years has been long anticipated by FABRITIUS and extensively cited and agreed to by FOERSTER. The existence in animals of a descending efferent pain-suppressing pathway in the posterolateral white matter of the cord has in the past 3 years become well established. Evidence for such a pathway in man was presented by the Finnish investigator FABRITIUS in a series of long papers in German between 1908 and 1912 (12,13). On the basis of a thorough analysis of 81 clinical cases, he correlated hyperesthesia with relatively abrupt involvement of the lateral corticospinal tract. If in an acute unilateral thoracic cord lesion the paralysis involved the hip joint either alone or as part of a more complete motor loss, hyperesthesia was likely to appear and to be due to involvement in the vicinity of the most posterior parts of the lateral corticospinal tract. FOERSTER (1936, 16), citing FABRITIUS, agreed that a portion of the ipsilateral hyperesthesia after a hemisection of the cord was due to the destruction of the posterolateral white matter.

To move now a little nearer to the present day, the important work of COLLINS, NULSEN and RANDT (9) had shown that awake patients experience pain only when small myelinated A-delta or unmyelinated C fibers are activated. This concept substantiating in man much previous work in animals has since received ample confirmation in other human observations. NOORDENBOS and WEDDELL found that in the intercostal nerves of patients with postherpetic neuralgia the absolute numbers of nonmedullated fibers increased and of large medullated fibers decreased as compared with normal nerves. This led NOORDENBOS to suggest an inhibitory role for the large diameter afferent fibers (35). The concentration of these afferents in the posterior columns and the possibility of activating them antidromicly has permitted much animal work to elucidate the basic mechanism of analgesia produced by stimulation of the primary afferent nerve.

The prolonged after-discharge in the midbrain tegmentum following maximal stimulation of a peripheral nerve has been shown by COLLINS and RANDT (10) to be due to stimulation of C fibers with a small early component related to A-delta stimulation (Fig. 1). The lower trace records the response through a so-called envelope detector. On the abscissa, time is recorded in 0.5-s intervals. A 0.5-s train at 500/s and 60 V to the forepaw, a really painful stimulus in man, causes a significant after-discharge for over 3 s. Nonnoxious stimuli cause an after-discharge lasting only circa 0.2 s.

SHEALY and colleagues in mid 1967, recording from this area of the mesencephalic tegmentum in cats, were able virtually to eliminate this after-discharge by continuous application of a 2 mA d.c. anodal current to the dorsum of the cervical cord via a single 3 · 3 mm platinum plate (41) (Fig. 2). A 50-s pulsed d.c. current similarly applied in awake behaving cats resulted in the animals allowing prolonged pinching and intense heat to the point of tissue damage with no apparent discomfort.

The cells in lamina 5 of the posterior horn of the cord usually respond both to noxious and innocuous stimuli, i.e., are polymodal neurons. HILLMAN and WALL (9) showed in decerebrate cats that stimulation of the dorsal columns exerted an extremely powerful inhibition here sufficient to turn off completely the high frequency of firing in a lamina 5 cell produced by damage to the most excitable part of the receptive field of that cell. Likewise ZIMMERMANN (49) at the Heidelberg meeting of this society in 1975 demonstrated suppression or abolition of the response of these polymodal neurons in the posterior horns to noxious heating of the skin when he excited antidromicly the dorsal column of the cord. A simultaneous excitation upon stimulation to this column was the more likely to be submerged by the competing inhibitory influence at frequencies of stimulation above 50 Hz (Fig. 3). He found similar inhibition of these polymodal neurons in the posterior horns of the cord upon direct stimulation of the large fibers in the peripheral nerves from the region of noxiously heated skin. FELDMAN (14) was the first to demonstrate quantitatively by the analysis of poststimulus time histograms the effect on the firing of lamina 5 cells of dorsal column stimulation (DCS). His low intensities of electric stimulation 0.05 ms at 4 5 were used intracutaneously in the cat (Fig. 4). They produced a light tactile sensation when similarly applied in man. His high intensities 0.5 ms at 20 V (Fig. 5) were painful in man and activated in the cats the full spectrum of afferent fibers including the smallest most slowly conducting ones. At individual lamina 5 cells, the low intensities evoked at short latency a brief 25 ms burst of high-frequency spikes; to these were added at the high intensity of stimulation a further train of spikes at decreasing frequency on out to 150 ms. The latter are presumably the electric insignia of pain. The intracutaneous stimuli were then applied on a background of high frequency ipsilateral stimulation on a posterior column. This produced an attenuation of the firing of lamina 5 cells much more striking in the late, pain-correlated portion of the response than in the earlier phase related to touch.

The most caudal supraspinal cluster of cell bodies responding primarily or exclusively to noxious stimuli or to activation of small-diameter afferent fibers is in the vicinity of nucleus gigantocellularis (NGC) in the reticular formation of the upper medulla (3,5,8,18). Moreover, studies in the alert behaving animal have shown that somatic stimuli from which the cat tries to escape increase NGC electric responses. Likewise, stimulation of NGC will elicit escape and behavior indicative of pain (6,7). All of this evidence that NGC has an important function in the aversive and motivational aspects of pain led SHETTER and ATKINSON (42) to study at that site the effects of stimulation of the dorsal column of the cord. They recorded from single cells the result of natural and of supramaximal electric stimulation to the contralateral forepaw of cats. The evoked response to the electric shock could be completely suppressed by dorsal column stimulation (DCS), whereas the response to a continuous forepaw crush could be markedly but not totally suppressed. The conditioning DCS (Fig. 6) was a train of ten pulses, each 0.3 s in duration, at 100/s, i.e., lasting only 0.1 s. The diminishing suppression it produced lasted only about 0.4 s (Fig. 7). The dorsal column was stimulated with a tiny bipolar concentric stainless-steel electrode only 1 mm in outside diameter; hence the stimuli were almost certainly confined to the dorsal columns. Evidence that this suppressor effect occurs at a spinal level was obtained by transecting or in some animals by removing both dorsal columns at the second cervical segment. To my surprise stimulation caudal to the cut produced an initial response, followed by subsequent inhibition to supramaximal peripheral stimulation as well as to further dorsal column shocks, whereas stimulation rostral to this cut provoked no response itself and as a conditioning stimulus was likewise ineffecitve (Figs. 8 and 9). Clearly the inhibition is taking place caudally at the posterior horn cells by antidromic conduction down the tract. Dorsal column collaterals are then presumably firing spinoreticular neurons projecting up the cord to nucleus giganto-cellularis.

In a somewhat similar type of study, EMMERS and RUDERMAN (11) recorded from the thalamic termination sites of the spinothalamic and spinocervicothalamic tracts in rats. Microelectrodes in the somesthetic thalamus were localized to neurons that responded with bursts of spikes to toe pinching. A conditioning stimulus via a 0.1-mm diameter electrode on the surface of the fasciculus gracilis completely abolished the response to this noxious stimulus on the same side if it preceded the test stimulus by 20-60 ms. The response to a similarly timed maximal electric stimulus to the cut rostral end of the sciatic nerve was likewise completely abolished. Cutting of the spinocervicothalamic pathway in the dorsolateral funiculus or of the spinothalamic tract in the ventral cord left only the alternate pathway intact. DCS was equally effective at suppressing the responses via either pathway. One must, however, point out that in this study in the rat nonnoxious mechanical stimuli were also suppressed with equal effectiveness, a major difference between this and the results of FELDMAN in cats.

Evidence for an intracerebral site of action of the suppression upon DCS was presented by NYQUIST and GREENHOOT (37). Records in the pain-related thalamic nucleus centrum medianum-parafascicularis complex (CM-Pf) yielded potentials of maximal amplitude from each of the four limbs at 20-30 V. Conditioning DCS was applied to the caudal part on one side only of the dorsal funicular surface at the thoracolumbar level. Such unilateral conditioning DCS pulses suppressed or abolished the late waves of the CM-Pf potential evoked from either side of the body *and from forelimbs as well as back limbs*. Moreover, when the dorsal columns were sectioned on both sides, the evoked CM-Pf potential was still effectively suppressed by unilateral DCS regardless of whether the dorsal column was stimulated rostral or caudal to the cut. So, contrary to the situation in NGC of the medulla, when one records from thalamus, an orthodromic as well as an antidromic inhibition is exerted by DCS, which is effective bilaterally in both cases from unilateral stimulation. In addition, it is effective when applied well caudal to the site of entry into the cord of the noxious afferent impulses from the periphery.

Effect of DCS in Man

I have described these animal studies at some length because they reveal such consistent suppression of acute pain behavior and its electric insignia. It is no wonder that many of us persisted so long in implanting electrodes in patients with chronic pain. The initial results were so frequently encouraging that substantial series soon accumulated. One delightful surprise was that in many of the patients relief long outlasted the duration of the stimulation. However, the cheering memory of a happy patient at hospital discharge was all too frequently dispelled by later problems. By October 1973, 5 1/2 years after my first implant of electrodes against the posterior columns, I had the lugubrious task of reporting disappointing results in 100 patients (44). Only 25% of 68 patients followed more than 6 months were classified as a success, i.e., their degree of relief permitted full productivity supported by no narcotic.

Before going into any more detail in the whole series I should like to present a case.

Patient C.S., 35 years old, housewife. 13 April 1973: rose thorn into tip of L. thumb - infection, incision, lymphangitis; 2-3 weeks later electric shock sensations upon touching distal thumb. Six months later slightest touch or cool air caused pain lateral two fingers, hand, and forearm. September 1974 to August 1976: ten operations - local neurectomies and excision neuromas superficial radial n. and thenar branches median n.; 12 progressively less successful nerve blocks.

March 1976: tegretol, transcutaneous nerve stimulation. June 1976: sympathectomy - transthoracic - eight upper L. thoracic ganglia.

14 October 1976: anxiety attack required short hospitalization. Four psychiatrists including one at Massachusetts General Hospital favor organic cause of pain. Continuing work as housewife, but L. upper limb almost useless.

Admission Massachusetts General Hospital July 1978: L. hand and distal 2/3 forearm wrapped in soft cotton batting; many layers cornified skin L. radial palm; analgesia and anesthesia distal phalanx thumb only; touch to proximal phalanx thumb or thenar eminence cause "electric shock" to shoot up arm to whole torso. Slight L. ptosis and miosis; no psychogalvanic reflex L. upper limb, i.e., sympathectomy complete.

7 July 1978: L. brachial plexus block in axilla (lidocaine) - anesthesia and analgesia entire forearm and hand; complete relief pain and hyperpathia 4 h. Recommendation of Professor R.D. ADAMS, Chief Neurological Service: L. posterior rhizotomy of cervical 5 - 8.

13 July 1978: operation: L. posterior interdural implant at cervical 3 of platinum electrodes whose final position was determined upon stimulation with patient awake.

16 July 1978: onset of stimulation 1 h every other waking hour - most comfortable at 150/s, 0.8 V, 200 μs pulse duration. Gradual reduction in stimulation until none 24 - 27 July 1978; then hyperpathia started to return. Used L. hand, filed finger nails, swam in cold water for first time in 5 years without pain. 20 October 1978: requires stimulation to stop pain in only two sessions per week - each 15 min at time of physical therapy to limber up joints of L. fingers.

I regret to emphasize that this result is far from typical of what I have accomplished by this operation. I present her as the kind of result that has led me to continue to work with this procedure. It may be that when extreme hyperpathia dominates the picture this operation has a better chance of success. You will recall that hyperpathia was the main feature of FOERSTER's two patients with surgical injury of the posterior columns. This component of the pain was relieved in 16 of the 23 patients who displayed it in our first group of 100 (p. 296, 44). Unfortunately, it was not relieved in the three patients in whom pain upon touching the area was a feature of postherpetic neuralgia.

The full extent of deterioration in the late results became clear at a Pain Symposium in Minneapolis in December 1973 at which 11 papers were given on dorsal column stimulation for relief of pain. Thus, SHEALY in March 1973 stated that "good to excellent control of pain can be achieved in 80% of chronic pain patients" (38) (by DCS). By the December 1973 meeting he said only 25% of his 80 patients had excellent relief (39), and this dropped to 15% when the delayed publication of the proceedings of the meeting occurred in July 1975 (40). Likewise LONG and ERICKSON with 30% excellent results at the December 1973 meeting (28) had this drop to 18% of 55 patients when the article appeared (29). NASHOLD and FRIEDMAN (32) after 1 year of follow-up had 40% good to excellent results in their 30 patients; at their 3-year follow-up this had dropped to 24% (31). Of the 130 patients of ADAMS and HOSOBUCHI, 69% were classified as good to excellent at the time of hospital discharge; 49% were so classified after an average follow-up of nearly 2 years. However, they did not require return to work as a criterion for success; only 12 of their patients returned to regular work (34).

One of the more encouraging series is that of WINKELMÜLLER and colleagues (48). In their 26 patients whose pain was due to benign causes, they achieved a 75% - 100% early relief of pain in 73% of them. This level of relief persisted for greater than 6 months in 46% of the 26 patients. They shared the general view that pain due to cancer should be treated by other more certain, even though higher risk methods.

There was a general reaction of discouragement most pronounced in Dr. SHEALY, the surgeon who carried out the first such operation in man. He has abandoned neurosurgery completely. Dr. LONG did no more dorsal column implants for over 2 years, and others of us did very few.

Although all of us had technical complications early in our series, these had largely been mastered by 1974. Electrodes are usually a pair of small platinum plates imbedded in silicone plastic less than 1 mm thick so that a minimal mass lies beneath dura. Almost everyone with a sizeable series had at least one patient awaken after operation with a severe neurological deficit from cord compression. Prompt removal of the electrodes was usually followed by major recovery; however, such sequelae have given rise to at least two malpractice law suits in the United States. Our tactic of awakening the patient on the operating table for final positioning of the electrodes permits repeated testing of motor function. We have had one single patient in whom an additional stitch in the dura caused weakness of dorsiflexion of a foot, which disappeared at once when that stitch was cut out. Cooperation of the awake patient is helpful on three other scores: (1) a more precise reference of sensation to the area of clinical pain may be achieved; (2) stimulation of a posterior root at the level of the electrodes can be eliminated by shifting them medially; and (3) rarely patients have such a huge dural sleeve that extra tucks in the dura may be helpful to secure sensation at a low voltage (44). KRAINICK and colleagues had a patient with C3 electrodes develop an acute paraplegia postoperatively while fully conscious; they thought this was probably due to buckling of the assembly against the cord because of muscular contraction. They reoperated promptly and immediate recovery occurred in a few hours (25). We have fixed the webbed silicone sheet to the outer leaf of dura by two vertical mattress sutures, which probably prevents buckling. Cerebrospinal fluid leaks and meningitis have been eliminated and possibly arachnoidal thickening minimized by creating an artificial pocket for the electrodes between inner and outer layers of dura, a tactic developed independently by the Freiburg group, BURTON, and me (24,4,44).

The use of a symmetric biphasic electric pulse to the electrodes (Fig. 10) should decrease tissue polarization but in our hands did not significantly improve the results (44). These and other technical improvements reduced the electronic failures. The main problem is biologic.

The logical tactic of trying some form of temporary test procedure included penetration of the dorsal funiculi by tiny electrodes introduced via a needle from laterally at C1-2 by HOSOBUCHI et al. (22). Such electrodes were left in position only a few hours - too short a time to be sure of the patient's response to stimulation. Many of us tried freely floating electrodes placed via percutaneous needles in the subarachnoid space, but the possibility of meningitis along the path of the leads precluded more than a few days observation of the effects of stimulation (23,44).

The development of tiny cylindric electrodes attached to long hollow leads through which a flexible wire stylet can be introduced has made possible the percutaneous introduction under fluoroscopic control of electrode pairs. The leads can be passed laterally under the skin and connected to another pair of leads that penetrate the skin at a distance from the connector site so that a protracted temporary trial of stimulation can be carried out (Fig. 12a and b). Possibly those patients, roughly 40%-50%, who leave the hospital dissatisfied with the result of DCS by permanent operation would be eliminated by this low-risk prolonged trial. Three groups in Montreal at the Second International Pain Congress reported on 1 September 1978 their experiences (2,36,45). They have kindly given me their manuscripts and I shall describe their and my results.

Before doing this, I shall summarize a 5 - 10 year follow-up on my personal series of 56 patients implanted at laminectomy and first reported in 1973. Only ten of them were securing total relief of pain at discharge from the hospital; the nine still living have all been rechecked in the last month and eight remain productive and completely free of pain. The tenth was pain free until her death from unrelated cause 8 months after operation.

Each of the ten had had an average of 4.2 previous operations for pain. In five of them the pain was referred to the distribution of the brachial plexus. Three had cervical spondylosis and/or protruded cervical disks; one had a post-traumatic neuropathy of the lower components of one brachial plexus and one pain in an upper limb phantom - not in the stump. Another had post-traumatic lateral femoral cutaneous neuralgia, two had the syndrome of many low-back operations with arachnoiditis by myelogram, and two had severe postcordotomy dysesthesias. One of the latter two was the one who died later. The other had relief for 3 years but always used his stimulator a great deal for the last 1 1/2 years at progressively increasing voltage until finally relief stopped.

Nearly all of these successful patients soon after operative implantation secured protracted relief following minutes to an hour of stimulation, and all but one now require no more than a few minutes of stimulation per day. Three need use the device only very few months and one, having needed it less and less for 4 years, remains pain free without it for 3 1/2 years. In each of the foregoing diagnostic categories with complete success, there were other patients who were either discharged pain free and had a later recurrence or who always had varying degrees of suboptimal or no relief.

The only diagnostic category to do somewhat better than the others is that of amputation stump and phantom limb pain. The Freiburg group have by far the largest experience: 52 patients. Of those with some or all of the pain in the stump, DCS reduced this in about two-thirds; likewise about two-thirds of the phantom pains were helped by DCS (25). Although their success rate after 1 year was an excellent 60%, this had dropped to about 30% by 1977 (26).

In some of these late failures, the area of stimulus-evoked paresthesia had changed and success was recouped by a reimplantation in nine of their amputees. NEILSON, ADAMS and HOSOBUCHI have also drawn attention to the good results of DCS for phantom limb pain. At follow-up 7 - 25 months after operation, five of their six patients were relieved - four almost totally. The sixth patient, despite excellent relief of the phantom limb pain, could not tolerate pain at the receiver site in the chest wall despite a surgical replacement (33).

Reports are now available on percutaneous implantation of spinal epidural electrodes in 133 patients (Table 1):

Table 1. Percutaneous implantation of spinal epidural electrodes

BLACK and NORTH	(22)	Follow-up	2-20 months
NORTH and LONG	(30)		21 months mean
URBAN and NASHOLD	(57)		6 months to 3 1/2 years
SWEET	(24)		2-28 months

As in the earlier series of implants at open operation, patients with a full range of types of chronic intractable pain were treated. NASHOLD has not reported full details of his results; in the other three series we are all running only 15%-25% good to excellent results after a year. For example, in my 24 cases relief was good or excellent without complications in only five and useful in one. Relief was good or excellent in three more whose wounds became infected, requiring removal of the assembly. In only one of these has the equipment been reimplanted as yet. She has recovered useful relief. In all three with infection, the tactic of a temporary implant in which wires emerge from the skin was followed by a second stage at which this whole assembly including the electrodes were removed and new electrodes reimplanted permanently at a different site.

This two-stage procedure having given rise to infection in 3 of the first 12 cases, we have in the next 12 internalized all of the apparatus at the first stage and have had no more infections. Independently LONG and NASHOLD have also decided to do a permanent implant at the first stage. The technical simplicity of the operation promoted at first in me a cavalier attidue toward it. The performance of the first part of the implantation in the radiographic suite and the amount of foreign material left in the patient actually demand unususually scrupulous attention to asepsis. In four patients, two of them underweight, the electrodes in the perhaps emaciated epidural space shifted position so readily as the patients moved about that after a second or third prompt replacement we gave up. In none of the four was there an adequate trial of stimulation. In general, change of position of the electrodes was a significant problem. It occurred in five other of my patients and required eight extra operations for correction. There were 47 such spontaneous electrode migrations in the NORTH-LONG series, and five in that of URBAN-NASHOLD. We now make it a point to have the electrode leads lie for several segments within the spinal canal in an effort to stabilize them. Malfunctions at the receiver, at the connection between electrode and receiver wires, at junctions of electrodes with their leads, or elsewhere along the leads can be localized by a combination of radiographs and recording of current densities at various places on the skin as the receiver is activated. We needed to reoperate for two such electronic breakdowns. Such failures were also a nuisance to the other three groups.

The principal problems, as with the implantation of flat platinum electrodes at laminectomy, have been: (1) the selection of patients who will derive sufficient benefit to begin with and (2) the recouping of relief in those patients who lose it for biologic rather than electronic reasons.

As in my first series, the good results include a few in all etiologic categories - two with neuropathic, three with rhizopathic, and three with myelopathic pain.

I fear that neither refinement of clinical criteria nor changes in the electronics are likely to achieve salient improvements. An avenue not intensively explored is that of placing one or more electrodes ventral to the cord as tentatively recommended by LARSON et al. (26) and by HOPPENSTEIN (20). I have lately realized that the epidural space often permits passage of the new steerable electrodes to the ventral aspect of the cord and am in the process of seeing if this may be fruitful (Fig. 12a and b). My tactic of using dorsodorsal, dorsoventral, and ventroventral electrodes of the Avery type implanted at open operation has not proved dramatically helpful. However, the development of tolerance to an initially effective dorsodorsal implantation has been repeatedly helped by reimplantation at a new site. I now leave in the initial assembly if it is yielding an acceptable paresthesia and implant an entirely new assembly. In one of these latter patients, the original assembly recovered its effectiveness after lying fallow for a year. The patient now uses the original set of electrodes during the day at work and the second set in the evening.

All four of the groups of neurosurgeons reporting recently have been tending not to implant epidural electrodes unless stimulus-evoked paresthesias were referred to the zone of clinical pain. This may be a mistake. Six of my patients in the original series derived excellent relief, for substantial periods, of pain referred to zones devoid of such paresthesias, and two of these are in the most favorable group of ten with very long-term relief. One of my five good results with epidural electrodes has a post-traumatic myelopathy with a total transverse lesion at lumbar 1 and no paresthesias referred to her painful legs. These results indicate that activation of intracranial structures by orthodromic conduction in the posterior columns can at times suppress pain, as also suggested by the work of NYQUIST and GREENHOOT in cats (35).

The complexity of many of the problems we are all seeing defies simple analysis. A single example will suffice. We first saw earlier this year a 65-year-old police sargeant with three pains: (1) a twisting knife-like pain at the right greater trochanter since an athletic injury 46 years earlier - it was intermittent, worsened gradually over the years until now it was provoked by any movement of the right leg. We presumed it was a post-traumatic peripheral neuropathy. Later a right sciatic pain beginning in mid-1971, was treated in August 1972, by removal of the two lowest lumbar disks on that side. The sciatic pain was eliminated but replaced by pain No. 2, a constant fiery type in the distal one-third of the right foot, presumably a post-traumatic rhizopathy. Open left C5-6 cordotomies in March 1975 and January 1976 yielded only transitory relief of this fiery pain and the second cordotomy was followed at once by pain No. 3: another constant fiery burn in the first two left fingers, hand, and forearm. A third open cordotomy on the right at C2-3 not only did not stop this new pain but extended it to include the entire left upper limb and scapula. There was now severe pain on light touch to the limb with at least daily episodes of spontaneous electric shock-like waves in the whole left upper limb lasting 10-60 min. We presume this is largely of myelopathic origin. Our experienced psychiatric consultant thought that psychological issues here were of minimal relevance. A medical regime of 5 mg of fluphenazine and 150 mg of amitriptyline/day reduced his resting pain to 20% of the previous level, but on even the mild activity of walking the pains returned. Epidural electrodes could be passed no higher than T1 probably because of the cordotomy scars. After protracted repositioning, stimulation of these electrodes yielded sensations in the entire lower limbs, the left scapular area, and the left triceps area but not below the elbow. Now 4 months later he is cheered by 75% relief, even when he is active, of all of the pain except that in the left hand and fingers where there is no reference of stimulus-evoked sensation. In this instance aspects of neuro-, radiculo-, and myelopathic pain have been usefully relieved. He carefully rations himself to 10 min of stimulation each waking hour. Note that although the electrodes are at T1 their activation has stopped most of the pain related to the right C2-3 cordotomy.

None of the electrophysiologic studies cited in the first part of the paper reveal inhibition lasting more than a few seconds. Hence, they do not account for two phenomena we have all observed in most of the patients with relief, namely a delay of minutes or hours before any relief appears and a continuation of relief for minutes to years after stimulation stops. Dr. NORTH has kindly given me his specific data on those scores (Table 2).

Table 2. NORTH and LONG (Personal communication)

Latency of relief after stimulation started	
0 - 1 min	8 patients
1 - 30 min	14 patients
30 - 120 min	4 patients
Persistence of relief after stimulation stopped	
0 - 1 min	6 patients
1 - 30 min	4 patients
0.5 - 1 h	5 patients
2 - 12 h	9 patients
> 12 h	1 patient

A remarkable example of both these features was an orthopedic surgeon I have already reported (44). His previous operations for his pain had included four cervical laminectomies and facetectomies, three cervical posterior rhizotomies, one open cervical cordotomy, and one bulbar spinothalamic tractotomy. These had neither relieved the pain nor produced analgesia throughout the painful zones. Despite excellent reference of stimulation-induced paresthesias to his painful upper limb and shoulder girdle, he began to have relief from daily stimulation for hours only during the second postoperative month. He discovered that when he stimulated only 15 min and then stopped his unabating pain would continue for a time but then be followed by partial relief for some hours. Another 15 min of stimulation would again give no immediate relief, but delayed relief became progressively better and longer lasting. After about 3 years of less and less need to stimulate, he stopped using the device and remains pain free 8 years after electrode implantation.

At the other extreme, I have had one patient with postmeningitic myelopathy whose pain disappeared instantaneously and completely the moment stimulation began.

Both the delay in appearance of relief and its persistence after stimulation are best explained on neurochemical grounds, for which supporting facts are now available. There are three newly discovered neuroanatomic systems, each with its own groups of cell bodies in certain parts of the brain stem and with an extraordinarily extensive system of axonal trees invading specific portions of cerebrum, diencephalon, cerebellum, and spinal cord. These are the monoaminergic systems that deliver the neurotransmitters dopamine, norepinephrine, and serotonin usually not only to synapses on individual cells but more diffusely to whole populations of cells in a nucleus. They function as modulators by which the brain regulates its own subsystems, one of wich is of course that related to pain. The roles of dopamine, norepinephrine, and serotonin in relation to electric stimulation-produced analgesia (SPA) have been studied by AKIL and LIEBESKIND (1). Via bipolar electrodes chronically implanted in the periaqueductal grey matter, one secures potent and reliable analgesic effects in animals. Dopamine and serotonin increase SPA, whereas norepinephrine inhibits it. When one specifically depletes serotonin with the drug p-chlorophenylalanine this reduces SPA, whereas increasing serotonin levels by administration of its precursors, tryptophane or 5-hydroxytryptamine, increases SPA. Similarly, dopamine receptor blockade by pimozide decreases SPA, while the precursor L-dopa or a dopamine receptor stimulator (apomorphine) increases SPA. Contrariwise, selective depletion of norepinephrine with disulfiram increases SPA. The combination of depressing norepinephrine and elevating dopamine levels is particularly effective in increasing SPA.

Moreover, these drugs do not in the absence of electric stimulation to the midbrain have any effect on pain thresholds. In man, WURTMAN, GROWDEN, and I have seen no effect on clinical pain by presumably increasing brain serotonin levels with a massive intake of L-tryptophan. We have not yet done this in patients using DCS. I suggest that we shall have to attack intractable pain simultaneously from a number of angles now open to us because of the newer knowledge. Direct electric stimulation of the descending serotonergic fibers in the dorsolateral funiculus is unlikely to succeed because they are tiny high threshold fibers close to large, low threshold motor fibers in the lateral corticospinal tract.

The neuropeptides represent still another avenue of attack we must be on the alert to exploit. At least six fully characterized oligopeptides have now been identified in the substantia gelatinosa, lamina 2, of the dorsal horn of the cord. Figure 13 shows the dense concentration in this region demonstrable by the immunocytochemical fluorescence methods of HÖKFELT and colleagues to whom I am indebted for these illustrations. Somatostatin is shown on the left and substance P on the right. In Figure 14, the diagram shows on the left the similarity between the dispositions of substance P and met and leuenkephalin in Rexed laminas 6 and 7 as well as 2. On the right, one sees that somatostatin and neurotensin do not occur in the deeper laminas. Likewise, angiotensin II has been found in high concentration in substantia gelatinosa both in the cord and in trigeminal nucleus caudalis (Fig. 15). We must learn to make use of these substances, their analogues, potentiators, or suppressors to enhance SPA in man.

Another lesson from the neuropeptides is the remarkably rapid development of tolerance to the intracerebroventricular injection of the naturally occurring substance β-endorphin. An initial dose into the cat's ventricle giving excellent analgesia has no such effect if repeated in less than 72 h even if ten times the original effective dose is given (21).

It seems apparent: (1) that homeostatic mechanisms have a remarkable capacity to restore the status quo ante and (2) that some change we are making in neurotransmitter and/or neuromodulator levels at critical sites is the basis for our few really good results with DCS. For the immediate future, we should perhaps concentrate our studies on the sizeable group of patients who lose initially good relief, seeking to tilt the neurochemical balance in favor of enhanced stimulation-produced analgesia. Put in the broadest terms, our basic problem is that we are working with the most complex system in the entire cosmos of which man is aware, namely, the mind of man himself. We have an advantage FOERSTER didn't have, to wit, thousands of neuroscientists in the Western world are eager to help us solve the problems of the human brain, if we will but seek them out and work with them. The initiative should come from us.

References

1. AKIL, H., LIEBESKIND, J.C.: Monoaminergic mechanisms of stimulation-produced analgesia. Brain Res. 94, 279-296 (1975)
2. BLACK, P., NORTH, R.B.: Experience with epidural electrical stimulation for intractable pain. Proceedings 2nd World Congress on Pain, Montreal, September 1, 1978, abstract p. 296, to be published
3. BOWSHER, D., MALLART, A., PETIT, D., ALBE-FESSARD, D.: A bulbar relay to the centre median. J. Neurophysiol. 31, 288-300 (1975)
4. BURTON, C.: Dorsal column stimulation: Optimization of application. Surg. Neurol. 4, 171-176 (1975)
5. CASEY, K.L.: Somatic stimuli, spinal pathways, and size of cutaneous fibers influencing unit activity in the medial medullary reticular formation. Exp. Neurol. 25, 35-56 (1969)
6. CASEY, K.L.: Responses of bulboreticular units to somatic stimuli eliciting escape behavior in the cat. Int. J. Neurosci. 2, 15-28 (1971)
7. CASEY, K.L.: Escape elicited by bulboreticular stimulation in the cat. Int. J. Neurosci. 2, 29-34 (1971)
8. CASEY, K.L., KEENE, J.J., MORROW, T.: Bulboreticular and medial thalamic unit activity in relation to adverse behavior and pain. Adv. Neurol. 4, 197-205 (1974)
9. COLLINS, W.F., NULSEN, F.E., RANDT, C.T.: Relation of peripheral nerve fiber size and sensations in man. Arch. Neurol. 3, 381-385 (1970)

10. COLLINS, W.F., RANDT, C.T.: Midbrain evoked responses relating to peripheral or "C" fibers in cat. J. Neurophysiol. 23, 47-53 (1960)

11. EMMERS, R., RUDERMAN, M.I.: Inhibition at the T-cells of the spinothalamic tract. A neurophysiological basis for electrically-induced analgesia. Proc. Soc. Exp. Biol. Med. 145, 1310-1316 (1974)

12. FABRITIUS, H.: Ein Fall von Stichverletzung des Rückenmarks. Zugleich ein Beitrag über die Leitungsbahnen im Rückenmark. Dtsch. Z. Nervenheilkd. 37, 415-454 (1909)

13. FABRITIUS, H.: Versuch einer Psychophysiologie des Gefühls. Monatsschr. Psychiatr. Neurol. 28, 400-410 (1910)

14. FELDMAN, R.A.: Patterned response of lamina V cells: Cutaneous and dorsal funicular stimulation. Physiol. Behav. 15, 79-84 (1975)

15. FÖRSTER, O.: Die Leitungsbahnen des Schmerzgefühls und die chirurgische Behandlung der Schmerzzustände. pp. 77-80. Berlin, Vianna: Urban & Schwarzenberg, 1927

16. FOERSTER, O.: Symptomatologie der Erkrankungen des Rückenmarks und seiner Wurzeln. In: Allgemeine Neurologie. Handbuch der Neurologie. BUMKE, O., FOERSTER, O. (eds.), Vol.V, p. 377. Berlin: Springer 1936

17. FOERSTER, O.: Symptomatologie der Erkrankungen des Rückenmarks und seiner Wurzeln. In: Allgemeine Neurologie. Handbuch der Neurologie. BUMKE, O., FOERSTER, O. (eds.), Vol. V, p. 639. Berlin: Springer 1936

18. GOLDMAN, P.L., COLLINS, W.F., TAUB, A., FITZMARTIN, J.: Evoked bulbar reticular unit activity following delta fiber stimulation of peripheral somatosensory nerve in cat. Exp. Neurol. 37, 597-606 (1972)

19. HILLMAN, P., WALL, P.D.: Inhibitory and excitatory factors influencing the receptive fields of Lamina V spinal cord cells. Exp. Brain Res. 9, 284-306 (1969)

20. HOPPENSTEIN, R.: Electrical stimulation of the ventral and dorsal columns of the spinal cord for relief of chronic intractable pain: Preliminary report. Surg. Neurol. 4, 187-194 (1975)

21. HOSOBUCHI, Y.: Personal communication Oct. 1978

22. HOSOBUCHI, Y., ADAMS, J.E., WEINSTEIN, P.R.: Preliminary percutaneous dorsal column stimulation prior to permanent implantation. Technical note. J. Neurosurg. 37, 242-245 (1972)

23. KRAINICK, J.-U., THODEN, V.: Electric stimulation of the spinal cord for the relief of pain. Adv. Neurosurg. 3, 210-215 (1975)

24. KRAINICK, J.-U., THODEN, U., RIECHERT, T.: Spinal cord stimulation in post-amputation pain. Surg. Neurol. 4, 167-170 (1975)

25. KRAINICK, J.-U., THODEN, U.: Schmerzphänomene bei Amputierten. Neurochirurgia (Stuttg.) 19, 72-80 (1976)

26. KRAINICK, J.-U., THODEN, U.: Postamputation pain and electrical stimulation. Reunion sobre Patologia de la Columna Vertebral. CONESA, H., SEIGNER (eds.). Vol. VI, pp. 99-108. Murcia: Ferrer Internacional 1977

27. LASRON, S.J., SANCES, A., Jr., CUSICK, J.F., MEYER, G.A., SWIONTEK, T.: Surg. Neurol. 4, 180-186 (1975)

28. LONG, D.M., ERICKSON, D.E.: Stimulation of the posterior columns of the spinal cord for relief of intractable pain. Pain Symposium. Minneapolis, 6-8 December 1973

29. LONG, D.M., ERICKSON, D.E.: Stimulation of the posterior columns of the spinal cord for relief of intractable pain. Surg. Neurol. 4, 134-141 (1975)

30. MELZACK, R., WALL, P.D.: Pain mechanisms: A new theory. Science 150, 971-978 (1965)

31. NASHOLD, B.S., Jr.: Dorsal column stimulation for control of pain. A three year follow-up. Surg. Neurol. 4, 146-147 (1975)

32. NASHOLD, B.S., Jr., FRIEDMAN, H.: Dorsal column stimulation for pain. A preliminary report on 30 patients. J. Neurosurg. 36, 590-597 (1972)

33. NIELSON, K.D., ADAMS, J.E., HOSOBUCHI, Y.: Phantom limb pain. Treatment with dorsal column stimulation. J. Neurosurg. 42, 301-307 (1975)

34. NIELSON, K.D., ADAMS, J.E., HOSOBUCHI, Y.: Experience with dorsal column stimulation for relief of chronic intractable pain 1968-1973. Surg. Neurol. 148-52 (1975)

35. NOORDENBOS, W.: Pain, pp. 68-88. Amsterdam: Elsevier 1959

36. NORTH, R.B., LONG, D.M.: Epidural dorsal column stimulation for chronic intractable pain. 21 month follow-up. Proceedings 2nd World Congress on Pain. Montreal, 1 September 1978, p. 296. (Abstract to be published). Advances in Pain Research and Therapy, Vol. 3, New York: Raven (in press)

37. NYQUIST, J.K., GREENHOOT, J.H.: Responses evoked from the thalamic centrum medianum by painful imput. Suppression by dorsal funiculus conditioning. Exp. Neurol. 39, 215-222 (1973)

38. SHEALY, C.N.: Pain suppression through posterior column stimulation. In: Neural Organization and its Relevance to Prosthetics. FIELDS, W.S., LEAVITT, L.A. (eds.), pp. 251-260. Miami: Symposia Specialists 1973

39. SHEALY, C.N.: Electrical stimulation of the human nervous system for the control of pain. Pain Symposium. Minneapolis, 6-8 December 1973

40. SHEALY, C.N.: Dorsal column stimulation: Optimization of application. Surg. Neurol. 4, 142-145 (1975)

41. SHEALY, C.N., TASLITZ, N., MORTIMER, J.T., BECKER, D.P.: Electrical inhibition of pain: Experimental evaluation. Anesth. Analg. (Cleve) 46, 299-305 (1967)

42. SHETTER, A.G., ATKINSON, J.R.: Dorsal column stimulation. Its effect on medial bulboreticular unit activity evoked by noxious stimuli. Exp. Neurol. 54, 185-198 (1977)

43. SWEET, W.H.: Lessons on pain control from electrical stimulation. Trans. Stud. Coll. Physicians Phila. 35, 171-184 (1968)

44. SWEET, W.H., WEPSIC, J.: Stimulation of the posterior columns of the spinal cord for pain control: Indications, technique, and results. Clin. Neurosurg. 21, 278-310 (1974)

45. URBAN, B.J., NASHOLD, B.S., Jr.: Percutaneous epidural stimulation of the spinal cord: Technique and complications. Proceedings 2nd World Congress on Pain. Montreal, 1 September 1978, p. 297. (Abstract) Advances in Pain Research and Therapy, Vol. 3. New York: Raven (in press)

46. WALL, P.D.: Presynaptic control of impulses at the first central synapse in the cutaneous pathways. Prog. Brain Res. 12, 92-115 (1964)

47. WALL, P.D., SWEET, W.H.: Temporary abolition of pain in man. Science 155, 108-109 (1967)

48. WINKELMÜLLER, W., DIETZ, H., STOLKE, D.: The clinical value of dorsal column stimulation (DCS). Adv. Neurosurg. 3, 225-228 (1975)

49. ZIMMERMANN, M.: Neurophysiological models for nociception pain and pain therapy. Adv. Neurosurg. 3, 199-209 (1975)

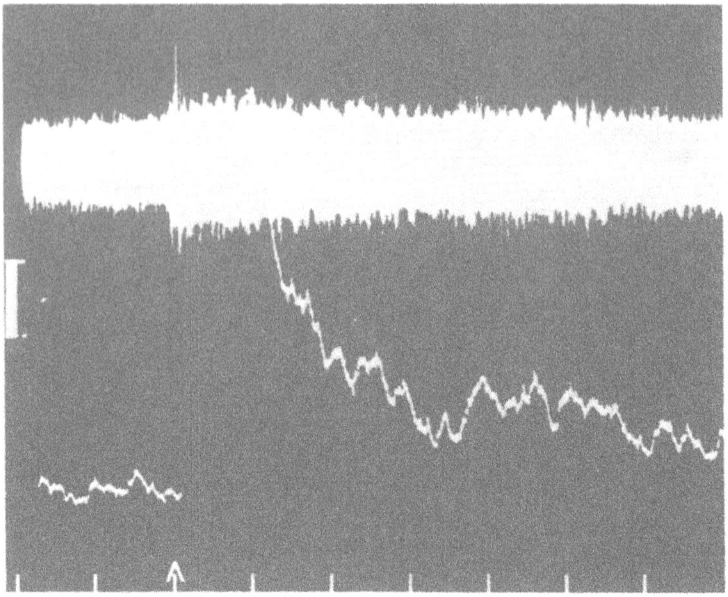

Fig. 1. Electrodes in midbrain tegmentum. Time on abscissa in 0.5-s intervals. Maximal electric stimulus to forepaw of cat at ↑ for 0.5 s, 500/s, 60 V. Lower trace records after discharge persisting in decreasing degree for over 3 s as compared with the baseline activity preceding the stimulus (41)

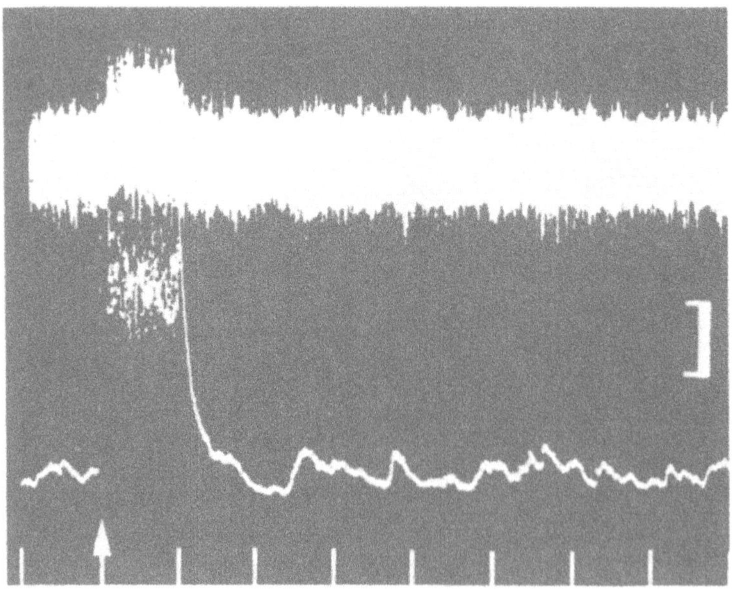

Fig. 2. Same recording conditions as Fig. 2 with addition of continuous application of 2 mA d.c. anodal current to dorsum of cat's cervical cord via a single 3 · 3 mm platinum plate electrode. This dorsal column stimulation virtually eliminates the after-discharge (41)

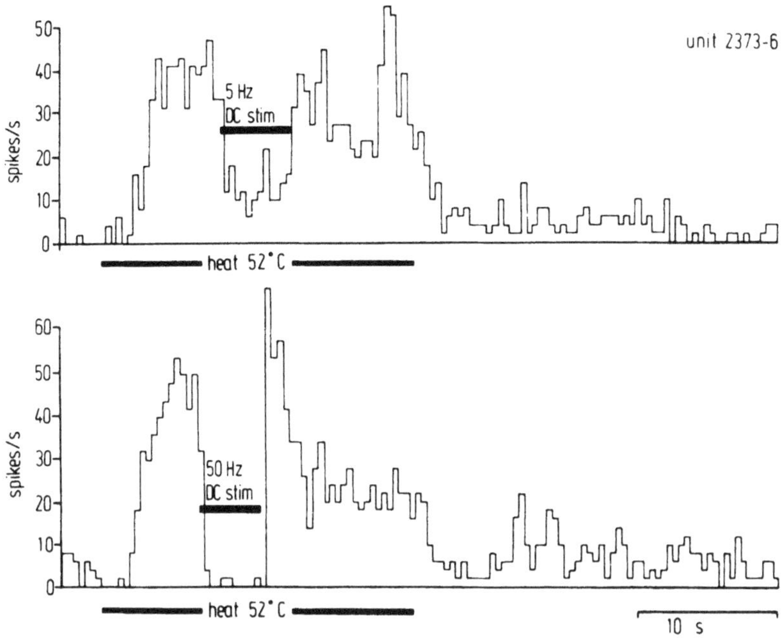

Fig. 3. Response of polymodal afferent neuron in posterior horn of spinal cord to noxious heating of skin to 52° C (continuous heavy back line *abscissa*). *Above:* Decrease in that response during stimulation of dorsal column at 5 Hz. *Below:* Abolition of that response during stimulation of dorsal column at 50 Hz. HANDWERKER, H.O., IGGO, A., ZIMMERMAN, M.: Pain 1, 147-165 (1975)

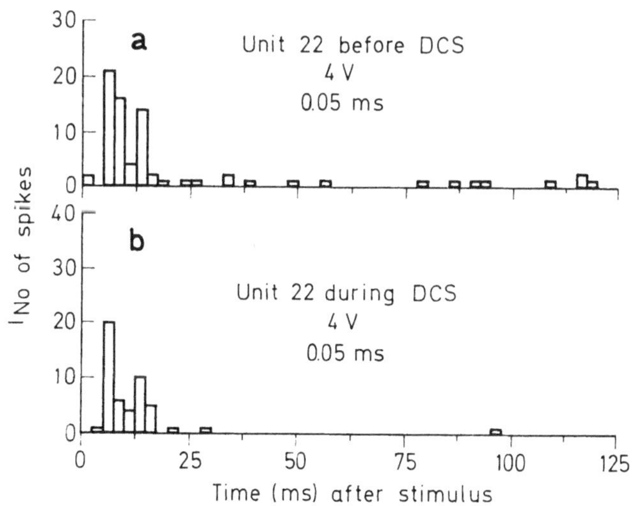

Fig. 4. Electric recording from a cell in lamina 5 of posterior horn. Response to low intensity intracutaneous electric stimulation in cat. The 25 ms burst of high-frequency spikes is decreased modestly when the stimulation of the skin is superimposed on a background of stimulation of an ipsilateral column. *DCS*, dorsal column stimulation

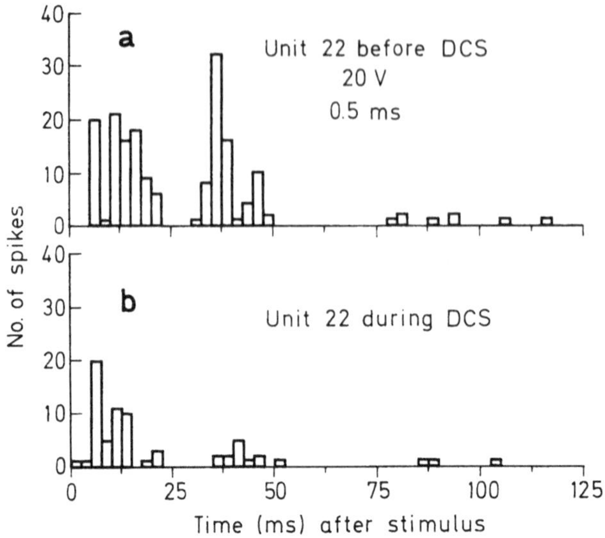

Fig. 5. Electric recording from a cell in lamina 5 of posterior horn. Response to high intensity intracutaneous electric stimulation of same cell. The new late burst of high-frequency spikes is reduced much more than the burst occurring in the first 25 ms. *DCS*, dorsal column stimulation (14)

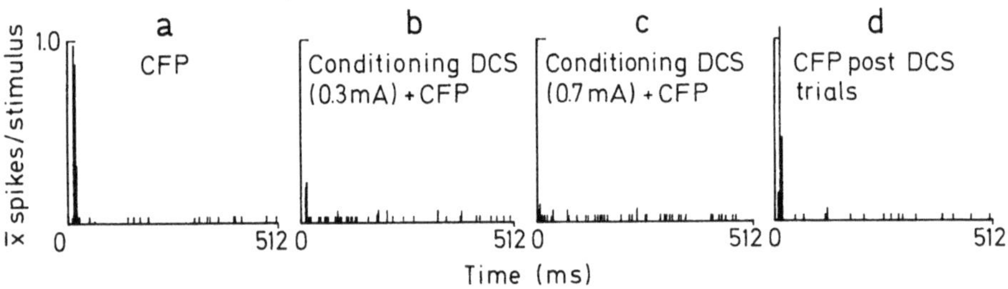

Fig. 6a-d. Recording from cells in nucleus gigantocellularis (NGC) in bulbar reticular formation. a Abrupt burst of high-frequency spikes after supramaximal electric stimulation to cat's contralateral forepaw (*CFP*). b Marked suppression of the response by a preceding (conditioning) dorsal column stimulation (*DCS*) at 0.3 mA. c Total suppression by such a conditioning stimulation at 0.7 mA. d Resumption of initial response without DCS

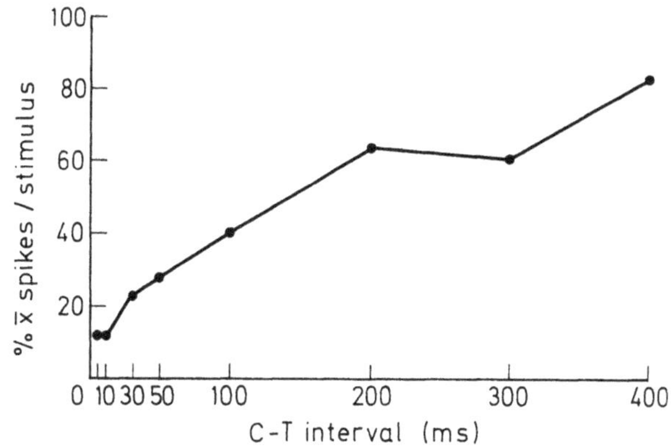

Fig. 7. Duration of effect of conditioning DCS. C-T interval between the 0.1-s train of conditioning DCS pulses and test stimulus to contralateral forepaw. The larger the C-T interval the less the suppression of the response of the cell in NGC

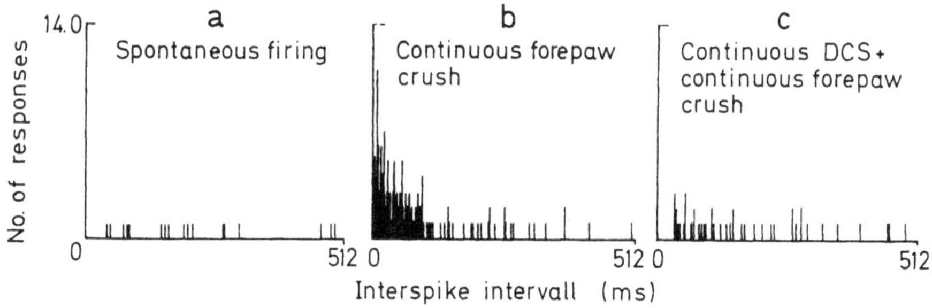

Fig. 8. Recording from cells in nucleus gigantocellularis (NGC) in bulbar reticular formation. Response of cell to continuous forepaw crush without and with continuous DCS. The suppression of this response during DCS is not as complete as that to a burst of supramaximal stimulation

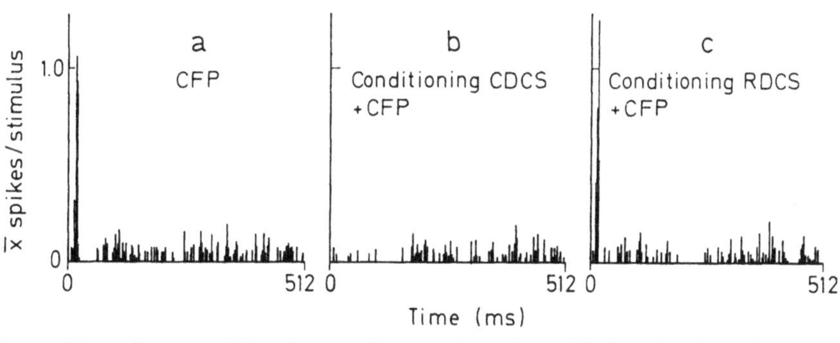

Fig. 9. Recording from cells in nucleus gigantocellularis (NGC) in bulbar reticular formation. Comparison of conditioning DCS when applied caudal to with effect when applied rostral to a transection of the dorsal columns at second cervical segment (42)

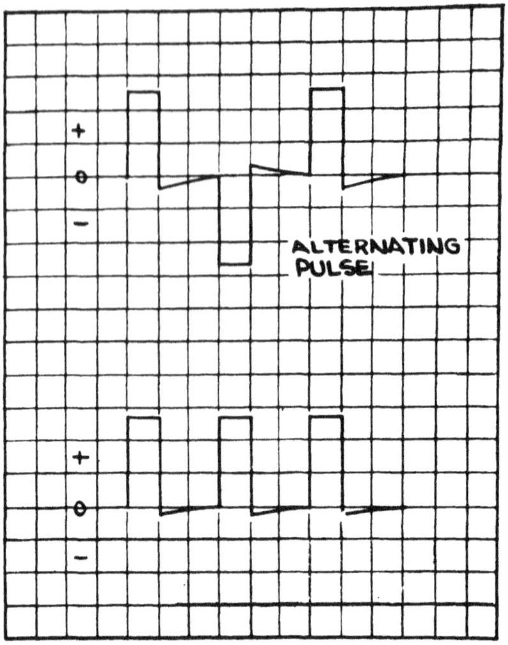

Fig. 10. Recording from cells in nucleus gigantocellularis (NGC) in bulbar reticular formation. *Upper trace*, the type of electric signal delivered by the later large receiver manufactured by Avery Laboratories. *Lower trace*, the asymmetric pulses delivered by earlier capacitance-coupled small Avery receiver (44)

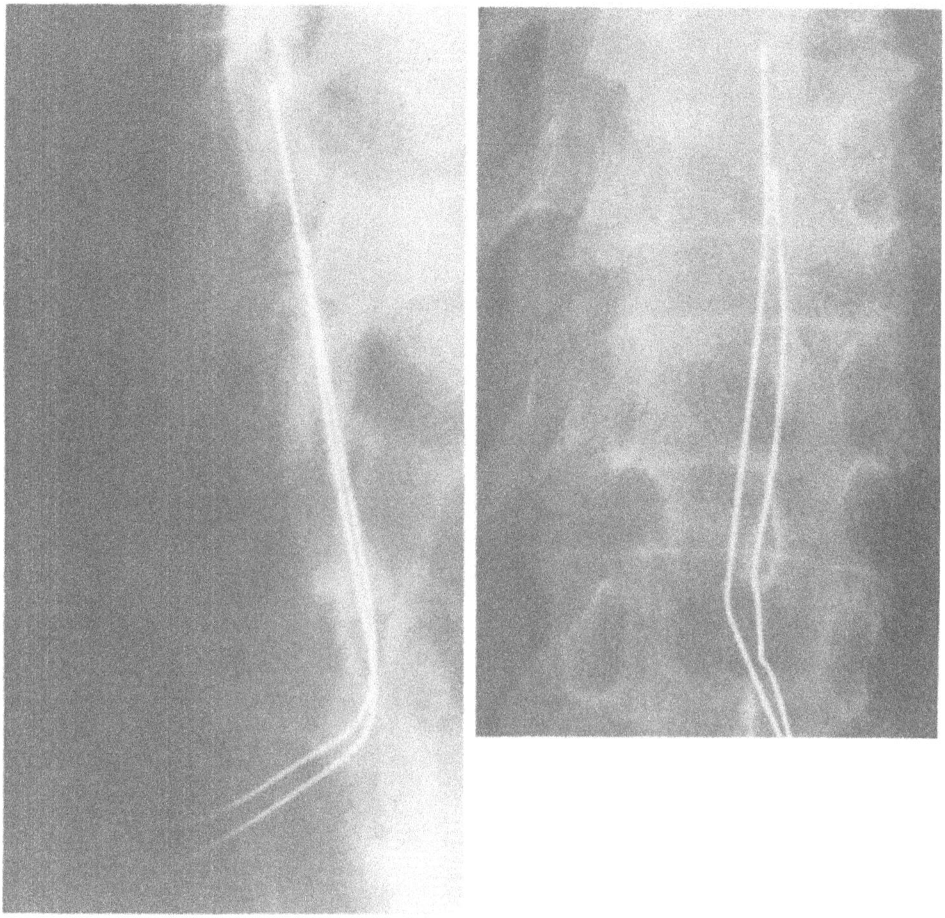

Fig. 11. Position of dorsal epidural electrodes placed via percutaneous needles introduced at T12-L1 interspace and passed rostrally for at least two vertebral bodies to lie slightly to one side of midline producing stimulus-evoked sensation to ipsilateral painful limb

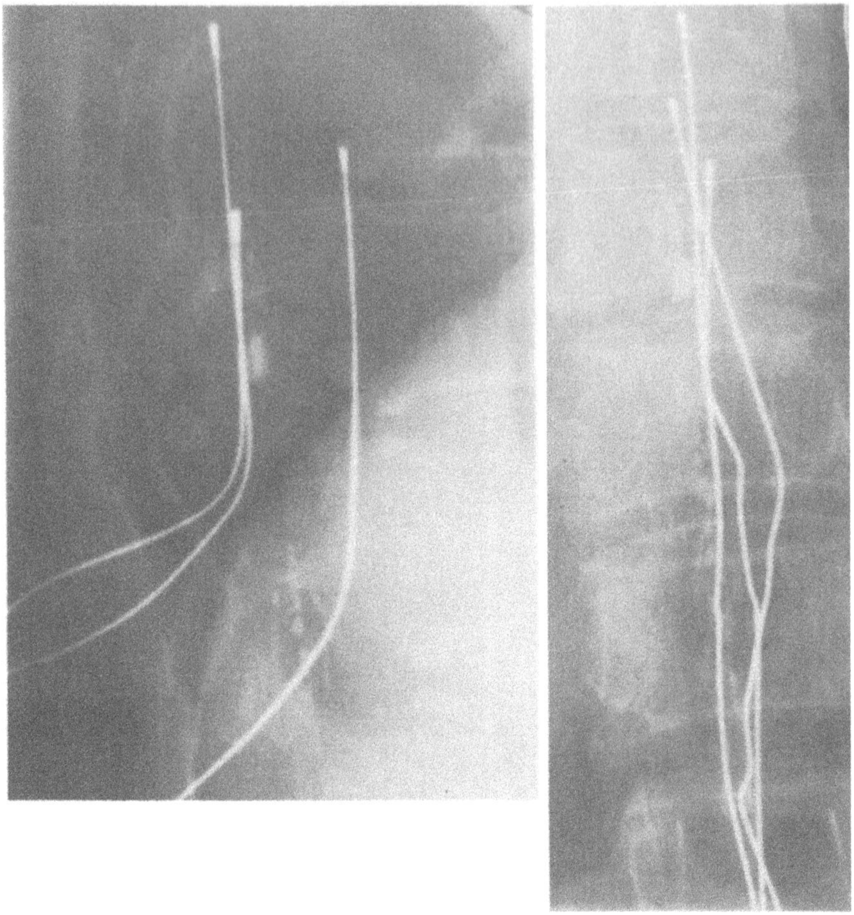

Fig. 12. Placement of one ventral and two dorwal electrodes in lower thoracic epidural space in successful effort to secure reference of stimulus-evoked sensation to saddle area

Fig. 13 A-D. Rat: immunocytochemical staining of posterior horn of spinal cord. *Above:* low magnification; *below:* high magnification of small rectangle indicated in upper view. A, C Somatostatin-like immunoreactivity; B, D substance P-like immunoreactivity
Note: Dense stain for substance P in D in Rexed's lamina 1 (to left of three *small arrows*; absence of stain for somatostatin in C in the same area. C and D are adjoining sections; extensive stain in lamina with both substances. HÖKFELT, T.: Neurosci. 1, 131-136 (1976)

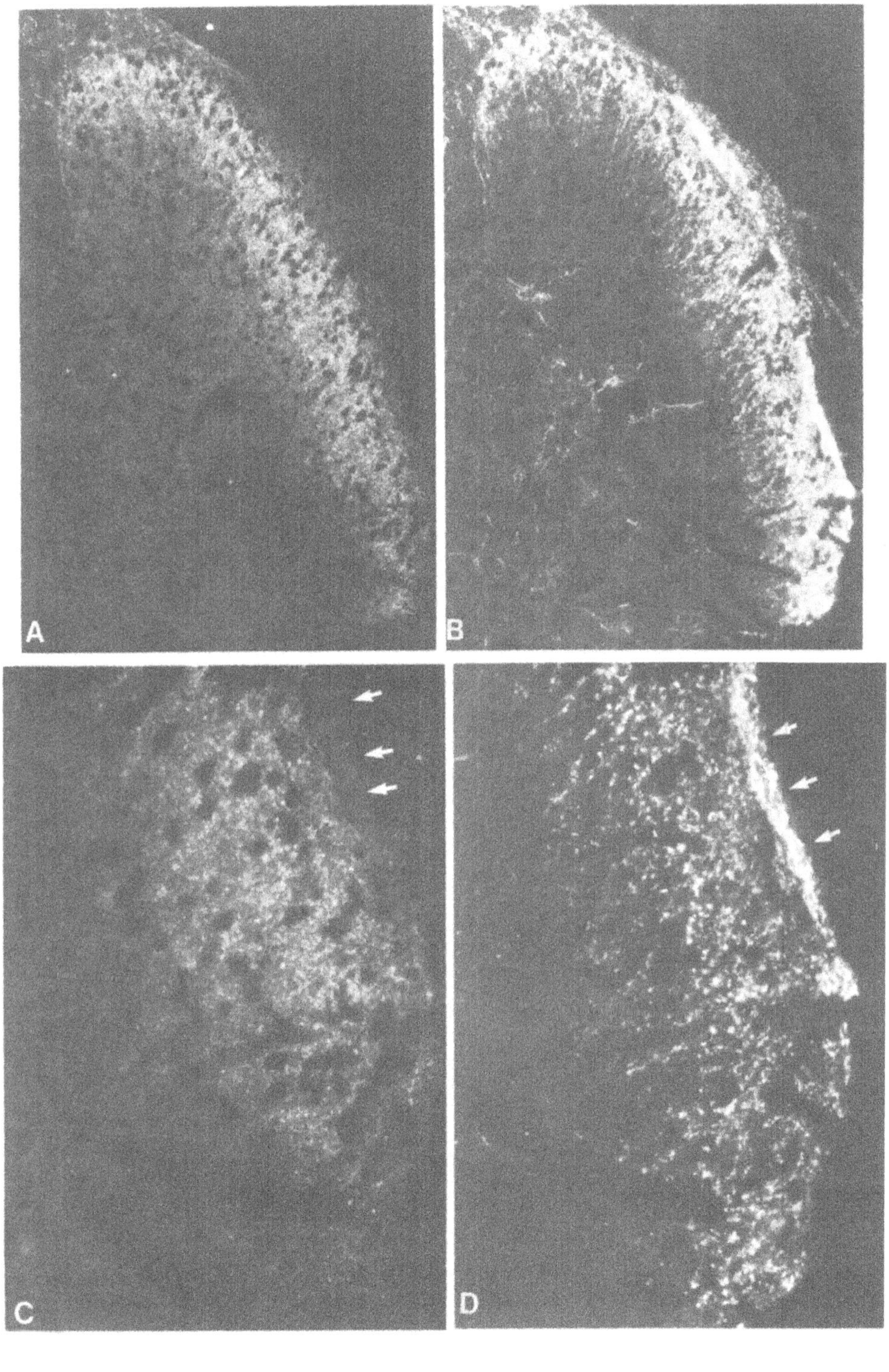
A
B
C
D

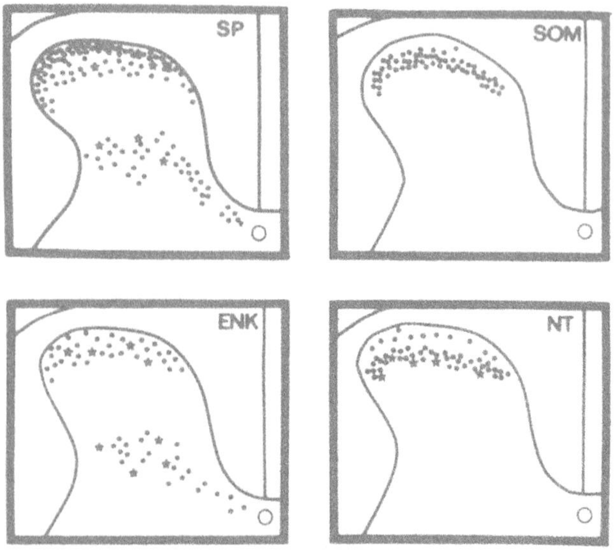

Fig. 14. Diagram of posterior horn of spinal cord to show disposition of fibers *(black dots)* and cells *(black stars)* with immunoreactivity for substance P (SP), somatostatin (SOM), enkephalin (ENK), and neurotensin (NT)

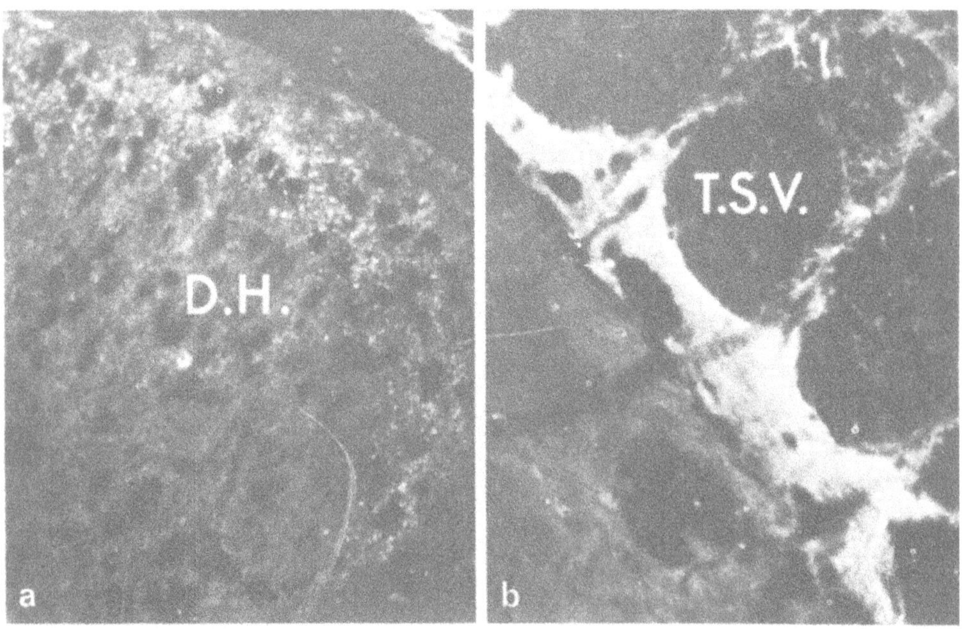

Fig. 15 a, b. Rat: angiotensin II-like immunoreactivity in substantia gelatinosa. In lamina 2 of dorsal horn of spinal cord; in nucleus caudalis of descending tract of trigeminal, nervus intermedius, glossopharyngeal, and vagus nerves D.H., dorsal horn; T.S.V., tract of spinal (descending) fifth cranial nerve. HÖKFELT, T.: Neurosci. Letters 2, 231 (1976)

Free Topics

Annual Academy Award Paper
Spinal Cord Blood Flow in Experimental Spinal Cord Trauma

H. J. SENTER

Introduction

The hypothesis that a portion of the neural dysfunction resulting from spinal cord trauma relates to pathophysiologic responses of the nervous system constitutes a basis for the hope that post-trauma therapy can reduce the cripling effects of spinal cord injury. Alterations in spinal cord blood flow (SCBF) may be one of the responses causing secondary injury in the traumatized spinal cord (16). The present study investigates the time course, quantitative alterations, and some of the factors responsible for changes in SCBF after severe experimental spinal cord injury. The data suggests that if altered blood flow contributes to the neural dysfunction, then therapeutic intervention instituted during the early post-traumatic period aimed at increasing SCBF may prove of value in preventing injury from secondary spinal cord ischemia.

Materials and Methods

The method used for measuring SCBF in these studies is the hydrogen clearance technique. This technique is based on the detection of the current generated by the oxidation of hydrogen at the surface of a platinum electrode implanted in tissue that is satured with inhaled hydrogen (3,4). Polarization of the platinum electrode against a silver reference electrode oxidizes the hydrogen at the surface of the electrode, and as the hydrogen is cleared from the tissue by blood and expired via the lungs, the clearance rate is reflected by a decreasing current (4,53). The relationship between the clearance rate and blood flow is described by the Fick equation as reviewed by AUKLAND and KETY (3,4,35). The major difficulties encountered with this technique when used to measure SCBF is the problem of obtaining reliable and reproducible results over a number of hours. To overcome this problem, the technique was refined as follows (64):

1) The use of electrolytically etched platinum microelectrodes
2) Standardization of electrode resistance, impedance, voltage, and current at each recording site and over the duration of the experiment
3) Modifications in amplifier and recording circuitry
4) Relatively atraumatic and stereotaxic placement of electrodes
5) Stabilization of the spinal column and decrease in respiratory movement

Materials and Methods

Electrodes are made from 250-μm diameter platinum wire etched with 15 V in a solution of 1.0 N NaOH and 0.6 N $NaNO_2$ to a 10-μm tip, 150 - 200 μm base diameter, and 700-μm taper length. The electrode is insulated by dipping into commercial nail hardener with nylon. The distal 0.7 mm is stripped of insulation under a dissecting microscope and the shaft calibrated at 0.5 mm intervals. Electrode impedance is determined and those with impedance greater than 25 kΩ are discarded. Electrodes are also bubble tested to check insulation. The amplifier has been modified after PASZTOR, DORSCH and BRANSTON (53) to sense ± 50 pA, with a maximum output of 5 mA, 0-1 Hz range and ability to detect microampere current changes. Gain and baseline are calibrated by an internal 110-mV source, and current is continuously monitored and matched when two or more electrodes are used simultaneously in different regions. The amplifier design with modifications is shown in Fig. 1.

Adult cats weighing 3 - 4 kg are anesthetized by intraperitoneal pentobarbital (35 mg/kg). The femoral artery and vein are cannulated and a tracheostomy performed. The animal is then paralyzed with gallamine triethiodide (Flaxedil) administered intravenously (1.5 mg/kg/h) and ventilated with oxygen-nitrous oxide gas (50%-50%) for the duration of the experiment. Arterial blood pressure, core and epidural temperature, and end-tidal CO_2 are continuously monitored and recorded. Arterial blood gases are obtained before, during, and after hydrogen saturation, and pO_2 and pCO_2 are maintained in a physiologic range (pO_2 > 90 and pCO_2 32-38 mm Hg). A dorsal laminectomy is performed from T4-T7. The cat is placed in a Kopf spinal stereotaxic holder in which the head, upper and lower thoracic spinous process, and pelvis are immobilized. Further diminution of motion is obtained by placement of a chest tube attached to a 20 cm^3 balloon, which dampens negative intrathoracic pressure. An Ag-$AgCl_2$ reference electrode is implanted subcutaneously adjacent to the laminectomy site. At the T6 level, using the operating microscope, the dura is incised 0.4 mm lateral to the dorsal root entry zone. On a micromanipulator, electrodes with a sharp 10-μm tip are advanced at a 45° angle to a depth of 1.25 mm without visible trauma to the cord. The laminectomy site is then filled with mineral oil and a microthermister placed in the epidural space to record temperature. Core and epidural temperature were both maintained within a range of 37.5° C ± 1.5° C.

The recording electrode is polarized with 650 mV for 15 min. Hydrogen, 6% of minute volume, is then added to the inspired gas until the tissue is saturated and a plateau is reached on the chart recorder. The hydrogen is turned off and the decreasing current recorded. Because of arterial recirculation, the first 45 s of every desaturation curve is disregarded (53). Time versus current is plotted on semilog paper, and the best fitting straight line determined. The T 1/2 is read off of this curve and used to calculate SCBF according to the Fick principle (3,35,53).

$$SCBF = \frac{69.31}{T\ 1/2}\ ml/100\ g/min.$$

In addition, a least squares and linear regression analysis is performed by computer.

The control series (group A) consisted of five cats that had SCBF measurements obtained at 45-min intervals for 6 h from two sites 1 cm apart. The trauma series (group B) consisted of ten animals prepared as above. Three to five control SCBF measurements were obtained on each cat from two electrode sites 1 cm above and 2 cm below the proposed site of trauma T6. Both electrodes were removed and 500 g/cm lesion (a 20 g weight dropped from a 25 cm height) was inflicted by the method of ALLEN (16), as modified by this laboratory (15). Electrodes were implanted in the dorsolateral funiculus at the level of trauma and 1 cm below trauma. SCBF measurements were obtained at 45-60 min intervals for the next 6 - 7 h.

The control autoregulation series (group C) consisted of five cats that had multiple blood flow measurements obtained at different levels of systemic arterial pressure (mSAP). After three to five flows had been obtained at normal blood pressure, mSAP was elevated by Harvard pump infusion or Aramine or lowered by infusion of nitroprusside.

The trauma autoregulation series (group D) consisted of five animals prepared as in the trauma series (group B) above. After the 500 mg/cm injury was inflicted at T6, the blood pressure was allowed to stabilize at its new lower level for 10 min, then was elevated back to its pre-trauma blood pressure by Aramine. SCBF determinations were obtained for 3.5 h. At this time, blood pressure was lowered with nitroprusside to 50 mm Hg, SCBF measured, then mSAP re-elevated with Aramine. Blood flow measurements were then obtained for another hour.

The control and GHB series (group E-1) consisted of three cats that had three to five control blood flow measurements obtained, then were given a bolus of gamma hydroxybutyrate (GHB) 300 mg/kg in 20 cc D_5W IV over 15 min, followed 1 h later by infusion of GHB 200 mg/kg/h. SCBF was recorded from both electrode sites for 6 h. The trauma and GHB bolus series (group E-2) consisted of five cats prepared as in group B (above). A single bolus of GHB (300 mg/kg) was given 0.5 h after cord trauma and blood flow recorded for 6 h. The trauma and GHB (bolus and infusion) series (group E-3) consisted of five animals prepared as in E-2 except that in addition to the initial GHB bolus given 0.5 h after trauma, a continuous infusion of GHB in D_5W (200 mg/kg/h) was begun 1 h after the bolus (1.5 h after trauma) and continued for 5 h. Blood flow was simultaneously recorded both at trauma and 1 cm below trauma for the 6-h recording period. Group E-4 consisted of four animals in whom dose response and time of administration response experiments were performed. Doses of 600 mg/kg and 150 mg/kg GHB were given to two cats respectively 0.5 h after cord trauma. An additional two animals were given GHB 300 mg/kg 2 h and 7 h, respectively, after 500 g/cm trauma was inflicted.

Group F consisted of five animals in whom the role of dopamine in post-traumatic blood flow patterns was investigated. Three animals were treated with haloperidol (a dopamine receptor antagonist) (26,70) in a dose of 0.35 mg/kg bolus 0.5 h after trauma and 0.36 mg/kg/h infusion 1.5 h post-trauma. Two animals received post-trauma treatment with apomorphine (a dopamine receptor stimulator) (26,70) in a dose of 2 mg/kg IP 0.5 h after trauma. Group G consisted of three animals in whom the treatment regimen consisted of aminophylline (a phosphodiesterase inhibitor) (20,26) doses of 3 mg/kg/h, 0,3 mg/kg/h, and 0.15 mg/kg/h with Isuprel (a β-adrenergic stimulator) (20,26) 3 μg/kg/h, 0.3 μg/kg/h, and 0.15 μg/kg/h respectively. In all series, the cat was sacrificed by perfusion with formalin and the cord removed for histologic examination of both electrode sites and cord trauma. The groups can be summarized as follows:

Group	Description	No. of animals
A	Control nontrauma	5
B	Control trauma	10
C	Control autoregulation	5
D	Trauma autoregulation	5
E-1	GHB control nontrauma	3
E-2	Trauma and GHB (bolus)	5
E-3	Trauma and GHB (bolus and infusion)	5
E-4	Trauma and GHB (dose response and time response)	4
F	Trauma and dopamine agonists and antagonists	5
G	Trauma and aminophylline plus Isuprel	3

Results

Control Series

A typical clearance curve from the control series is shown in Fig. 2a, which when transposed to semilog paper reveals a monoexponential decay (Fig. 2b), Figure 2c is the histologic demonstration of the recording site from which this curve was obtained. SCBF was 11.77 ml/100 g/min. For comparison, Fig. 3 a-c represents a traumatically placed electrode with its washout curve, biexponential semilog transposition, and histologic placement, respectively. Analysis reveals a slow clearance rate from A to B of 6.11 ml/100 g/min followed by a rapid phase from B to C of 11.66 ml/100 g/min. Such a biexponential function is one indication of technique failure in measuring white matter SCBF (34, 49,64). No such curves were included in any series. During hydrogen saturation, there was no detectable change in blood pressure, pulse rate, or pulse pressure. Although both end-tidal CO_2 and pCO_2 decreased slightly during the administration of hydrogen, both returned to normal within 20 s of cessation of hydrogen and remained at control levels during the time required for the hydrogen clearance.

Table 1 presents the control series for the present study. Based on 51 sequential determinations at eight electrode sites in five cats, the SCBF in the dorsolateral funiculus of T6 was 10.99 ml/100 g/min $\pm$ 0.89. Figure 4 presents the control series as percent change in SCBF against time over a 6.5-h recording period showing no significant change in SCBF during this period.

Trauma Series

1. Pretrauma Control Flows

Three to five pretrauma control flows were obtained in all cats. The average of the pretrauma control flows in this seires was 11.13 ml/100 g/min $\pm$ 1.29 (n = 38). The average of all control, pretrauma, and predrug administration flows from the total series of 50 animals was 11.59 ml/100 g/min $\pm$ 2.4 (n = 272). Both these values correlate well with each other and with the average SCBF from our initial control seires (above).

Table 1. Spinal cord blood flow (SCBF) utilizing the hydrogen clearance technique

Cat No.	No.[a]	SCBF[b]	SD[c]
1	4	12.15	± 0.80
	5	10.30	± 0.70
2	7	10.46	± 1.20
3	7	11.13	± 1.09
	7	13.28	± 1.81
4	8	9.96	± 0.96
5	8	10.09	± 0.97
	5	10.58	± 0.64
Mean	51	10.99	± 0.89[b]
Range		10.0	13.3[b]

a Number of consecutive blood flow determinations at each electrode site.
b SCBF, spinal cord blood flow in ml/100 g/min.
c SD, Standard deviation.

2. *Changes in Physiologic Parameters Due to Trauma*

In this laboratory, 500 g/cm injury at T6 has consistently produced complete paraplegia in 100% of animals, with no recovery during a 2-month follow-up period. In all cats, 500 g/cm injury induced profound but short lasting changes in physiologic parameters. Mean systemic arterial pressure (mSAP) nearly doubled, remained elevated for 45 s, then over 10 min gradually fell to a level of 30 - 40 mm Hg lower than the pretrauma blood pressure. The mSAP thereafter remained approximately at this level for the duration of the experiment. Pulse pressure increased and cardiac rate decreased during the same time period but returned to normal before the first SCBF determination.

3. *Changes in SCBF Due to Trauma*

Flows Observed at the Site of Trauma. Figure 5a demonstrates a typical white matter clearance curve from a pre-trauma control flow, and Fig. 5b is its monoexponential semilog transposition. The SCBF was 9.77 ml/100 g/min. Figure 5c is the clearance curve obtained from the same animal 4 h after 500 g/cm trauma recorded from the level of trauma. The SCBF was 6.90 ml/100 g/min. Figure 5d is its monoexponential semilog transposition, and Fig. 5e is the histologic demonstration of the recording site showing an electrode tract at a level that reveals the typical central hemorrhagic necrosis of experimental spinal cord trauma (14,18,16,56). Figure 6a presents the SCBF measurements obtained in each animal during the post-traumatic period. SCBF is shown as percent SCBF versus time with each animal's pretrauma SCBF measurements being taken as 100%. It is evident that nine of ten cats maintained blood flow to the injured cord segment during the 1st h after trauma and then developed ischemia. Only one animal (No. 6) became ischemic within the 1st hour after trauma. Additionally, three of the ten cats had return of blood flow by the end of the 6-h period.

Table 2. SCBF, pCO_2, and mSAP before and after trauma in ten cats, recorded at trauma

Before trauma				After trauma		
Cat No.	$\bar{X}$ SCBF[a]	pCO_2[b]	mSAP[c]	SCBF (6 h after trauma)	pCO_2[b]	mSAP[c]
1	11.62	31	100	13.41	32	65
2	9.89	36	140	6.62	34	110
3	13.30	36	110	12.44	34	85
4	11.36	34	140	7.22	34	75
5	9.29	36	150	5.11	33	65
6	13.84	38	150	5.73	35	65
7	8.90	31	150	8.32	32	65
8	9.71	35	125	4.64	34	75
9	10.98	32	120	6.31	37	100
10	10.64	32	100	6.50	33	100
Mean	11.13 $\pm$ 1.29 (n = 38)	34	125	7.62	34	80

a Spinal cord blood flow in ml/100 g/min.
b Measured as mm Hg.
c Mean systemic arterial pressure in mm Hg.

Table 2 presents SCBF, pCO_2, and mSAP at trauma for each of the ten cats before trauma and at the end of the 6-h recording period. Neither at the trauma site nor 1 cm away was there a consistent relationship between blood pressure, body weight, pretrauma SCBF, pCO_2, or histologic degree of tissue damage and the return of blood flow after 6 h. The single animal with early ischemia (No. = 6) did, however, demonstrate more extensive grey and white matter hemorrhages over a greater number of cord segments than did the other animals. Figure 6b shows the average SCBF measurements recorded at trauma in these ten cats (n = 62). Again, SCBF is presented as percent SCBF against time with each animal compared to its own pretrauma controls. The vertical lines indicate the standard deviation, and the two-tailed Student *t* test for each point is shown compared to control flows over a similar time period from the control series (Fig. 4). SCBF did not differ significantly from normal values for the 1st hour after trauma ($P > 0.1$) but was significantly reduced at subsequent time periods ($P < 0.005$). At 6.5 h however, $P < 0.03$, which reflects the fact that three animals did demonstrate a return of blood flow toward normal values. The average SCBF at 6.5 - 7 h after trauma was, however, still reduced by almost 40%. Below the SCBF is the graph of simultaneous blood pressure changes after trauma. The average mSAP before trauma was 125 mm Hg. After a short hypertensive response to trauma, mSAP fell an average of 30 - 40 mm Hg. It is important to note that although mSAP fell within 10 min of trauma, SCBF did not fall until 1 - 2 h later.

Flows Observed 1 cm Below Trauma. Figure 7a presents the SCBF in the same ten animals measured 1 cm below the site of trauma over the same 6.5-h recording period (n = 62). Again nine of ten animals demonstrated a period of time after trauma during which flow was maintained, then progressed to statistically significant ischemia. Four animals at this site demonstrated a return of blood flow after the 6th hour. Figure 7b sums the data from Fig. 7a. SCBF was not significantly decreased 1 cm away from trauma until over 2 h following injury, although mSAP fell within 10 min to 30 - 40 mm Hg below the pretrauma blood pressure.

Control Autoregulation

Figure 8 a-d represents blood flow measurements (and their monoexponential semilog transpositions) made at blood pressures of 50, 100, 150 and 200 mm Hg in a nontraumatized cat. Blood flow values were 8.72, 11.40, 13.27, and 17.85 ml/100 g/min, respectively.

Figure 9 presents the data obtained in five cats that had blood pressures manipulated as previously described. In two of the cats, only a single electrode was functioning. It is evident that all cats regulated blood flow fairly well below 90 mm Hg, but some animals had virtually no autoregulation above this blood pressure. Below 40 mm Hg, SCBF fell so precipitously that no accurate washout curve could be obtained in any animal.

Trauma Autoregulation Series

Figure 10a demonstrates a pretrauma clearance curve along with its semilog transposition. Figure 10b and c are blood flow determinations and their monoexponential transpositions at 1 h and 3.5 h, respectively, after trauma when blood pressure has been elevated to pretrauma levels by infusion of Aramine. Figure 10d is the histologic demonstration of the recording site for this experiment.

Figure 11a shows the average SCBF measurements recorded at trauma in these five cats. Again, SCBF is presented as percent SCBF against time with each animal compared to its own pretrauma controls. The vertical lines indicate standard deviation, and the two-tailed Student t test for each point is shown compared to the trauma series (group B) (Fig. 6b). Below the graph of SCBF is presented the average blood pressure at each time point with the post-traumatic hypotension indicated as well as the episode of nitroprusside-induced hypotension. It is evident that blood flow did not become significantly different from the non-blood pressure manipulated trauma series for over 1 h. Thereafter, SCBF in the normotensive series was significantly higher than in the non-blood pressure manipulated (trauma hypotensive) series ($P < 0.001$). When the blood pressure was lowered to 50 mm Hg by nitroprusside infusion, ischemia was reproduced, but the SCBF was so slow (less than 5 ml/100 g/min) that no exact value could be ascribed to this point. When blood pressure was again elevated, a return to the increased level of SCBF was seen ($P < 0.001$). After this episode of hypotension, there was no significant decrease in SCBF. Therefore, a postischemic "no-reflow" phenomenon was not seen in this model at the level of the most severe injury with this period and degree of hypotension.

Figure 11b presents data on the same five cats whose blood flow was simultaneously recorded 1 cm below the site of trauma. Again, SCBF is presented as percent SCBF against each cat's pretrauma blood flow measurements. At this site, SCBF was not different from the trauma series until nearly 2 h after trauma, then was statistically higher ($P < 0.001$). After the episode of nitroprusside-induced hypotension,

SCBF was transiently increased, but this was not statistically significant ($\underline{P} < 0.1$). In this model, postischemic hyperemia, therefore, did not occur at a site 1 cm below the point of maximum injury in the lateral column.

GHB Series

Group E-1: GHB Control

Figure 12 presents the data obtained in group E-1 where nontraumatized animals were treated with GHB, 300 mg/kg bolus followed in 1 h by a continuous infusion of 200 mg/kg/h. It is evident that there was a rapid and significant increase in SCBF when compared to the control series ($\underline{P} < 0.005$) (Fig. 4). After 3 h, however, despite continuous infusion of GHB, blood flow returned to normal and remained at the level for the duration of the experiment. During GHB administration, there was no significant change in pCO_2, pO_2, pH, end-tidal CO_2, core or epidural temperature, or mSAP to account for this finding. MACMILLAN also showed that GHB administration in doses of 500 mg/kg did not alter any of these physiologic parameters (46). All washout curves were monoexponential and had electrode placement confirmed histologically.

Group E-2: Trauma + GHB (Bolus)

Figure 13 presents the data obtained at the level of trauma in group E-2. A single bolus of GHB (300 mg/kg in 20 cc D_5W) was given 0.5 h after 500 g/cm trauma. Initially, an increase in SCBF was seen that less than 3 h ($\underline{P} < 0.005$) and then progressed to ischemia. After 3 h, the ischemia was the same as in the non-drug treated group ($\underline{P} < 0.5$). The hypertensive-hypotensive response to cord injury was not altered by the GHB administration. Additionally, no significant change was seen in pCO_2, end-tidal CO_2, core or epidural temperature, or mSAP due to the GHB bolus.

Group E-3: Trauma + GHB (Bolus and Infusion)

In this series of five animals, three to five pretrauma blood flow determinations were obtained and trauma inflicted at T6 in the usual manner. One-half hour after trauma, a GHB bolus (300 mg/kg) was given. One hour later (1.5 h after trauma), GHB infusion was begun at 200 mg/kg/h and continued for the duration of the experiment. Sequential blood flow determinations were recorded both at the level of trauma and 1 cm below trauma for the next 6.5 - 7 h. Figure 14 a-c presents a pretrauma blood flow, a 1-h and a 6-h post-trauma blood flow, respectively, and their semilog monoexponential transpositions. Blood flow values were 11.17, 12.83, and 10.50 ml/100 g/min, respectively. Figure 14d demonstrates the recording site from which these flows were obtained showing the typical feature of central hemorrhagic necrosis and scattered petechial white matter hemorrhages (16,56).

Figure 15 a and b present the SCBF at the level of trauma and 1 cm below trauma as followed for 6.5 h in these five animals. The SCBF of each animal is presented as percent —— of ——> its own pretrauma control flow. The time of trauma, GHB bolus, and GHB infusion are so indicated. It is evident that at the level of trauma (Fig. 15a) GHB caused a hyperemia in four of five animals and allowed only a 15% fall in SCBF in the fifth animal. The single cat with the nonhyperemic respone (—●—) had both a higher pretrauma blood flow (15 ml/100 g/min) and a slightly lower pCO_2 (31 mm Hg) than the other animals. One centimeter below trauma (Fig. 15b), four of five animals maintained blood flow in the normal range (± 15% of pretrauma SCBF), while only one animal demonstrated hyperemia. The two animals with a 15% fall in blood flow despite GHB (—*— and —◆—) had no significant difference in any physiologic parameter.

Figure 16a and b present the average of all SCBF measurements recorded at trauma and below trauma, respectively. Again SCBF is presented as percent SCBF ——→ against time with each animal compared to its own pretrauma controls. Standard deviation and two-tailed Student *t* test for each point are shown compared to the trauma (Fig. 16a), all blood flow determinations, including those within the 1st hour, were significantly different from the non-drug treated group ($P < 0.01$ or better). As long as the infusion was continued, blood flow remained normal or elevated and no post-traumatic ischemia occurred. Figure 16b demonstrated that 1 cm below trauma blood flow remained elevated for the duration of the experiment but was not statistically different from the non-drug trauma series for nearly 2 h. At no time during the bolus or infusion was there any significant change in pCO_2, end-tidal CO_2, temperature, or blood pressure that could account for these blood flow patterns. We were aware of the possible association between increased blood flow and increased grey and white matter hemorrhage (56) but were not able to make a definite association between the two parameters in this study.

Other Drug Studies

In two animals, the dose of the GHB bolus was changed. It was found that a 600 mg/kg bolus approached the LD_{50} and produced severe hypotension. A second cat was treated with a post-traumatic bolus of 150 mg/kg, which had little effect on the ischemia. It was concluded that a 600 mg/kg dose was too toxic and a 150 mg/kg dose ineffective. No further investigations were performed on bolus or infusion dose-response relationships. In two other animals, however, GHB (300 mg/kg bolus) was administered at 2 h and 7 h after cord trauma when ischemia was already seen. In both cases there was no increase in SCBF in the ischemic area. Alterations in dose or time of administration of GHB did not otherwise change the physiologic parameters described above.

Dopaminergic Active Drugs

Because GHB is known to inhibit the firing of nigrostriatal dopaminergic neurons and secondarily increase local dopamine stores (58,70), it was decided to investigate the effects of both a dopamine receptor antagonist (haloperidol) (26,70) and a dopamine receptor stimulator (apomorphine) (26,70) on post-traumatic SCBF. Figure 17a presents SCBF data obtained in three animals treated with a bolus (0.35 mg/kg) and infusion (0.35 mg/kg/h) of haloperidol during the same time periods as in the GHB trauma series (Fig. 16a). Similar doses of haloperidol have been shown to effectively block nigrostriatal dopamine receptors (70). At no point were there any significant differences between the trauma and trauma haloperidol groups ($P < 0.5$). Two other animals were given (apomorphine) 0.5 h after trauma in a dose capable of stimulating nigrostriatal dopaminergic receptors for up to 3 h (70). Once again, ischemia was reproduced in the same time pattern as the nontreated trauma series (Fig. 17b). No data points from this series were significantly different from the trauma series ($P < 0.5$).

Aminophylline Plus Isuprel

In a final series of three animals, aminophylline and Isuprel (a phosphodiesterase inhibitor and β-adrenergic stimulator) (20,26) were given by continuous infusion during the same post-traumatic period. Aminophylline doses administered were 3 mg/kg/h, 0.3 mg/kg/h, and 0.15 mg/kg/h with Isuprel doses of 3 μg/kg/h, 0.3 μg/kg/h, and 0.15 μg/kg/h, respectively. Similar doses of both these drugs in combination have been used to reverse experimental basilar artery spasm (20). The larger doses in the first animal caused a dramatic fall in blood pressure, but the two smaller doses caused no significant change in mSAP. Figure 17c shows that in all three animals, however, post-traumatic SCBF was unchanged from the non-drug treated trauma series ($P < 0.5$). In all series, the cat was sacrificed by perfusion with formalin and the cord removed for histologic examination of both electrode sites and cord trauma.

Discussion

There have been several studies designed to investigate the effect of trauma on SCBF (6,7,12,14,16,17,28,38,60,62,65). All studies agree that ischemia is the principal grey matter response, but there has been controversy as to the effect of trauma on white matter blood flow. The preservation of white matter integrity is of paramount clinical concern in maintaining long tract function. Because of previous criticisms of blood flow determinations by the hydrogen clearance method, we have modified the original technique extensively (64). The SCBF in the dorsolateral funiculus of cat thoracic cord was 10.99 ml/100 g/min + 0.89 in our control series (n = 51) and 11.59 ml/100 g/min ± 2.4 (n = 272) in all of our pretrauma and pre-blood pressure manipulation studies. Both these values correlate very well with autoradiographic measurements of thoracic cord white matter flow of 10.30 ml/100 g/min (59,61). As shown in Fig. 4, SCBF was not altered either by the number of blood flow determinations made at one site or the total time span of the experiment. The consistency, reliability, and reproducibility of our data compares favorably with the majority of techniques used by previous investigators (29,36). The ability to use each animal as its own control, plus the ability to record from one site over many hours, are significant advantages over methods that require the animal to be sacrificed to obtain a blood flow measurement.

In the trauma series of experiments, all animals demonstrated significant ischemia, both at the level of trauma and 1 cm below the site of trauma. Ischemia was, however, delayed in onset for 1 h at the level of trauma and below the site of injury; ischemia was delayed in onset for nearly 2 h after cord injury. Blood flow was maintained for 1 - 2 h after injury despite the fact that mSAP fell 30-40 mm Hg within 10 min after trauma. While the delay in onset of ischemia seemed uniform, there was a variable degree of return of blood flow at the end of the 7-h post-traumatic period in three of ten animals. There was no consistent correlation between return of blood flow and pCO_2, blood pressure, pretrauma SCBF, or the histologic degree of tissue damage. This return of flow does suggest, however, that cord vessels are not mechanically disrupted or occluded and are potentially able to carry adequate flow to the damaged cord segments. The correlation, in one animal, between the histologic severity of grey and white matter hemorrhages and the earlier onset of ischemia suggests that the degree of ischemia is proportional to the severity of the trauma. DUCKER has suggested that the degree of functional neurological recovery is dependent on the return of blood flow (16).

In one group of monkeys that recovered full neurological function after cord trauma, blood flow nearly doubled during the posttraumatic period (1 h up to 1 week). In animals that were paraparetic with partial preservation of function, SCBF during the post-traumatic period remained normal. In his completely paraplegic group, SCBF was significantly reduced during the post-traumatic period. He concluded that SCBF was the major determinant of neurological recovery in the post-traumatic period. Unfortunately, his technique, which measures argon clearance by a mass spectrometer, cannot differentiate grey from white matter flows and involves the insertion of a 1 mm probe into a 5 mm spinal cord, which may itself produce trauma (16,59,60).

Despite these studies, the precise relationship between spinal cord ischemia and neurological function is unknown. GOODING et al. have suggested that the combination of ischemia plus mechanical disruption is required to produce a severe myelopathy (25). In nontraumatized cord, they showed that severe ischemia alone failed to produce the permanent neurological deficit that compression plus ischemia produced. The exact percent decrease in blood flow necessary to produce neurological dysfunction in normal and traumatized cords is unknown, but our data suggests that a 40% decrease in SCBF in a severely traumatized cord is sufficient to produce a complete and permanent paraplegia.

In the cerebral vasculature, the ability to maintain blood flow despite changes in both intracranial pressure and blood pressure (autoregulation) is well known, although the mechanisms that mediate the compensatory changes in the vascular resistance in response to changes in blood pressure are not well understood (11). In the intact spinal cord, autoregulation has been documented by two investigators. KOBRINE et al. found a range of intact autoregulation between mSAP of 50 - 135 mm Hg (39). GRIFFITHS et al. recorded a range of intact autoregulation from 60 - 150 mm Hg (27). Both studies, however, induced hypotension by phlebotomy, which changes blood viscosity, hematocrit level, and circulating blood volume, all of which may influence vascular resistance and blood flow. Hypertension was induced either by norepinephrine, which is known to decrease cerebral blood flow, or angiotensin, which also has a direct sympathomimetic effect on the CNS (26). Aramine was used in this study because it is thought to act as a peripheral vasoconstrictor without CNS effects (26). Nitroprusside is believed to be a pure peripheral vasodilator with no known effect of blood viscosity (26). Our data is not in agreement with either previous study. Autoregulation in the dorsolateral funiculus of the thoracic cord was present only between blood pressures within the narrow range of 40 - 90 mm Hg. The response to blood pressures greater than 90 mm Hg was highly variable. Whether this represents different populations in our experimental groups or the influence of other factors during the experiment is not known. Unlike the cerebral vasculature with its blood supply by high volume, high pressure vessels (i.e., the carotid and vertebral vasculature), autoregulation in the spinal cord may not regulate blood flow to any but frankly hypotensive blood pressures.

The trauma autoregulation series of experiments demonstrate that autoregulation is intact during the initial post-traumatic period. Figure 18 schematically summarizes the data. Although mSAP fell 30-40 mm Hg within 10 min after trauma, SCBF was maintained for over 1 h. If mSAP was elevated back to normal during this time, SCBF did not increase further. This implies that in the trauma hypotensive and trauma normotensive series, autoregulation is intact during the 1st hour at the level of trauma and for nearly 2 h 1 cm below trauma. After this point, however, if the blood pressure was elevated with

Aramine, SCBF increased dramatically ($P < 0.001$) at both electrode sites, indicating loss of autoregulation. Four hours later, nitroprusside-induced hypotension reproduced severe ischemia in all cats. Return of mSAP to normal did not induce either thrombosis (the no-reflow phenomenon) at the level of trauma nor reactive hyperemia 1 cm below. The data, therefore, suggests that, in our model, autoregulation is lost on a delayed basis after experimental cord trauma and may be a factor responsible for post-traumatic white matter ischemia.

What happens in vivo to the resistance vessel when autoregulation is lost is currently not known. The vessel may be fixed in a mid-position or dilated state or may in fact be responding passively to changes in transmural pressure. Figure 18 suggests one possible mechanism. In the spinal cord, where negligible venous pressure is assumed, the relationship between flow, pressure, and resistance is described by (11):

$$\text{Flow} = \frac{\text{Pressure}}{\text{Resistance}} \quad \text{or} \quad \text{SCBF} = \frac{\text{mSAP}}{\text{R}}.$$

During the first 60-90 min after trauma (phase 1), autoregulation is intact. Flow is constant, but blood pressure has fallen, so resistance must be decreased (i.e., vasodilation of the resistance vessel has occurred). After this initial period, autoregulation is lost (phase 2). Flow is decreased, blood pressure remains low, so vascular resistance must be greater than during phase 1 (i.e., mid-position or vasoconstriction of resistance vessel). This explanation supports the ischemic concept of post-traumatic SCBF (60). How these vascular changes are mediated is unknown. Both REIVICH (57) et al. and BRUCE (11) et al. have shown that after cerebral trauma autoregulation is lost in a highly focal pattern, implying local control of autoregulation. KOBRINE et al. have demonstrated no significant loss of autoregulation after cervical cord section, implying local control of autoregulation (i.e., metabolic or myogenic) in the spinal cord (40). Further studies suggested α- and β-adrenergic innervation of spinal cord resistance vessels (41,42). In the present study, the loss of autoregulation at different intervals after cord trauma at the two electrode sites also suggests local control of autoregulation. The delay in onset of ischemia coincident with the loss of autoregulation might be explained on the basis of release of certain vasoactive substances (13,30,32,31,52) Norepinephrine (52), serotonin (10), and dopamine (50) have been suggested as mediators of post-traumitc ischemia. These same substances might be involved in the loss of autoregulation. It is also possible that the delayed loss of autoregulation is secondary to decreased metabolic activity of the injured cord (16,55). In both the nontraumatized cord and within the first 60-90 min after cord trauma, intact autoregulation to low blood pressures may involve an active, energy-dependent vasodilatation, while the loss of autoregulation after trauma may involve a passive, energy-independent response to transmural pressure. At normotensive blood pressures, the resistance vessel may be in mid-position, similar to what has been proposed for the cerebral vasculature. The same dependency of blood flow on systemic arterial pressure has been demonstrated in cerebral ischemia (9,33, 71,72) and vasospasm studies (44).

The role of blood pressure in post-traumatic patterns of SCBF has not been investigated nor emphasized previously in the literature, nor has the loss of autoregulation after spinal cord injury been demonstrated (56,60). It is clear that studies, which do not specify blood pressure alterations and manipulations, are subject to misinterpretation and confusion. Possibly, differences in mSAP in different animal models may account for some of the conflicting literature on post-traumatic alterations in SCBF. If alterations in post-traumatic SCBF do constitute a cause of secondary injury, then, as suggested by RAWE at al. (56), the maintenance of blood pressure within the normal range during the post-traumatic period of "spinal sympathetic shock" might be indicated in selective cases.

The consistent delay in onset of decreased blood flow after trauma suggested that therapeutic intervention within the first 60 - 90 min after cord injury might prove of value in reversing or limiting some elements of long tract dysfunction due to the secondary ischemic insult. The current study suggests that gamma-hydroxybutyrate may alter the ischemic response to trauma.

Gamma-hydroxybutyrate (GHB) is an analogue of GABA, itself known to extend inhibitory actions on some neural systems (58,70). GHB has been shown to act as a central nervous system depressant with specific suppressant action on nigrostriatal dopaminergic neurons and on spinal cord reflexes (58,70). It can cross the intact blood-brain barrier and has been found in normal mammalian brain. The half-life of an anesthetic dose of GHB is about 1 h, and a single dose can abolish the righting reflex in rats for 3 h. While its precise mechanism is unknown, two effects have been identified. GHB inhibits the release of dopamine from dopaminergic neurons resulting in an increase in local tissue dopamine content (58,70). It is also a potent CNS depressant, although its mechanism in this respect is completely unknown. GHB has been used clinically as an anesthetic agent, and it has been investigated for possible beneficial effects in head-injured patients (19). In one study, at a relatively low dose of 60 mg/kg, GHB decreased cerebral metabolic rate ($CMRO_2$) 27% and cerebral A-V O_2 difference by 33% with no effect seen on cerebral blood flow (CBF). The same study, however, found that if a barbiturate was used, a comparable decrease in $CMRO_2$ was associated with a fall in CBF. Relative to the barbiturates, therefore, GHB was able to lower cerebral metabolism while maintaining adequate CBF (19).

In this series of experiments, GHB exerted a significant effect upon blood flow in both the normal and traumatized spinal cord. A single dose produced an increase in post-traumatic SCBF that lasted 2-3 h, thereafter returning to its normally post-traumatic ischemic pattern. If a continuous infusion of GHB was begun 1 h after the single dose, the ischemic response was altered for the duration of the drug infusion. This effect was seen both at the trauma site and 1 cm below the site of trauma. Because of GHB's inhibitory effect on dopaminergic neurons, we attempted but failed to modify the ischemic response with a dopamine receptor blocker reported to have no activity as a CNS depressant (haloperidol) (26). A dopamine receptor stimulator (apomorphine) (26) similarly failed to alter the ischemic response to trauma. This suggests that the effect of GHB on SCBF was not just due to dopamine receptor stimulation or block. However, to confirm the inability of either dopamine receptor stimulators or blockers to alter post-traumatic ischemia, a larger series is needed.

Several studies have attempted to quantify alterations in vasoactive substances occurring after both cerebral ischemia (23,30,43,45,69) and experimental spinal cord injury (13,32,31,37,50,52). Increased levels of norepinephrine (52), histamine (37), serotonin (10), and dopamine (50) have all been reported after cord injury, but results have frequently been contradictory and no single substance has been conclusively linked to post-traumatic blood flow alterations (18). Although both hypothermic irrigation (1,34,68) and the use of specific vasoactive amine blockers have their respective proponents (16,31,34,52), no treatment protocol to date has been shown to alter cord pathology. It is entirely possible that the combination of several vasoactive substances, all released in small amounts after cord injury, could contribute to the ischemia. There is data in both clinical and experimental studies to suggest that small amounts of one vasoactive substance will potentiate the vasoconstrictive properties of other substances (8,23,47, 48,63,67,69). Attempts to increase post-traumatic blood flow should not, therefore, be directed at single vasoactive blocking agents. Several studies in cerebral ischemia (22,24,43,45) and spinal cord trauma (16) have suggested that a cruical time period of 1 - 2 h exists after the insult during which irreversible biochemical (10,16) vascular (2,10, 14,17,16), electrophysiologic (16), and pathologic processes occur (14,16). If the ischemic response to cord injury constitutes a secondary insult, then attempts to increase blood flow during the early post-traumatic period may prove of value in reversing some elements of long tract dysfunction.

The mechanism of GHB-induced hyperemia is unknown. GHB, by acting as a CNS and metabolic depressant (58), may be interfering with the release or activation of several vasoactive substances, possibly through depressed enzymatic activity. MACMILLAN has recently demonstrated that GHB, like the barbiturates, is able to normalize tissue levels of high energy phosphates in hypoxic rat brain and decrease postischemic lactate accumulations (46). A similar mechanism in the ischemic spinal cord could account for the maintenance of blood flow in our GHB-treated traumatized cords. GHB may also be acting as a direct vasodilator; however, preliminary studies in this lab show no effect of GHB on experimental vasospasm, nor did aminophylline and Isuprel, a popular vasodilating regimen (20), have any effect on post-traumatic spinal cord ischemia.

The concept of increasing blood flow while decreasing metabolic activity, thereby protecting ischemic tissue from secondary injury, is not new. In several clinical and laboratory studies, metabolic inhibitors, especially the barbiturates, have demonstrated the ability to minimize neural dysfunction caused by an ischemic insult (5,19,21,46,51,54,66, 73). MACMILLAN has demonstrated that GHB has the ability to alter metabolism in both normoxic and hypoxic models. During prolonged cerebral hypoxia, GHB was able to maintain the cerebral energy state and markedly improve survival from the ischemic-hypoxic insult (46). Other studies suggest that the early return of blood flow to ischemix cortex can restore lost electric activity, normalize metabolic function, improve synaptic transmission, and improve neurological function (9,22, 24,33,71,72). A similar situation may exist in the ischemic spinal cord. Gamma-hydroxybutyrate, by decreasing the metabolic requirements of the injured tissue and simultaneously increasing blood flow, may prove of value in reversing or limiting some elements of long tract dysfunction due to secondary injury.

Conclusions

1) The predominant lateral white matter vascular response to severe experimental spinal cord injury is ischemia when systemic hypotension is present.
2) The ischemia is delayed in onset for over 1 h at the site of trauma and for over 2 h 1 cm below trauma.
3) Autoregulation is intact during the initial hour of the post-traumatic period and is then lost coincident with the onset of ischemia.

The alteration in autoregulation progresses from the site of trauma to 1 cm from trauma within 2 h.

4) The ischemic response may be mediated both by lost autoregulation and by relative vasocinstriction of the resistance vessels.

5) When given during the early post-traumatic period, gamma-hydroxybutyrate prevents the ischemic response and may therefore protect the injured cord from secondary injury.

References

1. ALBIN, M.S., WHITE, R.J., ACOST-RUA, G., YASHON, D.: Study of functional recovery produced by delayed cooling after spinal cord injury in primates. J. Neurosurg. 29, 113-120 (1968)
2. ALLEN, W.E., D'ANGELO, C.M., KIER, E.L.: Correlation of microangiographic and electrophysiologic changes in experimental spinal cord trauma. Radiology 111, 107-115 (1974)
3. AUKLAND, K.: Hydrogen polarography in measurement of local blood flow; theoretical and empirical basis, Acta Neurol. Scand. (Suppl.) 14, 26-29 (1965)
4. AUKLAND, K., BOWER, B.F., BERLINER, R.W.: Measurement of local blood flow with hydrogen gas. Circ. Res. 14, 164-187 (1964)
5. BARKER, J.L.: Central nervous system depressants: Effects on post-synaptic pharmacology. Brain Res. 92, 35-55 (1975)
6. BINGHAM, W.G., GOLDMAN, H., FRIEDMAN, S.J., MURPHY, S., YASHON, D., HUNT, W.E.: Blood flow in normal and injured monkey spinal cord. J. Neurosurg. 43, 162-171 (1975)
7. BINGHAM, W.G., SIRINEK, L., CRUTCHER, K., MOHNACKY, C.: Effect of spinal cord injury on cord and cerebral blood flow in monkey. Acta Neurol. Scand. (Suppl.) 56, 238-239 (1977)
8. BOISUERT, D.P., WEIR, B.K., OVERTON, T.R., REIFFENSTEIN, R., GRACE, M.G.: Cerebrovascular responses to subarachnoid blood and serotonin in the monkey. Acta Neurol. Scand. (Suppl.) 64, 322-323 (1977)
9. BRANSTON, N.M., SYMON, L., STRONG, A.J.: Measurements of autoregulation impairment and low-reflow related to cortical CBF in acute experimental ischemia in baboons. Acta Neurol. Scand. (Suppl. 64) 56, 370-371 (1977)
10. BRODNER, R.A., DOHRMANN, G.J., ROTH, R.H., RUBIN, R.A.: Elevated cerebrospinal fluid levels of 5-hydroxy-tryptamine following experimental spinal cord trauma. Brain Res. 118, 348-351 (1976)
11. BRUCE, D.A., LANGFITT, T.W., MILLER, J.D., SCHURZ, H., VAPALALITE, M.P., STANCK, A., GOLDBERG, H.: Regional cerebral blood flow, intracranial pressure and brain metabolism in comatose patients. J. Neurosurg. 38, 131-139 (1973)
12. CRAWFORD, R.A., GRIFFITHS, I.R., McCULLOCH, J.: The effect of norepinephrine on the spinal cord circulation and its possible implications in the pathogenesis of acute spinal trauma. J. Neurosurg. 47, 567-576 (1977)
13. De la TORRE, J.C., JOHNSON, C.M., HARRIS, L.H.: Monamine changes in experimental head and spinal cord trauma. Surg. Neurol. 2, 5-11 (1974)

14. DOHRMANN, G.J., ALLEN, W.E.: Microcirculation of traumatized spinal cord: a correlation of microangiography and blood flow patterns in transitory and permanent paraplegia. J. Trauma 15, 1003-1013 (1975)

15. DOHRMANN, G.J., PANJABI, M.M., WAGNER, F.C.: An apparatus for quantitating experimental spinal cord trauma. Surg. Neurol. 5, 315-318 (1976)

16. DUCKER, T.B.: Experimental injury of the spinal cord. In: Handbook of clinical neurology. VINKEN, P., BRUYN, G.W. (eds.), Vol. 25, pp. 9-26. Amsterdam: North Holland 1976

17. DUCKER, T.B., PEROT, P.L.: Spinal cord oxygen and blood flow in trauma. Surg. Forum 22, 413-415 (1971)

18. DUCKER, T.B., KINDT, G.W., KEMPE, L.G.: Pathological findings in acute experimental spinal cord trauma. J. Neurosurg. 35, 700-708 (1971)

19. ESCURET, E., ROQUEFEULD, B., FRER BEAU, P., BALDY-MOULINER, M.: Effect of hyperventilation associated with administration of central nervous depressants in brain injuries. Acta Neurol. Scand. (Suppl. 65) 56, 154-155 (1977)

20. FLAMM, E.S., YASARGIL, M.G., RANSOHOFF, J.: Alteration of experimental cerebral vasospasm by adrenergic blockage. J. Neurosurg. 37, 294-301 (1972)

21. FLAMM, E.S., DEMOPOULUS, H.B., SELIGMAN, M.L., RANSOHOFF, J.: Possible molecular mechanisms of barbiturate-mediated protection in regional cerebral ischemia. Acta Neurol. Scand. (Suppl. 65) 56, 150-151 (1977)

22. FRASER, R.A., YOSHIDA, J., PATTERSON, R.H.: Focal cerebral ischemia and the no reflow phenomenon Acta Neurol. Scand. (Suppl. 64) 56, 120-121 (1977)

23. GILBERT, J.C., GOLDBERG, L.I.: Characterization by cyproheptadine of the dopamine-induced contraction in canine isolated arteries. J. Pharmacol. Exp. Ther. 193, 435-442 (1975)

24. GINSBERG, M.D., REIVICH, M., GIANDOMENICO, A.: Regional brain glucose metabolism during recovery from transient cerebral ischemia. Acta Neurol. Scand. (Suppl. 64) 56, 128-129 (1977)

25. GOODING, M.R., WILSON, C.B., HOFF, J.T.: Experimental cervical myelopathy. J. Neurosurg. 43, 9-17 (1975)

26. GOODMAN, L.S., GILMAN, A. (eds.): The pharmacologic basis of therapeutics. New York: MacMillan 1970

27. GRIFFITHS, I.R.: Spinal cord blood flow in dogs: The effect of blood pressure. J. Neurol. Neurosurg. Psychiatry 36, 914-920 (1973)

28. GRIFFITHS, I.R.: Spinal cord blood flow after acute experimental cord injury in dogs. J. Neurol. Sci. 27, 247-259 (1976)

29. GRIFFITHS, I.R., ROWAN, J.O., CRAWFORD, R.A.: Spinal cord blood flow measured by a hydrogen clearance technique. J. Neurol. Sci. 26, 529-544 (1975)

30. HADLY, F.J., SCOTT, J.B.: Metabolically linked vasoactive chemicals in local regulation of blood flow. Physiol. Rev. 48, 688-707 (1968)

31. HEDEMAN, L.S., SIL, R.: Studies in experimental spinal cord trauma. Part II. J. Neurosurg. 40, 44-52 (1974)

32. HEDEMAN, L.S., SHELLENBERGER, M.K., GORDON, J.H.: Studies in experimental spinal cord trauma. Part I: Alterations in catecholamine levels. J. Neurosurg. 40, 37-44 (1974)

33. HOPE, D.T., BRANSTON, N.M., SYMON, L.: Restoration of neurologic function with induced hypertension in acute experimental cerebral ischemia. Acta Neurol. Scand. (Suppl. 64) 56, 506-507 (1977)

34. KELLY, D.L., LASSITER, K.R., CALOGERO, J.A.: Effects of local hypothermia and tissue oxygen studies in experimental paraplegia. J. Neurosurg. 33, 554-563 (1970)

35. KETY, S.S.: Theory of blood-tissue exchange and its application to measurement of blood flow. In: Methods of Medical Research. BRUNER, H.D. (ed.), Vol. 8, pp. 223-233. Chicago: Year Book Publisher 1960

36. KOBRINE, A.I., DOYLE, T.F., MARTINS, A.N.: Spinal cord blood flow in the rhesus monkey by the hydrogen clearance method. Surg. Neurol. 2, 197-200 (1974)

37. KOBRINE, A.I., DOYLE, T.F.: Role of histamine in post-traumatic spinal cord hyperemia and luxury perfusion syndrome. J. Neurosurg. 44, 16-20 (1976)

38. KOBRINE, A.I., DOYLE, T.F., MARTINS, A.N.: Local spinal cord blood flow in experimental traumatic myelopathy. J. Neurosurg. 42, 144-149 (1975)

39. KOBRINE, A.I., DOYLE, T.F., RIZZOLI, H.V.: Spinal cord blood flow as affected by changes in systemic arterial blood pressure. J. Neurosurg. 44, 12-15 (1976)

40. KOBRINE, A.I., DOYLE, T.F., NEWBY, N., RIZZOLI, H.V.: Preserved autoregulation in the rhesus spinal cord after high cervical cord section. J. Neurosurg. 44, 425-428 (1976)

41. KOBRINE, A.I., EVANS, D.E., RIZZOLI, H.V.: The effect of alpha adrenergic blockade on spinal cord autoregulation in the monkey. J. Neurosurg. 46, 336-341 (1977)

42. KOBRINE, A.I., EVANS, D.E., RIZZOLI, H.V.: The effects of beta adrenergic blockage on spinal cord autoregulation in the monkey. J. Neurosurg. 47, 57-63 (1977)

43. KOGURE, K., SCHEINBERG, P., MATSOMOTO, A., BUS, R., REINMUTH, O.M.: Catecholamines in experimental brain ischemia. Arch. Neurol. 32, 21-43 (1975)

44. KOSNIK, E.T., HUNT, W.E.: Post-operative hypertension in management of patients with intracranial arterial aneurysms. J. Neurosurg. 45, 148-154 (1976)

45. LAVYNE, M.H., MOSKOWITZ, M.A., LARIN, F., ZERVAS, N.T., WURTMAN, R.J.: Brain catecholamine metabolism in experimental cerebral ischemia. Neurology 25, 483-5 (1975)

46. MACMILLAN, V.: The effects of gamma-hydroxybutyrate and gamma-butyrolactone upon the energy metabolism of the normoxic and hypoxic rat brain. Brain Res. 146, 177-187 (1978)

47. MEIER, R., TRIPOD, J., STUDER, A.: Comparison of peripheral vascular properties of different vasoconstrictors. Arch. Int. Pharmacol. 117, 185-196 (1958)

48. MEIER, R., TRIPOD, J., WIRT, A.: Classification of serotonin antagonists and sites of peripheral action. Arch. Int. Pharmacol. 109, 55-57 (1957)

49. MEYER, J.S., FUKUUCHI, Y., KANDA, T., SHIMAZU, K.: Regional measurements of cerebral blood flow and metabolism using intracranial injection of hydrogen with comments on intracerebral steal. In: Brain and Blood Flow. RUSSELL, R.W.R. (ed.), pp. 71-80. London: Pitman 1971

50. NAFTCHI, N.E., DEMENY, M., DeCRESCITO, V., TOMASULA, J.J., FLAMM, E.S., CAMPBELL, J.B.: Biogenic amine concentrations in traumatized spinal cord of cats. J. Neurosurg. 40, 52-57 (1974)

51. NICOLL, R.A., ECCLES, J.C., OSHIM, T., RUBIN, I.: Prolongation of hippocampal post-synaptic potentials by barbiturates. Nature 258, 625-627 (1975)

52. OSTERHOLM, J.L., MATHEWS, G.J.: Altered norepinephrine metabolism following experimental spinal cord injury. Part 1. Relationship to hemorrhagic necrosis. J. Neurosurg. 40, 3-34 (1974)

53. PASZTOR, E., SYMON, L., DORSCH, N.V.V.C., BRANSTON, N.M.: The hydrogen clearance method in assessment of blood flow in cortex, white matter, and deep nuclei of baboons. Stroke 4, 556-567 (1973)

54. RANSON, B.R., BACKER, J.L.: Pentobarbital modulated transmitter effect on mouse spinal neuron growth in tissue culture. Nature 254, 703-715 (1975)

55. RAWE, S.E., PEROT, P.L.: Autoradiographic metabolic studies in experimentally produced spinal cord trauma. Surg. Forum 28, 453-455 (1977)

56. RAWE, S.E., LEE, W.A., PEROT, P.L.: The histopathology of experimental spinal cord trauma. The effect of systemic blood pressure. J. Neurosurg. 48, 1002-1007 (1978)

57. REIVICH, M., MARSHALL, W.J.S., KASSELL, N.: Effects of trauma on cerebral vascular autoregulation. In: Cerebravascular diseases. Seventh Conference. TOOLE, J.F., MOOSSY, J., JANEWAY, R. (eds.), pp. 63-69. New York: Grune & Stratton 1971

58. ROTH, R.H.: Striatal dopamine and gamma-hydroxybutyrate. Pharmacol. Ther. (B) 2, 71-88 (1976)

59. SANDLER, A.N., TATOR, C.H.: Review of the measurement of normal spinal cord blood flow. Brain Research 118, 181-198 (1976)

60. SANDLER, A.N., TATOR, C.H.: Review of the effect of spinal cord trauma on the vessels and blood flow in the spinal cord. J. Neurosurg. 45, 638-646 (1976)

61. SANDLER, A.N., TATOR, C.H.: Regional spinal cord blood flow in primates. J. Neurosurg. 45, 647-659 (1976)

62. SANDLER, A.N., TATOR, C.H.: Effect of acute spinal cord compression injury on regional spinal cord blood flow in primates. J. Neurosurg. 45, 660-676 (1976)

63. SAVINI, E.C.: The antagonism between 5-hydroxytryptamine and certain derivatives of lysergic acid. Br. J. Pharm. 11, 313-317 (1956)

64. SENTER, H.J., BURGESS, D.L., METZLER, J.: An improved technique for measurement of spinal cord blood flow. Brain Res. (In Press) 1978

65. SMITH, A.J.K., McCREERY, D.B., BLOEDEL, J.R., CHOU, S.N.: Hyperemia, CO_2 responsiveness, and autoregulation in the white matter following experimental spinal cord injury. J. Neurosurg. 48, 239-251 (1978)

66. SMITH, A.L.: Barbiturate protection in acute focal cerebral ischemia. Stroke 5, 1-7 (1974)

67. SVENGAARD, N.A., EDVINSON, L., OWMAN, C.: Changes in sensitivity of cerebral vessels to noradrenaline and 5-hydroxytryptamine in the presence of subarachnoid blood. Acta Neurol. Scand. (Suppl. 64) 56, 318-319 (1977)

68. THIENPRASET, P., BANTEL, H., BLOEDEL, J., CHOU, S.: Effect of delayed local cooling on experimental spinal cord injury. J. Neurosurg. 42, 150 (1975)

69. TODA, N.: Influence of dopamine and noradrenaline on isolated cerebral arteries of the dog. Br. J. Pharmacol. 58, 121-126 (1976)

70. WALTERS, J.R., ROTH, R.H.: Dopaminergic Neurons: An in vivo system for measuring drug interactions with presynaptic receptors. Arch. Pharmacol. 296, 5-14 (1976)

71. WALTZ, A.G.: Effect of blood pressure on blood flow in ischemic and nonischemic cortex. Neurology 18, 613-621 (1968)

72. WISE, G., SUTTER, R., BURKHOLDER, J.: Treatment of brain ischemia with vasopressor drugs. Stroke 3, 135-142 (1972)

73. YATSU, F.M.: Protective effects of barbiturates on cerebral ischemia. In: Head injuries. McLAURIN, R.L. (ed.), pp. 185-187. New York: Grune & Stratton 1976

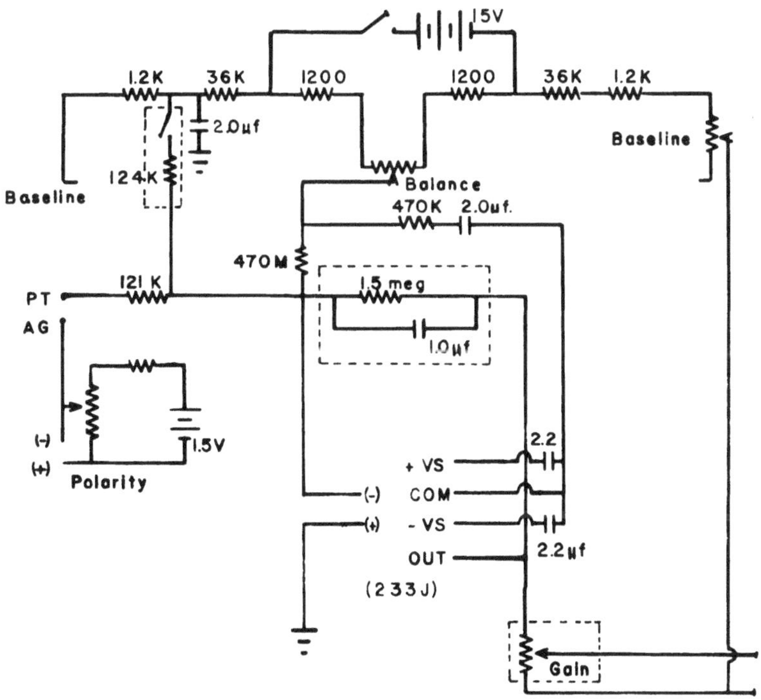

Fig. 1. Amplifier design with modifications outlined

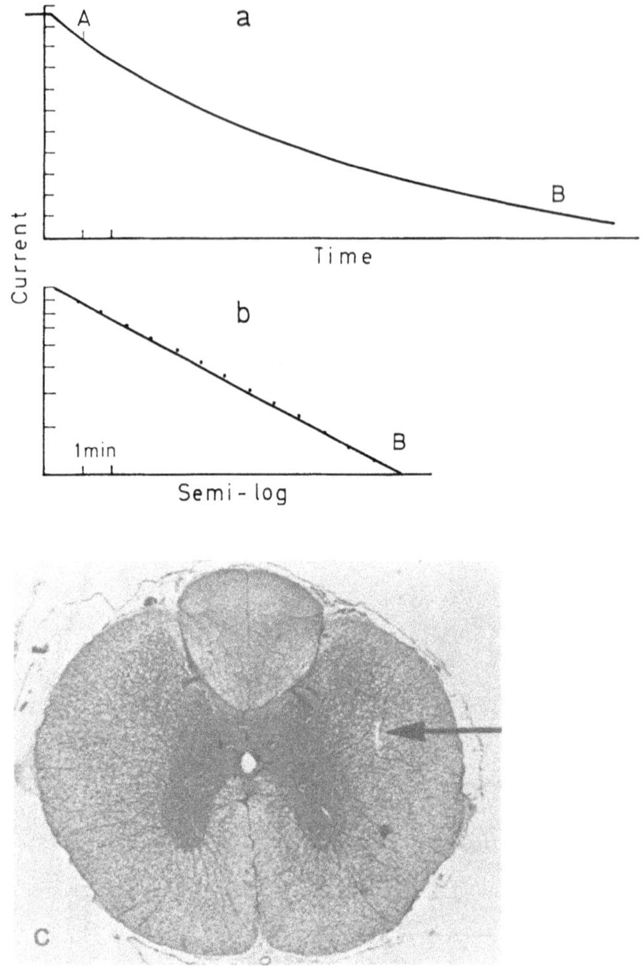

Fig.2. a Typical hydrogen washout curve from the control series. SCBF was 11.77 ml/100 g/min. b Semilog transposition of Fig. 2a demonstrating a monoexponential decay. c Histologic demonstration of the recording site from which Fig. 2a was obtained. The *arrow* indicates the electrode tract. Bodian stain, · 25

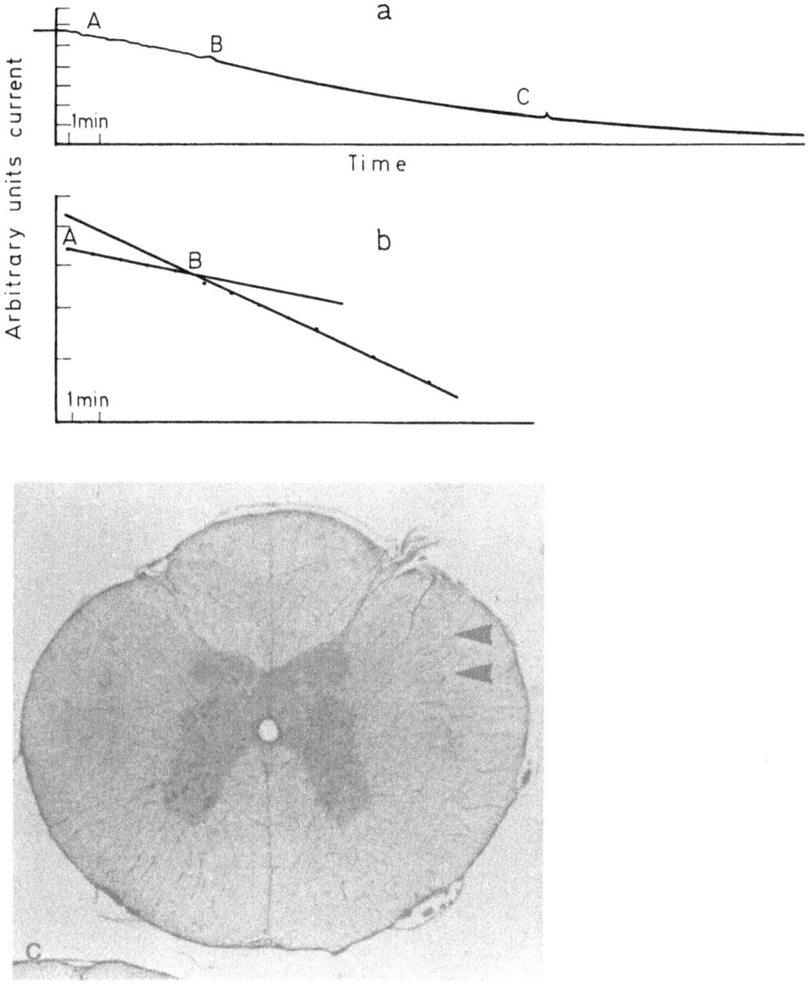

Fig. 3. a Washout curve of a traumatically placed electrode. b Semi-log transposition of Fig. 3a demonstrating a biexponential decay. The SCBF from A to B is 6.11 ml/100 g/min, and the SCBF from B to c is 11.66 ml/100 g/min. c Histologic demonstration of the recording site from which Fig. 3a was obtained showing traumatized tissue around the electrode recording site. The *arrows* indicate the electrode tract

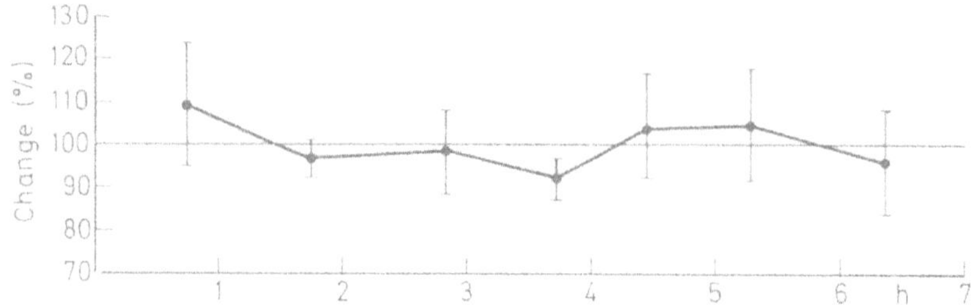

Fig. 4. Control (nontrauma) series of SCBF in the dorsolateral funiculus presented as percent SCBF against time. In this group, SCBF was 10.99 ml/100 g/min $\pm$ 0.89 (n = 51)

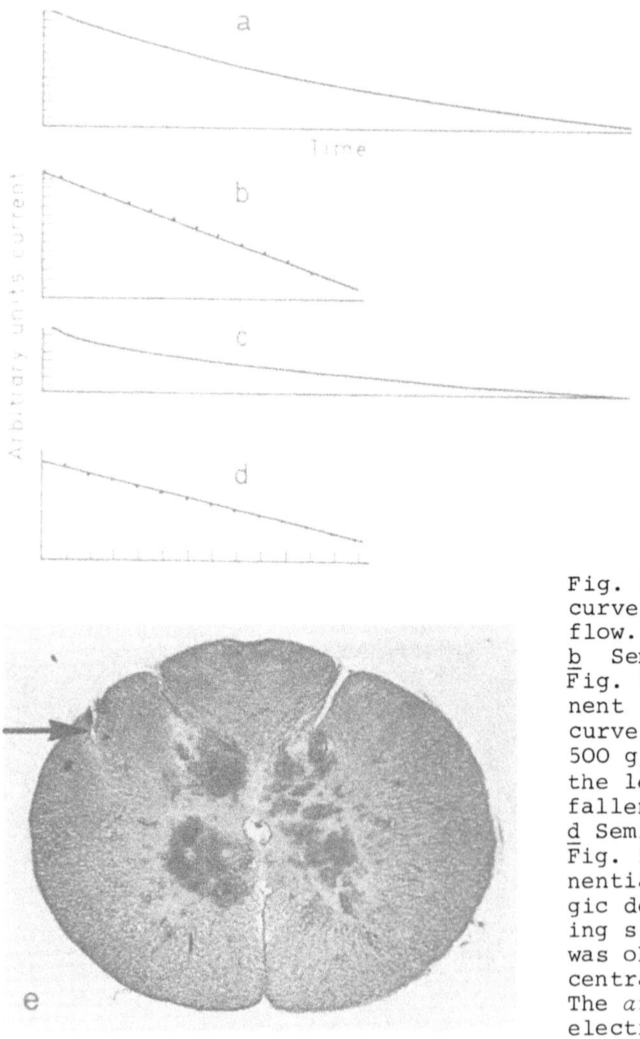

Fig. 5. a Typical washout curve of a pretrauma control flow. SCBF was 9.77 ml/min. b Semilog transposition of Fig. 5a showing a monoexponent function. c Washout curve recorded 4 h after 500 g/cm trauma recorded at the level of trauma. SCBF had fallen to 6.90 ml/100 g/min. d Semilog transposition of Fig. 5c showing a monoexponential function. e Histologic demonstration of recording site from which Fig. 5c was obtained showing typical central hemorrhagic necrosis. The *arrow* indicates the electrode tract

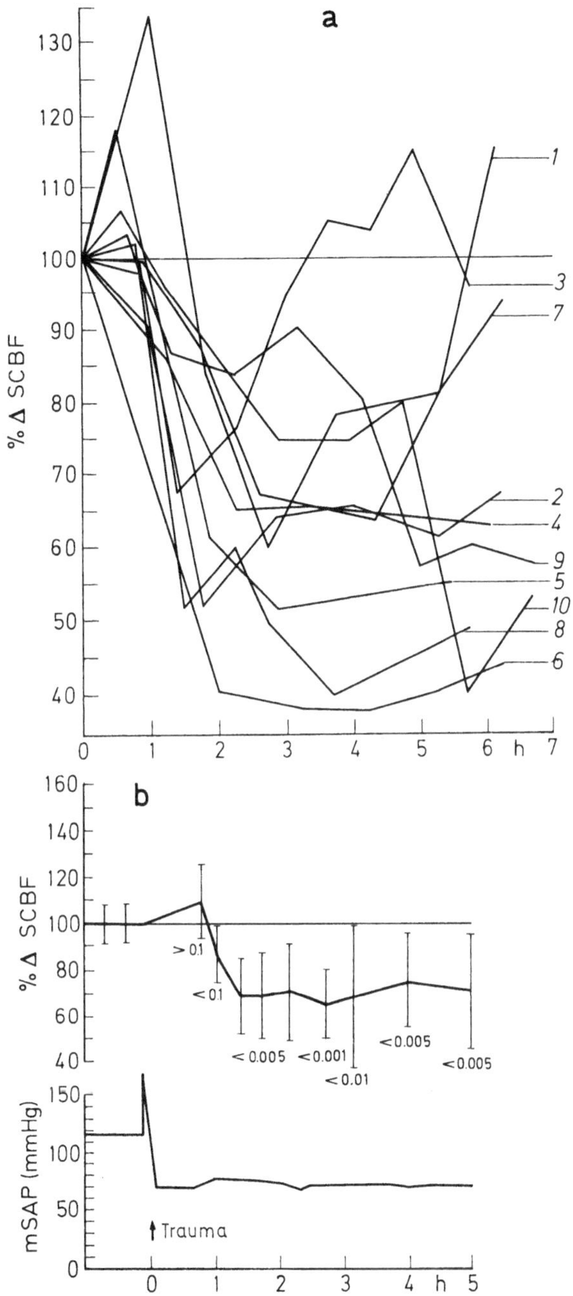

Fig.6. a SCBF at the level of trauma as followed for 6.5 h. The SCBF of each animal is represented as percent of its own pretrauma control flows; 500 g/cm trauma was produced at time 0. b Percent SCBF recorded at the level of trauma with each animal compared to its own pretrauma blood flow value; 500 g/cm trauma was inflicted at time 0. Average values for mSAP at 15-min intervals before and after trauma are represented below SCBF. *Vertical lines* represent standard deviations, and P values compare SCBF against data from the control series during the same time after electrode implantation (Fig. 4)

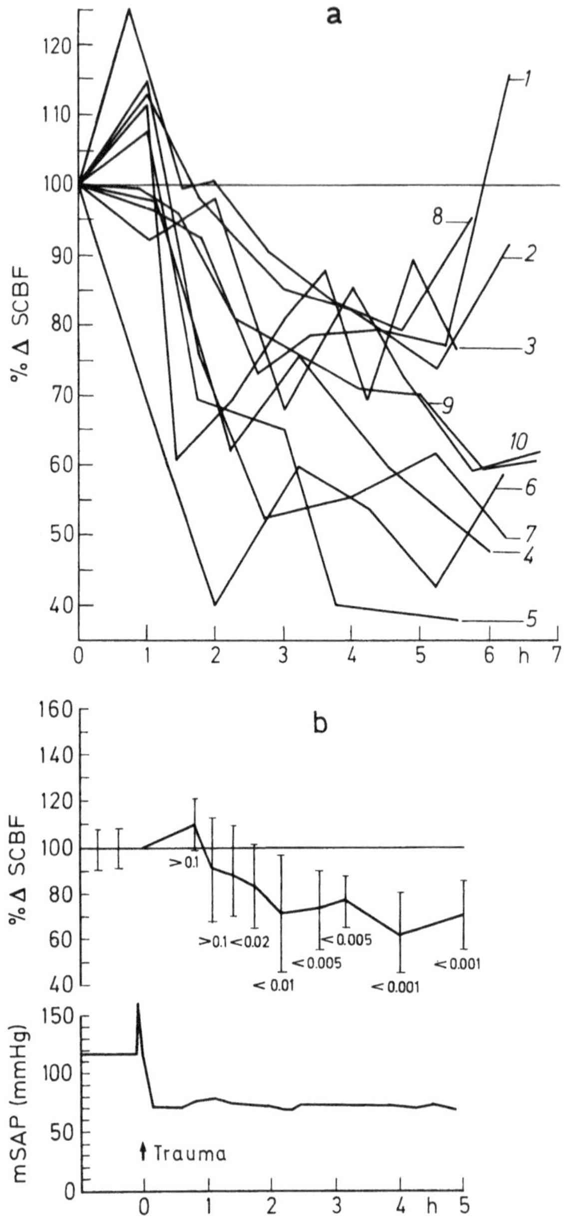

Fig.7. a SCBF 1 cm below trauma as followed for 6.5 h. SCBF of each animal is represented as percent of its own pretrauma control flows; 500 g/cm trauma was produced at time 0. b Percent SCBF recorded 1 cm below trauma; 500 g/cm trauma was inflicted at time 0. Average values for mSAP at 15-min intervals are represented below SCBF. *Vertical lines* represent standard deviations, and P values compare SCBF against data from the control series during the same time after electrode implantation.

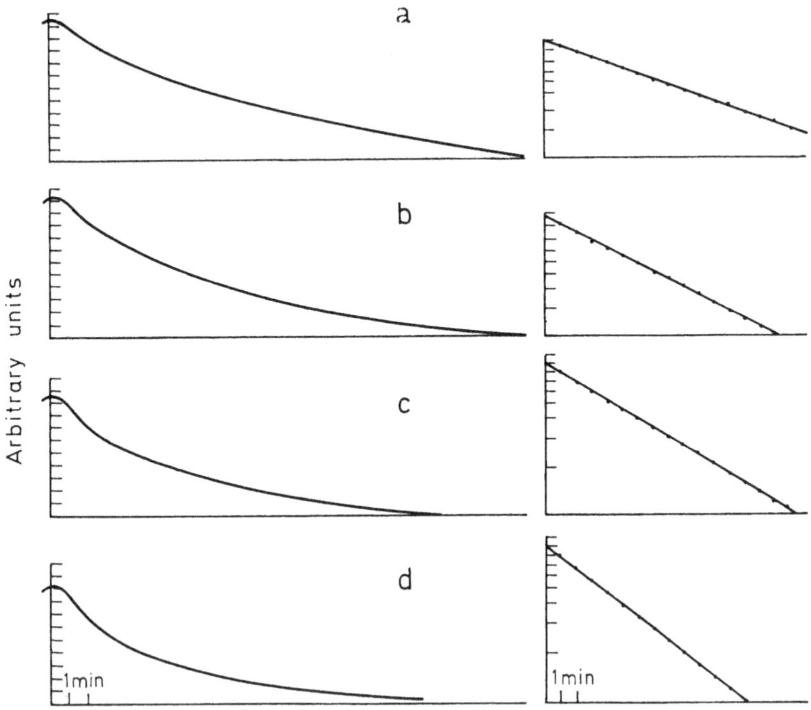

Fig.8. a Clearance curve and semilog transposition at mSAP of 50 mm Hg. The SCBF was 8.72 ml/100 g/min. b Clearance curve at mSAP of 100 mm Hg in the same animal. The SCBF was 11.40 ml/100 g/min. c Clearance curve at mSAP of 150 mm Hg. The SCBF was 13.27 ml/100 g/min. d Clearance curve at mSAP of 200 mm Hg. The SCBF was 17.35 ml/100 g/min

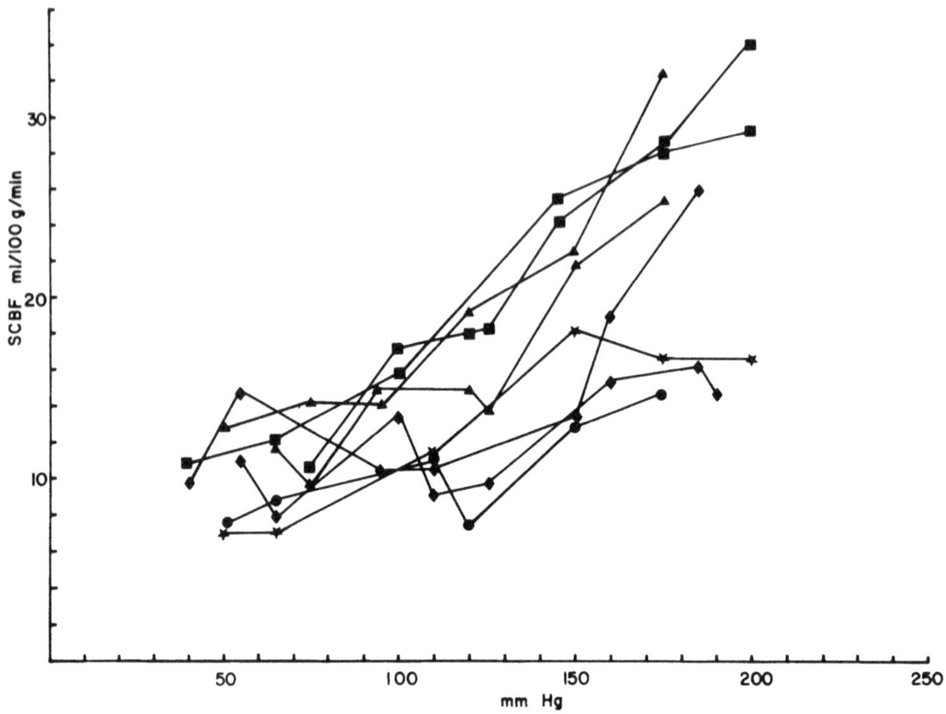

Fig. 9. SCBF in ml/100 g/min against mSAP in mm Hg for the individual cats in the control autoregulation series. Similar symbols represent different electrode sites in the same animal. Two animals had only one electrode recording blood flow

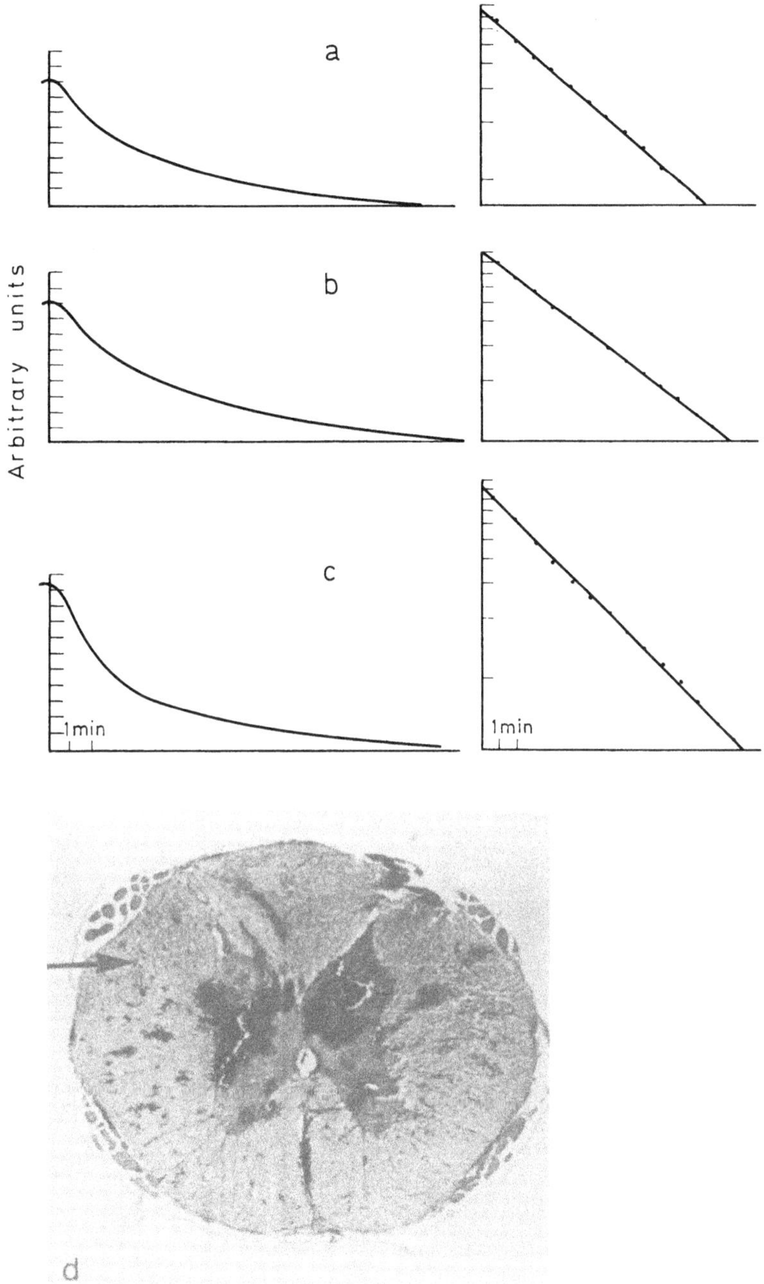

Fig.10. a Clearance curve and monoexponential semilog transposition recorded before 500 g/cm injury. The SCBF was 16.54 ml/100 g/min. b Clearance curve and transposition recorded 1 h after trauma when the mSAP has been maintained at pretrauma levels by infusion with Aramine. The SCBF was 16.06 ml/100 g/min. c Clearance curve and semilog transposition recorded 4 h after trauma with the blood pressure elevated. The SCBF was 19.82 ml/100 g/min. d Histologic confirmation of recording site and of central hermorrhagic necrosis. The *arrow* indicates the electrode tract

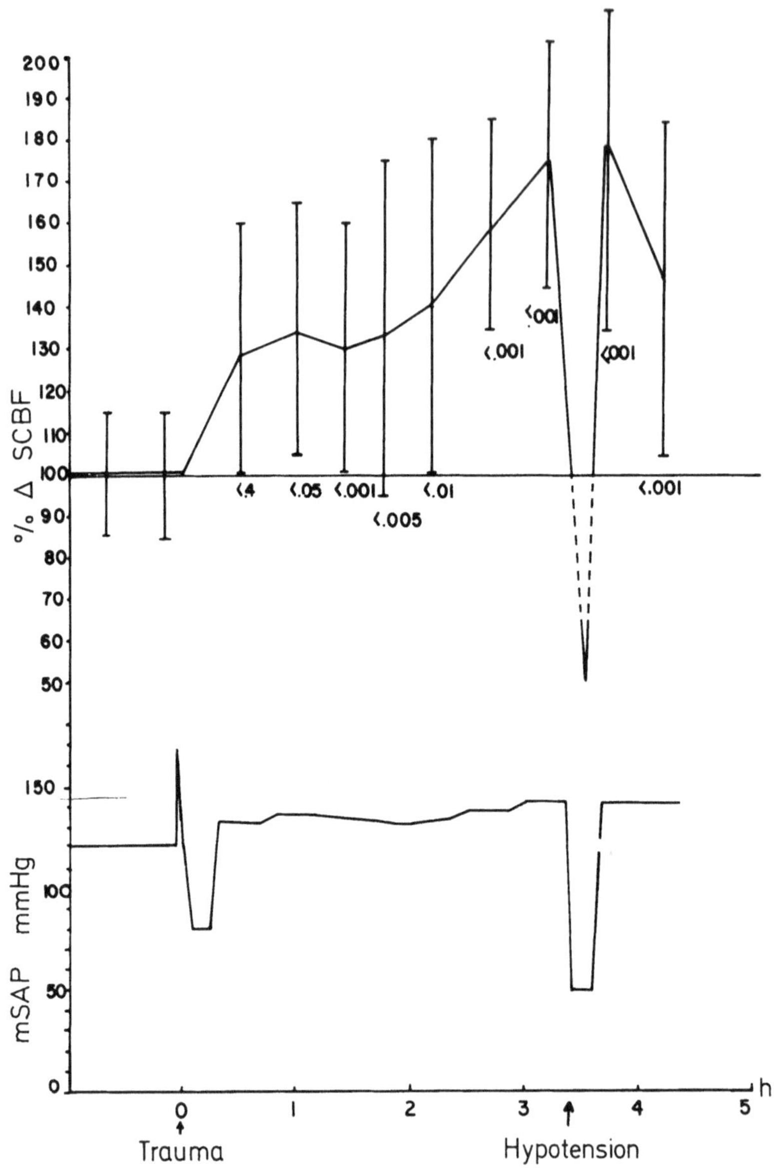

Fig.11. a Percent SCBF at the level of trauma when the post-traumatic blood pressure has been returned to normal with Aramine. Trauma was inflicted at time 0. The average values for mSAP at 15-min intervals are presented below SCBF. The episode of nitroprusside-induced hypotension and re-elevation of blood pressure with Aramine are also indicated. The *vertical lines* represent standard deviation, and P values compare SCBF against data from the trauma series (without blood pressure manipulation) (Fig. 6b)

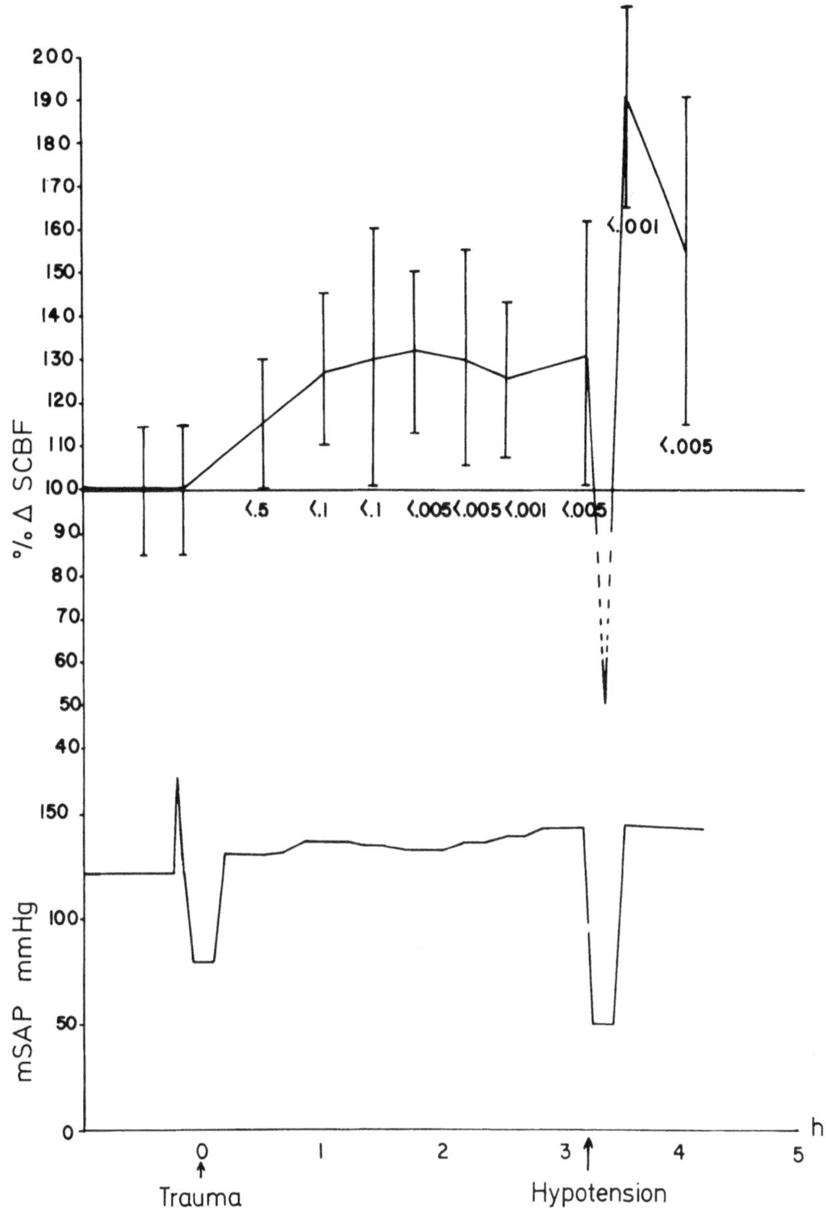

Fig. 11. b Similar presentation as Fig. 11 a for data recorded 1 cm below trauma. The P values compare SCBF against data from the initial trauma series (Fig. 7 b)

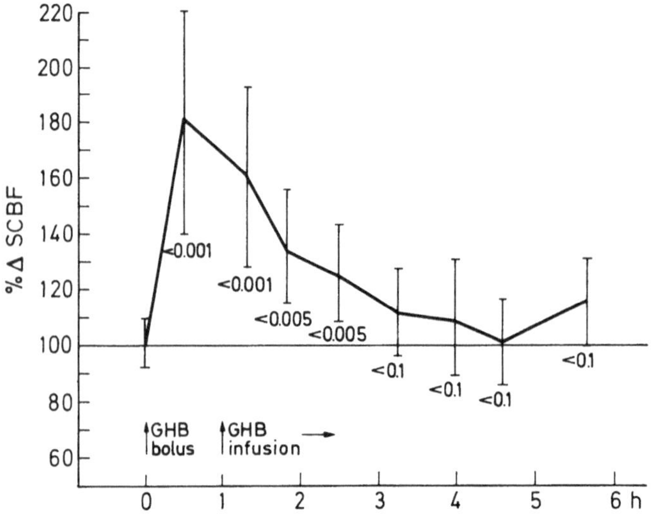

Fig. 12. Control (nontrauma) + GHB (300 mg/kg bolus and 200 mg/kg infusion) series of animals. Each cat's blood flow is compared to its own pre-drug control flows and is graphed as percent SCBF. Standard deviations are shown, and *P* values compare SCBF against data from the initial control series (Fig. 4) during the same time periods.

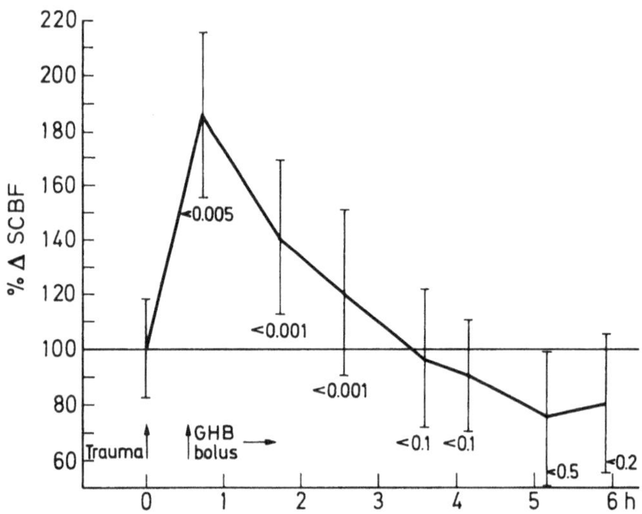

Fig. 13. Same presentation as Fig. 6b except for a single dose of GHB (300 mg/kg) given 0.5 h after 500 g/cm injury. The *P* values compare SCBF to data from the trauma series (Fig. 6b) during the same time after cord injury

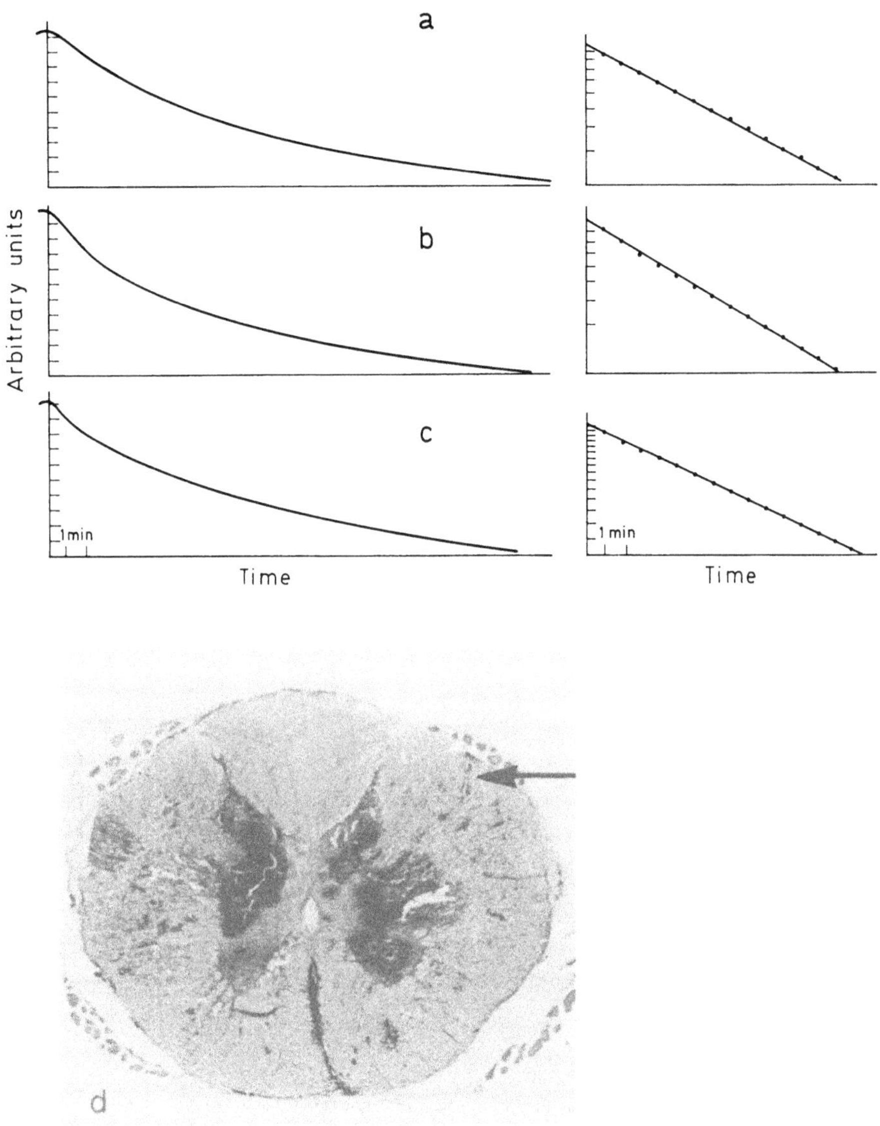

Fig. 14 a-c. Hydrogen washout curves of a pretrauma, 1-h, and 6-h post-trauma flows from an animal treated with GHB (bolus + infusion). Also shown are their semilog transpositions demonstrating monoexponential decays. The SCBF values were 11.17, 12.83, and 10.50 ml/100 g/min, respectively. d Histologic demonstration of recording site from which these curves were obtained. The *arrow* indicates the electrode tract, and the cord shows the typical changes of post-traumatic central hemorrhagic necrosis

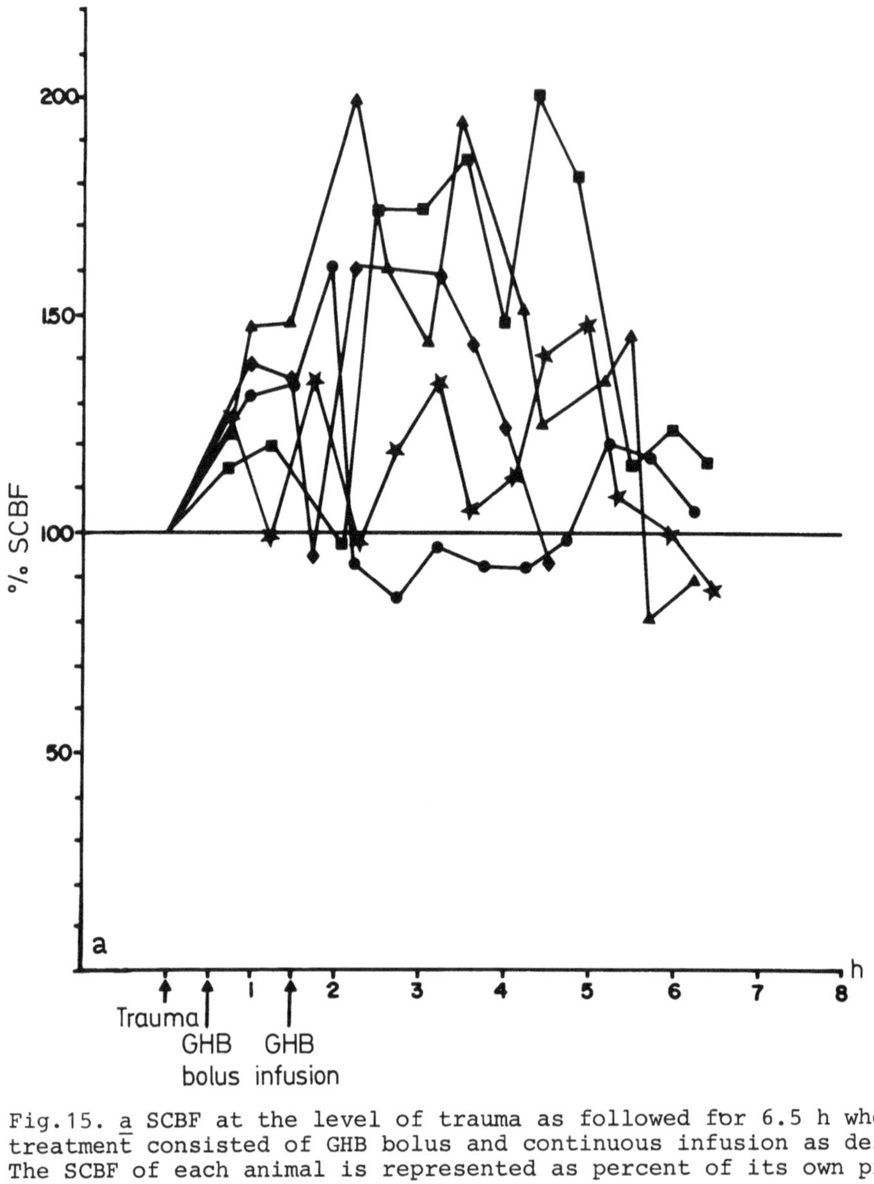

Fig.15. a SCBF at the level of trauma as followed for 6.5 h when treatment consisted of GHB bolus and continuous infusion as described. The SCBF of each animal is represented as percent of its own pre-trauma control flows

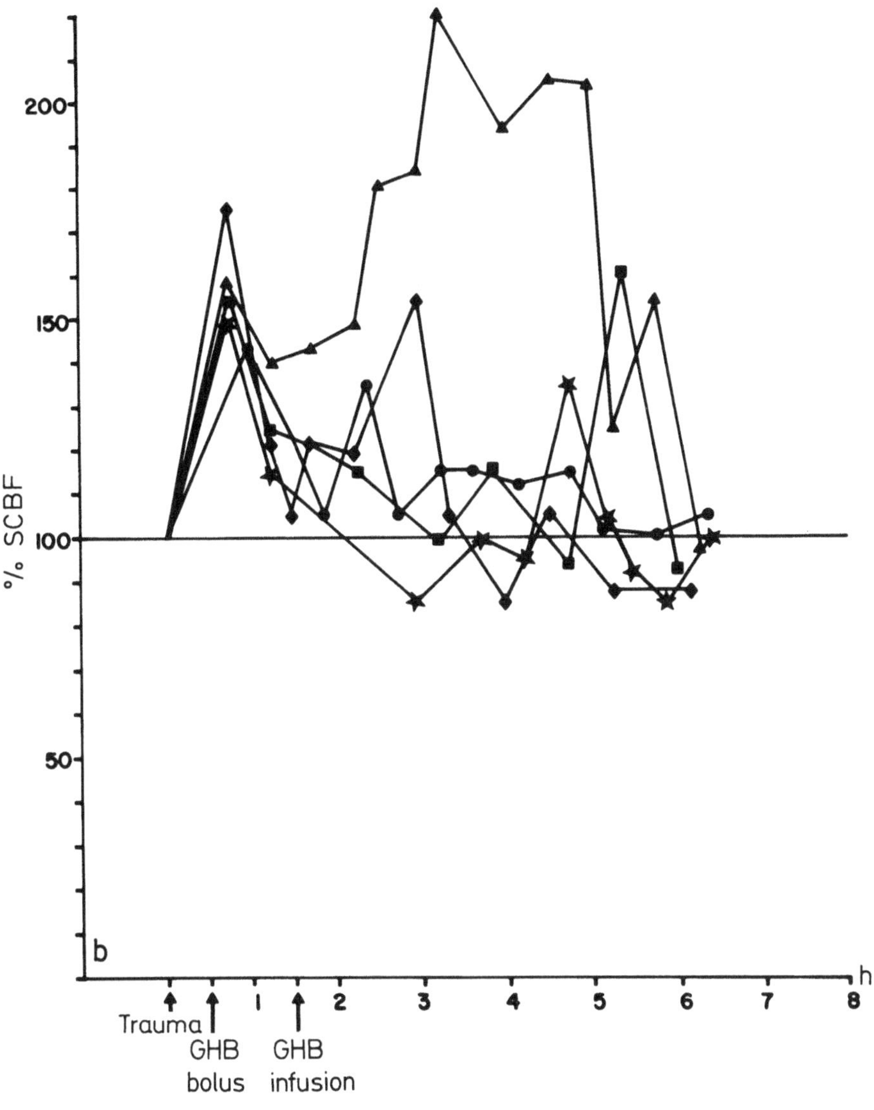

Fig. 15 b. SCBF recorded 1 cm below the level of trauma with data presented similarly to Fig. 15 a. At trauma and below trauma recordings from the same animal are indicated by identical symbols

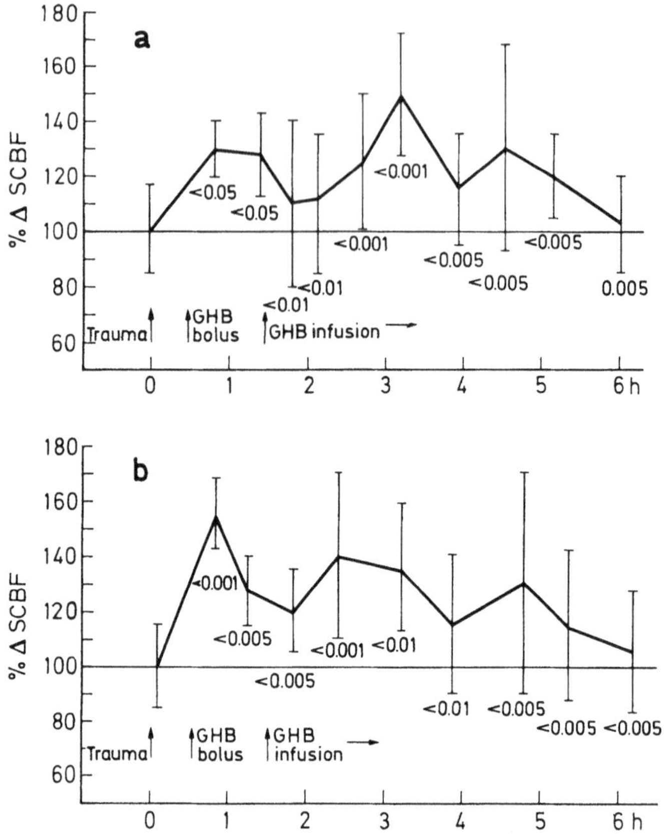

Fig.16. a Summation of all data from Fig. 15a showing percent SCBF recorded at the level of trauma. The GHB bolus and infusion time markers are so indicated. *Vertical lines* indicate standard deviation, and P values (two-tailed Student t test) compare SCBF against values obtained from the control trauma series during the same time period (Fig. 6b). b Similar presentation as Fig. 16a for data recorded simultaneously 1 cm below trauma

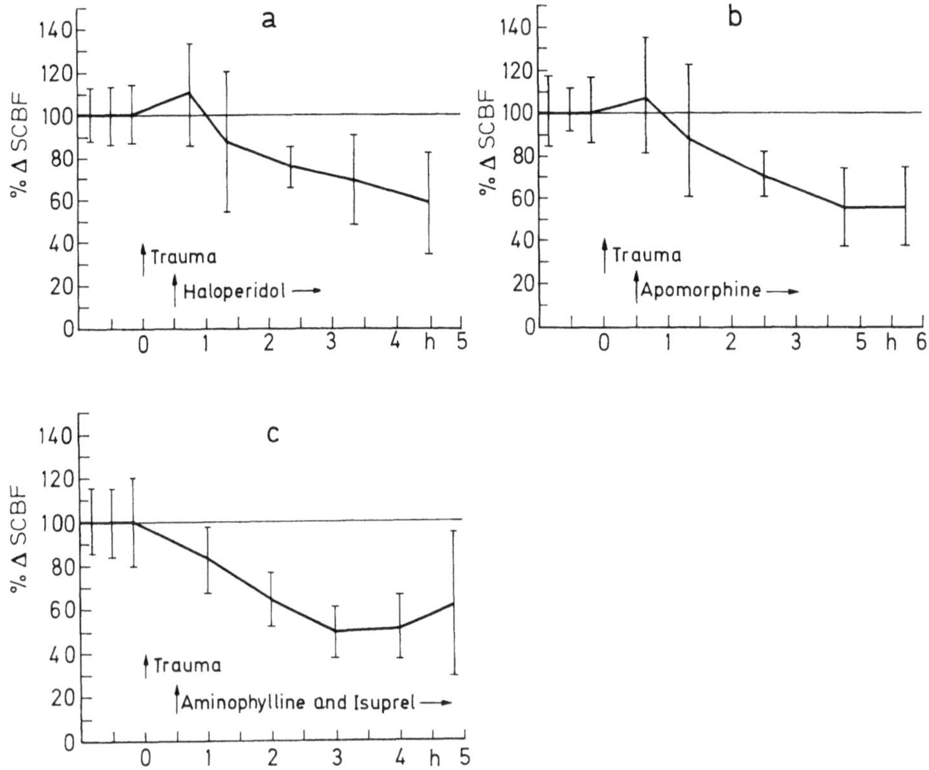

Fig.17. a SCBF after 500 g/cm injury when treatment consisted of haloperidol (bolus and infusion) begun 0.5 h after cord injury and continued for the duration of the experiment. No data points were statistically different from the nontreated trauma series (Fig. 6b) ($P < 0.5$). b Same presentation as Fig. 17a except that therapy consisted of apomorphine given during the same post-traumatic period. No points were statistically different from the nontreated trauma series (Fig. 6b) ($P < 0.5$). c Same presentation as Fig. 17a except that therapy consisted of administration of aminophylline and Isuprel given during the same post-traumatic period. No points are statistically different from the nontreated trauma series (Fig. 6b)

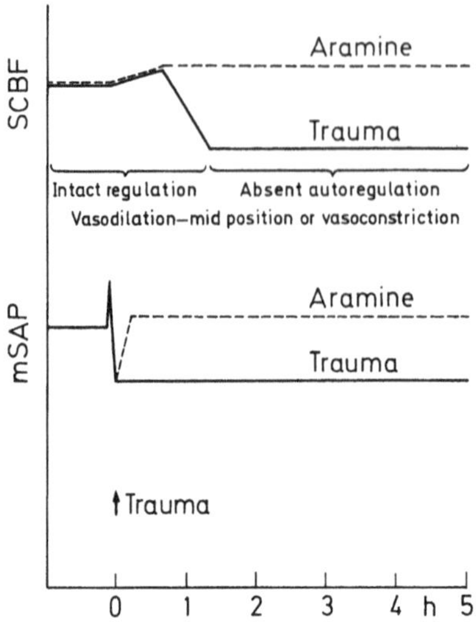

Fig. 18. Schematic summary of the relationship between SCBF and mSAP during the post-traumatic period. Phase 1 is the period of intact autoregulation lasting 60-90 min after trauma. Phase 2 is the subsequent period of absent autoregulation during which ischemia occurs

Recovery in Spinal Cord Injuries

J. T. LUCAS and T. B. DUCKER

Introduction

The first recorded evidence of the classification of spinal cord injuries is contained in the famous Edwin Smith papyrus, which was copied by an unknown scribe around 1700 B.C. The author is thought to be Imhotep who was a physician to Pharoah Zoser III of Egypt. The author classified the injuries into three subdivisions depending on the severity of the lesion: "A disease I shall treat", "A disease I shall fight", and "A disease which cannot be treated". Centuries later Galen (130-200 A.D.) was reported to have been the first to recognize differing levels of injury. Since that time numerous clinical syndromes and classifications have been introduced by both anatomists and clinicians. None of the proposed classifications up to the present time allow precise mathematic summary for statistical analysis.

We have subsequently developed a system of classification for patients with spinal cord injuries, based on the level of vertebral trauma and the resulting motor examination. This new classification was initially used to evaluate over 800 patients collected by our 1973-1975 Nationwide Spinal Cord Injury Registry (NSCIR). This classification, as well as the resulting statistical inferences, will be presented in this paper.

Methods

Between the years 1973 and 1975, the NSCIR collected information on over 800 patients with spinal cord injuries. To study these 800 patients, a meaningful classification had to be developed that would lend itself to statistical analysis. This classification has two primary subdivisions: (1) that of the level of vertebral trauma documented by radiologic exam and (2) the resulting neurological pathology. The resulting cord injury was documented immediately after injury and again at approximately 1 year after injury by neurological examinations.

The level of vertebral trauma was subdivided into single sites, multiple sites, and no evidence of vertebral trauma. This paper will deal with those patients suffering only one level of vertebral trauma (698 patients). A single level of vertebral trauma is defined as the subluxation of two adjacent vertebra and/or fracture of the caudal vertebra of the pair. As seen in Table 1, the single sites of trauma are also arranged according to the groups of muscles tested in the neurological exam. For example, those patients who suffered fracture dislocations of T-1 on T-2 and/or fractures of T-2 (T-1/T-2, T-2)

Table 1

Subluxations and/or	fractures	Designations	Root(s)	Motor group tested
	C1	C1	C1	
C1/C2	C2	C1/C2-C2	C2	Diaphramatic muscles (FEV_1 T.V.)
C2/C3	C3	C2/C3-C3	C3	
C3/C4	C4	C3/C4-C3	C4	
C4/C5	C5	C4/C5-C5	C5	Shoulder abduction
C5/C6	C6	C5/C6-C6	C6	Elbow flexion
C6/C7	C7	C6/C7-C7	C7	Elbow extension
C7/T1	T1	C7/T1-T1	C8	Small hand muscles
T1/T2-T8/T9	T2-T9	T1/2-T8/9	T1-T8	Intercostals
T9/T10 T10/T11	T10 & T12	T9/10-T10/11	T9-T10	Upper abdominalis
T11/T12 T12/L1	T12 & L1	T11/12-T12/L1	T11 & T12	Lower abdominalis
L1/L2 L2/L3	L2 & L3	L1/2-L2/3	L1 L2	Psoas
L3/L4 L4/L5	L4 & L5	L3/4-L4/5	L3 L4	Quadriaceps
L5/S1	S1	L5/S1-S1	L5	Plantar extension
			S1	Plantar flexion

through T-8/9, T-9 are grouped together because the only clinical test of cord or root motor function is that of the intercostal muscles.

The entire neurological exam for each patient was evaluated. However, for statistical reasons, only the resulting motor exam is presented in this paper. The motor function of the muscle groups listed in Table 1 is graded on a scale of 0-5, with 5 normal, 4 functional, 3 fair, 2 poor, 1 trace, and 0 absent. Figure 1 is a graph of motor function for all patients with a cord injury secondary to fracture dislocation of C-5/6 and/or fracture of C-6. As seen in Fig. 1, certain patterns of motor dysfunction below the level of injury can be determined from the graph of the mean motor function of each muscle group arranged in a cephalad to caudal progression. Asymmetric, root, and normal motor exams are not graphed in Fig. 1. Asymmetric lesions, not covered in this paper, are essentially combinations of partial loss uniform, partial loss with caudal gain, and partial loss with caudal loss motor lesions with one type of pattern predominating on one side of the body or the other. These patterns of motor dysfunction allow for grouping of patients into subdivisions. This grouping results in our new motor classification (Table 2).

Table 2

Classification of motor dysfunction	Motor pattern
Motor complete at bony level of trauma (CBL)	a
Graded complete (CG)	b
Partial loss at site of trauma with a secondary caudal cord segment loss in motor function (PCL)	c
Partial loss at site of trauma with caudal sparing of motor function (PCS)	d
Partial loss of uniform nature at site of vertebral trauma (PLU)	e
Asymmetric motor loss	
PLU and PCL	e and c
PLU and PCS	e and d
PCL and PCS	c and d
Root single	
multiple	
Normal	

For analytic purposes, we divided spinal cord lesions into two types of complete lesions and three types of partial lesions. The five groups are (1) complete at bony level (CBL), (2) graded complete (GC), (3) partial with caudal loss (PCL), (4) partial with caudal gain or caudal sparing (PCS), and (5) the uniform partial lesions (PLU). Motor complete lesions or complete at bony level (CBL) are defined as those cord lesions with a complete loss of motor function within two cord segments below the cord segment corresponding to the nerve root that exits at the site of vertebral trauma. The reason for this two-cord segment allowance is to accomodate for the cord and vertebral body anatomic disalignment. This motor pathologic pattern is represented in Fig. 1. Graded complete lesions (GC) are defined as those lesions with a caudally displaced complete loss of motor function and includes those motor complete lesions that occur from two to four cord segments below the cord segment corresponding to the nerve root that exits at the site of vertebral trauma. Partial loss at the site of vertebral trauma with a secondary caudally displaced loss in motor function (PCL) is the next motor pattern and classification. This secondary loss in motor function may be partial or complete in nature and by definition occurs in at least four cord segments below the level of bony trauma. Partial motor loss at the site of vertebral trauma with caudal sparing of motor function (PCS) are lesions similar to the previously described central cord syndrome (1). Partial motor loss of uniform nature (PLU) is self-explanatory and similar to but not secondary to cortical motor loss. This type of motor loss is predominantly associated with asymmetric lesions.

After all patients with one level of vertebral trauma were classified according to the bony level of trauma and the above-described motor classification, the patients were further screened by the authors (both physicians) for a complete medical audit. Only those patients with complete medical audit are included in this study (436 patients). Each patient with complete medical audits, motor classification, and single level of vertebral trauma was then summarized by the mathematic indices below: motor index initial (*MIi*), motor index current (*MIc*), and recovery rate (*RR*).

Motor index initial is defined as the sum of motor function (graded 0-5) for each muscle group tested (Table 1) divided by the number of motor units tested on the initial exam:

$$MIi = \frac{\text{Motor function for each muscle group}}{\text{Number of muscle groups tested}} .$$

Motor index current is calculated the same way as motor index initial with the exception of using the current or 1-year after injury neurological examination. Recovery rate is defined as the fraction of lost motor function that is regained over a given time span (1 year):

$$RR = \frac{MIc - MIi}{5 - MIi} \text{ or } \frac{\Delta\ MI}{5 - MIi}$$

Expressed as percentage: % recovered = $\frac{MI}{5-MIi}$ x 100.

The next stage of statistical analysis included that of finding the mean and standard deviation of *MIi* and *RR* for the various motor classifications at each level of vertebral trauma (see below) - (3,4).

$$MIi \text{ mean} = \overline{MIi} = \frac{\Sigma\ MIi}{N_{MIi}};$$

$$MIi \text{ standard deviation} = \sqrt{\frac{\Sigma(MIi - \overline{MIi})^2}{N_{MIi}}};$$

$$RR \text{ mean} = \overline{RR} = \frac{\Sigma\ RR}{N_{RR}};$$

$$RR \text{ standard deviation} = \sqrt{\frac{\Sigma\ (RR - \overline{RR})^2}{n_{RR}}}.$$

The *MIi* and standard deviation for each level and motor classification are listed in Table 3 and the RR is listed in Table 4.

Table 3. Motor index initial

		C1 /2-2	C2 /3-3	C3 /4-4	C4 /5-5	C5 /6-6	C6 /7-7	C7 T1 /T1-	T1 T8 /2 /9	T9 T10 /10 /11	T11 T12 /12 /L1	L1 L2 /2 /3	L3 L4 /4 /5	L5 /S1
CBL	mean	-	-	0.0	0.0	.32	.58	1.46	2.06	2.49	2.73	NS	-	-
	τ	-	-	0.0	0.0	.26	.28	.37	.60	.1	.1	NS	-	-
CG	$\bar{m}$	-	NS	.37	.25	.71	1.35	-	2.70	-	3.13	NS	-	-
	τ	-	NS	.30	.17	.20	.56	-	.47	-	.38	NS	-	-
PCL	m		1.64			1.09		3.03	-	-	NS	-	-	-
	τ	"	.55	"	"	1.0		.64	-	-	NS	-	-	-
PCS	m		2.48			2.85		3.22	NS	-	NS	NS	-	-
	τ	"	2.04	"	"	1.61		1.37	NS	-	NS	NS	-	-
PLU	m			3.25					NS	-	NS	NS	-	-
	τ			.67					NS	-	NS	NS	-	-

Table 4. Recovery rates

		C1 /2-2	C2 /3-3	C3 /4-4	C4 /5-5	C5 /6-6	C6 /7-7	C7 /T1-1	T1 T8 /2 /9	T9 T10 /10 /11	T11 T12 /12 /L1	L1 L2 /2 /3	L3 L4 /4 /5	L5 /S1
CBL	$\bar{m}$	-	-	.07	.19	.10	.10	.21	.07	.05	.14	NS	-	-
	τ	-	-	.2	.26	.20	.14	.26	.14	.07	.2	NS	-	-
CG	$\bar{m}$	-	NS	.12	.11	.12	.27	-	.20	-	.67	NS	-	-
	τ	-	NS	.14	.20	.17	.30	-	.34	-	.26	NS	-	-
PCL	$\bar{m}$	.08				.24	.61		-	-	NS	-	-	-
	τ	±.10				.24	.38		-	-	NS	-	-	-
PCS	$\bar{m}$	.80				.73	.69		NS	-	NS	NS	-	-
	τ	.24				.33	.34		NS	-	NS	NS	-	-
PLU	m			.64					NS	-	NS	NS	-	-
	τ			.31					NS	-	NS	NS	-	-

To determine if classification by bony level of trauma and resulting motor patterns produce statistically different groups of patients, the *MIi* of adjacent groups in Table 3 were compared for variance by using the *F* test (3). In Table 3, the motor classifications that are significantly different to a P value of $P < 0.01$ are connected by a single hash mark. The groups not significant to this level but to a P value of P 0.05 are connected by double hash marks.

Results

Table 3 lists the mean *MIi* and the corresponding standard deviation for the patients classified by level of vertebral trauma and motor classification. For example, a patient with a fracture dislocation of C-5/6 or fracture of C-6 classified as complete at bony level (CBL) would have a *MIi* between 0.06 and 0.58 in 68% of the cases and between 0.06 and 0.84 in 95.5% of the cases. Of the above cases with fracture dislocations of C-5/6, C-6 and classified as complete at bony level, 68% have at least 88% loss of motor function, and 95.5% of this group of patients have at least an 83% loss of total motor function, whereas patients injured at the same level but classified as partial loss with caudal gain have at least an 82% loss of the motor function in 68% of the cases. By using Table 3, the *MIi* can be predicted within the normal limits of variance if the level of fracture and type of lesion are known. Therefore, Table 3 shows an expected morbidity of motor function.

Since each motor classification for a single vertebral level was compared for significant variance by the *F* test, one may classify with reasonable certainty a patient by his motor index initial into partial, graded complete, or transverse complete (CBL) categories if the level of vertebral trauma is known.

The expected recovery rates for each group of patients classified by motor pattern and by level of bony injury are listed in Table 4. For example, a patient with C-5/6, C-6 fracture dislocation and CBL would be expected to recover a maximum of 0.24 of lost motor function at least 17.5% of the time or 0.34 of lost motor function in at least 2.25% of the cases.

The number of patients in each positive category of variance for *RR* is indicated in Table 5. No patient was found to be above four standard deviations of the mean. Five patients or 1.6% of the total patients were found three standard deviations above the mean *RR*, and 13 patients were found between the second and third standard deviations of the mean recovery for a percentage of 4.2% of the entire population under study. These 18 patients (5 + 13) had one of the two types of complete lesions, and all patients classified as partial lesions had *RR* less

Table 5

	Number of patients (CBL)	CG	Partial	Total
$> 4\ \sigma$ RR	0	0	0	0
$> 3\ \sigma$ RR $< 4\ \sigma$ RR	4	1	0	5
$> 2\ \sigma$ RR $< 3\ \sigma$ RR	3	5	0	8
Total	7	6	0	13

than two standard deviations of the mean. Tables 6 and 7 contain summaries of pertinent treatment regimens for those patients with *RR* better than two and three standard deviations of the mean.

As seen in the above formulas, the *MIi* is directly related to the recovery rate. This relationship is supported when *MIi* is graphed in conjunction with percent recovery as seen in Fig. 2. Note that this graph is asyntopic at both the lower (motor complete) and the upper end (normals). In addition, this relationship, when tested by Chi-square, produces a P value of $P < 0.001$.

Table 6. Patients with recovery rates greater than three standard deviations above the mean

Level	Motor classification	Patient number	Summary of major treatments
C5/6	CBL	5118	Patient placed in cervical tongs immediately on admission; underwent a myelography and discoidectomy with anterior fusion, 1 day post-injury
		8196	Patient placed in cervical traction with tongs immediately on admission and closed reduction achieved within 24 hours post-injury
C6/7	CBL	8190	Patient placed in cervical traction on admission with myelography carried out within 2 hours post-injury. Complete block found anteriorly and patient underwent discoidectomy and anterior fusion post myelogram
T11/12 T12/L1	CBL	8153	Patient underwent myelogram on admission and block was decompressed within 24 hours post-injury by laminectomy
C4/5	CG	3983	Closed reduction achieved within 13 hours post-injury by cervical traction. High doses of steroids started on admission. Patient underwent anterior fusion 12 days post-injury

Discussion

The prognostic evaluation of a patient with spinal cord injury as to degree of motor recovery can be approached in basically two ways: (1) individually or (2) by comparison of one patient to a group. The individual evaluation, of course, requires a thorough neurological examination, including all modalities and subsequent interpretation of the findings based on the time-honored principles of "the less the injury the greater the recovery", or partial lesions recover and

Table 7. Patients with recovery rates greater than two standard deviations but less than three standard deviations above the mean

Level	Motor classification	Patient number	Summary of major treatments and/or procedures
C3/4	CBL	8101	Tongs placed on admission with reduction, myelogram and discoidectomy with anterior fusion 48 hours post injury
C4/5	CBL	8174	Tongs placed on admission for stability; myelogram performed 15 days post injury with subsequent discoidectomy and anterior fusion
C7/T1	CBL	8214	Closed reduction on admission with tongs and negative myelogram
C4/5	CG	6001	Closed reduction with tongs 6 hours post injury and negative myelogram performed 8 hours post injury
C5/6	CG	6822	Closed reduction 14 hours post injury with tongs. Posterior fusion performed 10 days post injury
C6/7	CG	2512	Closed reduction on admission with tongs
C6/7	CG	7030	Stability maintained with tongs on admission, no reduction needed
T1-T8/9	CG	4539	Laminectomy performed 10 hours post injury

complete lesions do not. This method is in reality a comparison of that patient under study to one of past experience with other patients. This method can be statistically analyzed by using linear regression techniques as done by MANGUM (5) on our earlier data. With this technique, one essentially ascribes numeric coefficients to neurological findings, such as the presence or absence of reflexes, bladder function, sensory findings, and motor function. By computations described in her thesis, a prognostic coefficient can be ascribed to each modality under study. The neurological modalities with the highest prognostic index or ability to predict the final outcome as to recovery are, of course, those indices with an all-or-none character. In other words, if the bladder is intact, the patient has a partial lesion and is likely to recover to a greater degree than a patient would with a neurogenic bladder. Reflex examination follows a similar pattern but is more complicated as to the time of examination in relation to the degree and duration of spinal shock.

The sensory exam depends on modality tested. Position sense is again of an all-or-none character but with a lower prognostic index (anterior cord). Pain and temperature with a lower prognostic coefficient are complicated by the findings in our study that patients with sensory levels primarily maintain that level at 1 year after injury and only vary in the intensity of the sensory deficit, which was unmeasured in this study. MANGUM's study did not differentiate the prognostic coefficent of the above group from those few with receeding sensory levels.

The motor index with a prognostic coefficient slightly below the sensory coefficient is probably the most accurate clinical tool at present for predicting return of motor function if certain limitations are imposed. First, the assessment must be made within the first 24 h after injury. The motor function is graded on a 5-0 scale as used by American physiatrists. The initial motor function is used to group patients in the motor classification presented above. Lastly, one recognizes these are groups with variance from the expected mean as measured by the standard deviation of that group.

Based on the above early findings, patients with spinal cord injuries can be classified accurately from their motor exam, and subsequently this exam can be summarized in a meaningful way with mathematic indices. The summary indices (*MIi*, *MIc*, *RR*) can then be used in statistical equations to determine the significance of variables under study.

The uses of the *MIi* are multiple. As shown, it can be used as an aid in the classification of patients if the bony level of trauma is known. For example, a patient with *MIi* of 0.89 and C-6/7 C-7 fracture dislocation could be considered a complete at bony level lesion because the patient is within two standard deviations of the mean for that level (0.58 + 2 (0.28) = 1.14). However, the patient's motor index is within one standard deviation of graded complete lesion for that level (1.35 - 1 (0.56) = 0.76). Therefore, this patient is more likely to be a graded complete lesion than a complete at bony level lesion.

The *MIi* can also be used to predict the morbidity of a particular lesion at each level of vertebral trauma. A patient with a motor complete lesion at C-5/6 vertebral level should have a *MIi* of 0.32 $\pm$ 0.26. In other words, the patient's *MIi* should be between 0.86 and 0.58, 68% of the time or between 0.0 (-0.2) and 0.84, 95.5% of the time. To state morbidity in another way, 84% of the time *MIi* should be below 0.58 for a patient with a C-5/6 fracture dislocation classified as motor complete, and similarly, for 97.75% of the patients the *MIi* should be 0.84 or below.

To express *MIi* in terms of percent loss of function initially, the below equation is used:

$$\frac{5 - MIi}{5} \cdot 100\%.$$

Therefore, 97.75% of the motor complete patients with C-5/6 fracture dislocation will have 83% loss of motor function.

Recovery rates listed in Table 4 can be used as a prediction of motor gains at 1 year after injury, evaluations of present treatment regimes, and when used in conjunction with *MIi*, as controls for new treatment regimes.

To predict the expected percent of gain in motor function at 1 year after injury, the below formula is used:

$$\left[RR \pm (\mathrm{SD})\right] \cdot 100\% = \text{Percent expected gain.}$$

For example, a motor complete patient (CBL) with a C-5/6, C-6 fracture and/or dislocation will be expected to recover over 70% of loss motor function in only 0.15% of the cases, 50% of loss motor function in 2.25% of the cases, 30% in 16% of the cases, and finally 10% in 50% of the cases. On the other hand, 50% of the cases will have a recovery rate less than 10%; in addition, at least 16% will be expected to show a deterioration in motor function (negative recovery rate) when a normal distribution is present.

Recovery rates can be used to evaluate present treatment regimes by studying the treatment of patients with recovery rates greater than two or three standard deviations above the expected mean recovery rate. The number of patients found within various positive ranges of the standard deviation is listed in Table 5. Note that no patient classified as a partial lesion was found above two standard deviations above the mean. This is secondary to the upper limit (1.0) in recovery rate, being less than two standard deviations. Also the large variance of *RR* in partial lesions is probably a factor secondary to grouping of the patients in Table 3. For graded complete and complete at bony level lesions, five patients were found above three standard deviations. This comprises 1.5% of the total population and 1.9% of the transverse or sharply demarcated complete and graded complete populations. Both percent are above the expected percent of 0.15% for a normal distribution. If one considers graded complete lesions and complete or CBL lesions separately, it is evident that this higher than expected percent above three standard deviations of the mean is primarily due to the sharply demarcated transverse complete lesions. Patients 5118 and 8190 with motor complete lesions on admission had traumatic soft herniated discs found with myelography and documented at surgery. BROOKE (4) was the first to report complete transverse myelitis secondary to a herniated nucleus pulposis. The authors of this paper found this to be of significant incidence in an earlier study of anterior decompression and fusion in complete lesions and have documented the statistical findings in an earlier work (5). The remaining three patients in Table 6 received aggressive therapy, yet these patients can be matched patient per patient with recovery rates not as significant. However, these patients in conjunction with those in Table 7, support the concept of early and aggressive bony decompression either by closed or open reduction. Between two to three standard deviations above the mean recovery, there are eight patients. While 8 of 436 are within the expected percent of occurrence, the cases should be studied. All patients in this group (Table 7) received early decompression of bony elements or removal of soft disc (case 8101).

Due to the direct relationship of *MIi* and *RR*, the *MI* at 1 year after injury can be predicted by using the below formula:

$MIc = RR\ (5 - MIi) + MIi.$

However, the standard deviation of *RR* must be considered and would give the expected gains within the limits of the standard deviation. For example, a patient classified as a C-5/6 motor complete with a *MIi* of 0.32 would be expected to have *MI* at 1 year after injury between -0.14 and 1.72 in 68% of the cases, if the *RR* (0.1 ± 0.2) in Table 4 is applied.

Lastly, recovery rates in conjunction with *MIi* can be used as controls for new treatment regimes. This can be accomplished both qualitatively and quantitatively. Qualitative evaluation consists of comparing the *RR* of patients properly classified and receiving a new treatment regime, with the recovery rates of those patients in the same classification not receiving that method of treatment. If the recovery rate value for the treatment group is consistently higher than two or three standard deviations above the mean recovery rates listed in Table 4 and the motor index initial is not significantly higher than the classification under study, then the treatment should be recognized as suggestive.

The quantitative method of study involves comparing two groups of patients similar in classification but dissimilar in treatment. In this case the *MIi* of the two groups of patients should not be significantly different by the *F* test. If the treatment under study is significantly better, then the treatment group under study should have a significantly better *RR* than the control group by the *F* test.

A significant number of patients must be studied in both of the above methods, for otherwise erroneous conclusions may result. For example, it is possible for 16 of 100 patients classified as CBL with C-5/6, C-6 fracture dislocations to have a *MIi* of 0.58 or better, and the same number to have a recovery rate of 0.30 or better. In other words, it is possible for 16 of 100 patients to go from a *MIi* of 0.58 to a maximum *MIc* of 2.04 and yet still not be one standard deviation above the mean.

Presently, we are carrying out a randomized prognostic study using the above motor classification system of analysis and the modified neurological examination form depicted in Table 5. The spinal cord motor index is composed of 14 representative muscles with a numeric grade (0 - 5) for testing the patients muscle power at each site. A normal score in all muscles of the index is 100 points. The extremities are graded on a scale of 0 - 5, according to the standards used in physical therapy (5 normal; 4 good; 3 fair; 2 poor; 1 trace; 0 none), while the axial muscles are graded on a simpler scale of 2 - 0 (2 strong; 1 weak; 0 absent). Note that the diaphragm, intercostals, upper and lower abdominals will also be evaluated by vital capacity (VC), force expiratory volume/s (FEV), and tital volume (TV).

Summary

In this paper we have presented a new motor classification of patients with spinal cord injuries. This system of classification provides statistically discrete subdivisions. The patients in each of the subdivisions of the classification can be mathematically summarized with numeric indices that then may be accurately analyzed statistically. This allows the clinical researcher in spinal cord injuries to evaluate current treatments and assess the potential of new treatment regimes. In addition, tables of *MIi* and recovery rates have been presented to aid in the correct classification of new patients and in the prediction of their present chances of motor recovery. Lastly, the data presented indicates the need for early aggressive bony decompression either open or closed and illustrates the need to suspect traumatic soft disc in complete lesions.

References

1. HUNTSBERGER, D.V., WEAVERTON, P.E., BACON: Statistical interference in the biomedical Sciences 1970
2. LUCAS, J.T., DUCKER, T.B.: Spinal cord trauma. A comprehensive study of classification treatment and prognosis (in press)
3. SCHNEIDER, R.C., CHERRY, G.L., PANTEK, H.E.: The syndrome of acute central cervical spinal cord injury. J. Neurol. Sc. II, 546 (1954)
4. WEINBERG, G., SCHUMAKER, J.A.: Statistics: an intuitive approach. 3rd ed. Wadsworth 1974

5. LIDE, M.T.M.: A prognostic index for motor ability in cervical spinal cord injuries. Graduate Thesis, Medical University of South Carolina 1973

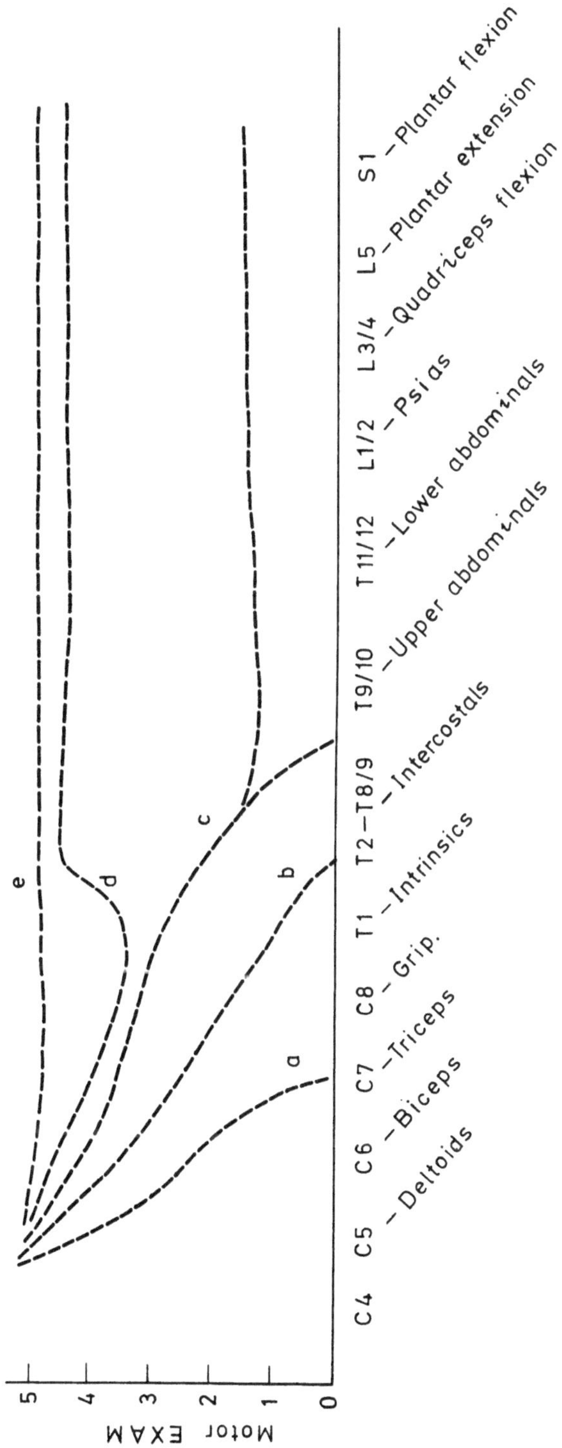

Fig. 1. Classification of patients (motor) (biological continuum - C5/6)

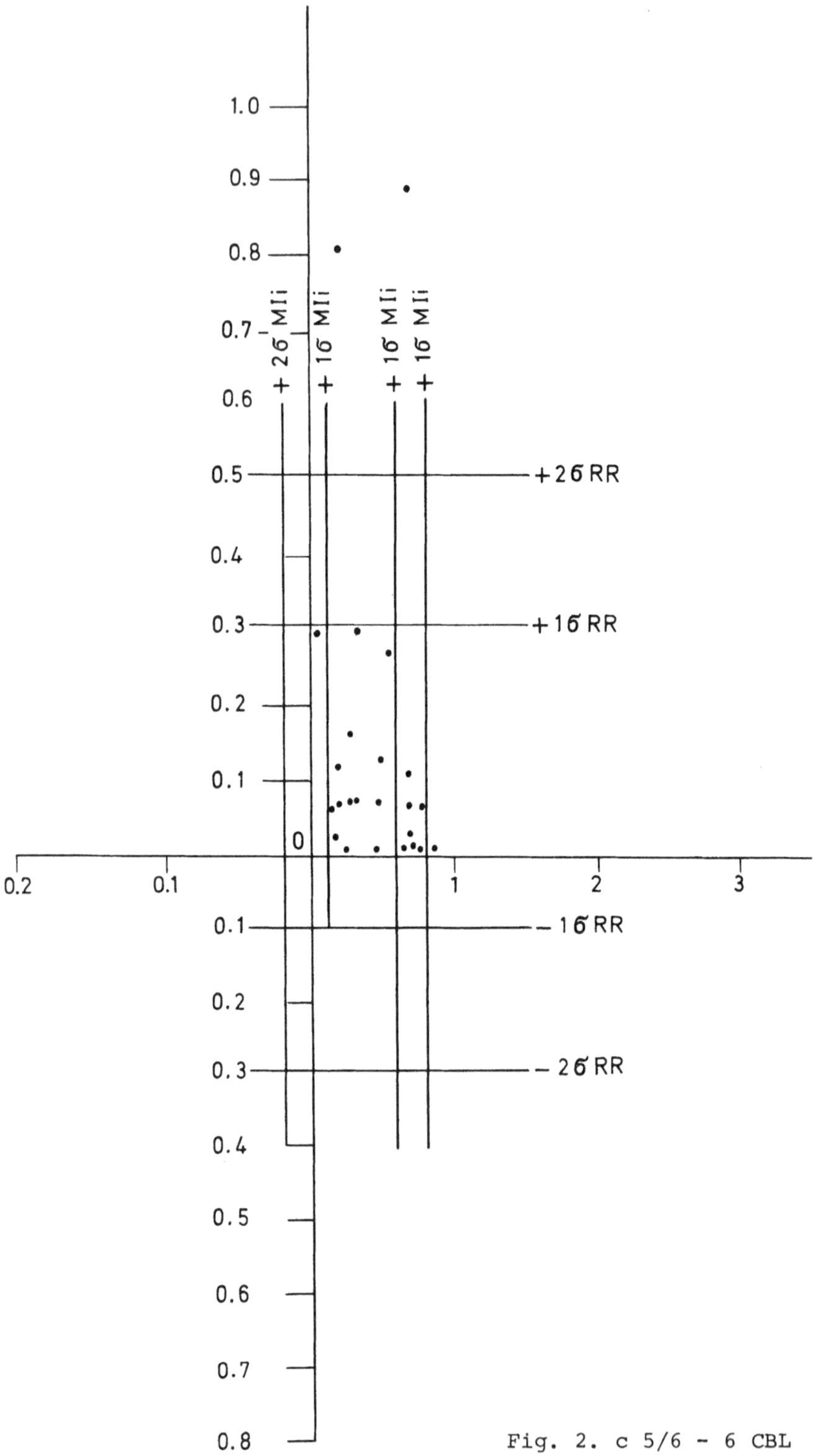

Fig. 2. c 5/6 - 6 CBL

Ventricular CSF Pulse Pressure Amplitude: an Index of Intracranial Compliance

E. L. FOLTZ and S. LEDERHAUS

Introduction

The precise dynamic etiology of ventriculomegaly in hydrocephalus has not been conclusively demonstrated. The need for such understanding is clear, however, for several reasons: (1) as a basis for the continued search for treatment of hydrocephalus by other than CSF shunting techniques; (2) for application in our continued efforts at early diagnosis of adult occult hydrocephalus in the presence of normal mean CSF pressure; and (3) as basic data in our continued search for a simple, quantitative method to differentiate arrested from active hydrocephalus without relying on extended observation times.

As background, intracranial pulse pressure of CSF was implicated by BERING as etiologic for ventricular enlargement in hydrocephalus (2, 3,4). Subsequent studies of CSF pressures by various scientists have failed to clearly prove this relationship (1,5,6,7), but a concept has developed wherein the expansile and pulsatile arterial in-thrust in the choroid plexus produces a pulsatile distension of CSF spaces (ventricles and subarachnoid spaces) during cardiac systole, which in turn compresses cerebral veins, especially cortex surface veins, and thus causes volume venting of venous blood from the head (Fig. 1). This effect produces the pulsatile flow of jugular venous blood. No CSF volume venting of significance occurs in this sequence because of the short time base of the pulse beat. The time base of CSF bulk flow out of the head is much too long to respond immediately to systolic in-thrust from the choroid plexus, but CSF space distension does occur producing pulsatile compression of those intracranial veins that are in proper anatomic position to produce an immediate outflow of venous blood. As demonstrated in Fig. 1, this phenomenon is presumed present in the normal state with the CSF pulse wave, or pulse pressure, having the characteristics of a damped wave, i.e., the force involved in the CSF pulse wave is reduced or damped by the "moving resistance" of the venous volume venting effect. If the volume venting effect were to be reduced or lost, this CSF pulse wave should theoretically become "undamped" with amplitude increase and an increase in the slope of the systolic wave incline, indicating an "unmoving resistance".

The formula for calculating the force that results from the arrest of a volume of moving fluid is:

$$F = mv^2/2\Delta t;$$

mv^2 = kinetic energy of moving fluids;
m = mass of the fluid;
v = velocity of movement of the fluid;
t = time from velocity stated to motion arrest.

Thus, shortening the t by converting the moving resistance of venous volume venting toward a rigid resistance without volume venting will increase the force of the pulse wave.

Such an effect could theoretically be achieved experimentally if one accepts the concept that the force of the systolic choroid plexus pulse is transmitted through the distensible CSF compartment to compress the venous compartment and thus cause a volume venting of venous blood from the head via the jugular venous system. Two maneuvers which can shorten t in the force formula are:

1) obliterate critical intracranial venous volume, thus destroying the moving resistance and producing more rigid resistance;
2) remove the CSF volume which is interspaced between the pulsatile force source (the choroid plexus) and the compressible venous structures, thus interrupting the pressure transference sequence with loss of venous venting thereby.

The mass (m) and fluid velocity (v) of the force equation are directly proportional to cardiac output and systemic blood pressure. Thus, if blood pressure and pulse rate are constant, changes in t by manipulating intracranial venous and CSF volume would produce significant force changes. This equation can be calculated for absolute values, but relative values are satisfactory for the emphasis of the current experiments reported.

Experimental Design

A single experimental manipulation which could conceivably produce these two effects separately was considered (8). Obviously, such a manipulation must conform to the Monro-Kelley doctrine though on a time base of the pulse rate, and the effect must be contributing to intracranial compliance (initial intracranial compensation to pressure increase, etc.) (10,11,12,13).

Extensive efforts at changing intracranial venous volume had been done in our experimental laboratory whereby the intracranial venous compartment was loaded by jugular compression, head elevation, and head depression (9,10,15). The effects were more difficult to interpret than previous work on mean intracranial pressure effects (13, 14,18). On the other hand CSF volume loading could theoretically achieve the ends desired if both positive loading (15,17)(infusion into CSF spaces to produce high mean pressure) and negative loading (withdrawal of CSF to produce low mean pressures) were investigated. No vascular reflex responses or metabolic effects would be activated under this protocol. Presumably the high mean pressure by CSF infusion would reduce intracranial venous volume by extrusion, and CSF withdrawal might simply interrupt the CSF compression of veins. The simplicity of this design was attractive.

Methods

Eighteen healthy mongrel dogs were selected for comparable weight and size (6 - 8 kilo body weight). Surgical anesthesia levels were accomplished by intravenous pentobarbital and intubation with artificial respiration by the Harvard pump technique. End-expiratory CO_2 and O_2 were measured constantly by Beckman gas analyzer; these values were kept at normal levels throughout the experiments. Inspiratory tracheal pressures were adjusted to 12-15 cm of water and the respiratory rate was varied from 30 to 40 as needed to maintain normal end-expiratory CO_2 and O_2 levels. Blood pressure was recorded throughout and remained normal and unchanged (femoral artery catheter).

After anesthesia stabilization, the animal was placed in the Wells stereotactic dog apparatus, with moderate anteflexion of the occipito-cervical junction. Under sterile conditions, stereotactic cannulation of the right frontal horn was accomplished using a 7/64 twist drill skull perforation and a 20 blunt needle type metal cannula. This cannula was connected by a short, rigid tubing filled with Elliott's B Solution to a Statham P-23 or P-50 transducer with hard copy write-out on a Grass Model 7A polygraph and simultaneous recording with a TEAC magnetic tape recorder.

In most of these preparations, subdural pressure was likewise recorded from the right frontal area through a 1 cm trephine done under sterile conditions through which a 0.25 cc silicone rubber balloon was inserted into the subdural space and connected to a hydraulic system for measurement of subdural pressure simultaneously with intraventricular pressures. This aspect of the procedure is not critical to this report.

Under similar sterile conditions, a 20 sharp needle was then introduced into the cisterna magna for purposes of infusing artificial CSF (Elliot's B Solution) and withdrawing CSF via a standard infusion-withdrawal mechanical pump. Some of these infusions and withdrawals were done by a 2 cc tuberculin syringe under manual control (Fig. 2).

Ventricular pressures were recorded at high gain to clearly amplify the pulse pressures and wave forms of the ventricular CSF and subdural pressures. The recording on magnetic tape allowed subsequent playback for more discrete analysis.

The protocol for the infusion and withdrawal of CSF under these circumstances was:

1) At homeostatic or normal CSF pressures, ten minutes baseline record of mean CSF and pulse pressure CSF was recorded (hard copy and magnetic tape).
2) CSF was slowly withdrawn from the cisterna magna until no more could be obtained, producing a mean CSF pressure which at times went as low as -100 mm of CSF in the right lateral ventricle; pressures were recorded for 5 min.
3) The CSF was then slowly infused back into the cisterna magna until homeostatic or normal CSF pressures were reattained and recordings made for 10 min.
4) Artificial CSF was slowly and steadily reinfused (5-7 cc) to achieve an intracranial pressure of up to +500 mm of CSF; CSF pressures were then recorded for 5 min.
5) CSF then slowly and steadily withdrawn until the CSF mean pressure was again at homeostatic or normal levels, and pressures recorded for an additional 5 min.

This protocol in a multistage experimental design was concluded with instillation of kaolin suspension into the cisterna magna to produce hydrocephalus in these animals over the ensuing 4 to 6 weeks. This entire procedure was done under sterile technique and all animals survived this recording sequence.

Results

In all 18 animals the effects were similar (Figs. 3, 4 and 5):

1) Resting or homeostatic CSF mean pressure was 100 - 120 mm of water; the resting or homeostatic CSF pulse pressure was 10 - 14 mm of water.

2) CSF withdrawal to maximum possible (variable from animal to animal) produced a mean pressure fall as low as -100 mm of CSF but often no lower than 0 mm CSF; *the CSF pulse pressure augmented* significantly when mean pressure approached one-half the resting level, increasing then to *18 - 38 mm of water*.

3) CSF reinfusion to former resting CSF pressures and pulse pressures often required 1 to 3 cc more fluid reinfused than had been withdrawn.

4) Continued infusion of Elliott's B Solution to produce elevated CSF mean pressure up to +500 mm of water produced reappearance of *augmented pulse pressure amplitudes*, usually parallel to the increasing mean pressure.

5) Withdrawal of CSF to reproduce the resting mean pressure also produced the resting pulse pressure seen at first (10 - 14 mm of water). These maneuvers did not seem to impair the system under measurement, and there was no difference in their responses if the sequence was reversed, i.e., high intracranial pressures (ICP) produced first followed by the low pressures, etc.

Discussion

These results support the basic thesis presented since both maneuvers (withdrawal and infusion), augmented pulse pressure amplitude. This strongly suggests that the resting or normal pulse amplitude of CSF was converted from a damped pressure wave to an undamped wave with consequent increase in amplitude, reflecting increased force as related to the force equation.

This CSF pulse pressure augmentation occurred as mean CSF pressure rose above normal and also as CSF mean pressure was forced below normal. This CSF pulse pressure augmentation in high ICP may be based on loss of volume venting of venous blood since maximal extrusion of such had occurred as a result of the high CSF mean pressure that had compressed the cortical veins (13). Such maximal extrusion of venous blood out of the head obviated volume venting and converted the moving resistance to hard resistance with a small t value in the force equation involving kinetic energy of moving fluids ($f = mv^2/2\Delta t$).

Explanation of the CSF pulse pressure augmentation (and therefore force increase) when mean CSF pressure is forced below normal is not immediately obvious, but certainly the CSF compartment is largely exhausted by the withdrawal, and choroid plexus pulsations may therefore not be transmitted to the cerebral surface veins, which may, in fact, be distended. This combination of loss of CSF interface and increased venous volume inertia may prevent venous volume venting, however, and CSF pulse pressure amplitude is again augmented *even though the mean pressure is low*. Clinical application of this phenomenon to adult occult hydrocephalus is attractive.

Current use of terms involved in ICP include compliance, resistance, and elastance. Compliance and resistance are related primarily to volume venting capacity of intracranial contents, referring primarily to blood volume or CSF volume changes, whereas elastance relates more to the ability of the brain mass itself to conform geometrically in a manner which compensates for increasing pressure.

Compliance (K) is considered as the reciprocal of resistance (11,16) when considering ICP on an indefinite time base. If the time base is constricted to pressure phenomena related to the time base of the pulse, then the resistance can be equated to the pulse amplitude of the CSF wave and probably the systolic slope or gradient. Therefore, at normal ICP the K equals 1/r. Under normal conditions as measured, the pulse amplitude of this CSF wave varies from 10 to 18, whereas increased mean pressure produces a high pulse pressure value of 20 to 30. Therefore, compliance at normal level is equal to 1/10, or 0.1, whereas at increased pressures as shown in this work, compliance is equal to 1/30, or 0.03, - indicating a significant loss of compliance. From a semantic standpoint, this is an interpretation from mean pressure observations and seems logical. The single entity involved in this K reduction, again limiting this to CSF pulse pressure measurements only, must be the intracranial venous volume available for volume venting on the time base of the pulse.

The concepts are in concert with those presented by MARMAROU (16) and HAKIM (11), in which the mathematical evaluations are based only on mean pressure.

The observations reported here may further a more precise definition of *"normal"* CSF pressure. Reports vary widely as to what normal CSF mean pressure level is, largely because of variabilities in the methods of recording and a certain impreciseness in reference points. If the CSF pulse pressure *wave* form reported here in dogs were to be used as a guide in human recordings, it is likely that an index of CSF pulse pressure amplitude could easily be identified which will reflect the truly normal mean pressure (i.e., a fully damped wave). Increased mean pressure would show an undamped wave with high amplitude even though mean pressure might be within current limits of normal. Such studies are in progress. This is particularly applicable to hydrocephalus in the adult.

Conclusions

1) CSF pulse pressure amplitude may reflect the intracranial status of factors damping this CSF pulse wave under normal conditions.
2) Increased mean CSF pressure and lowered mean CSF pressure both produce augmentation of this CSF pulse amplitude.
3) Such CSF pulse pressure amplitude augmentation is probably due to loss of volume venting from the cranium of venous blood and may be a major component of the brain compliance reaction to intracranial pressure elevations as well as lowered mean intracranial pressure.
4) Application of this phenomenon to the study of ventriculomegaly in hydrocephalus is warranted. Such studies are currently under way.
5) These observations may aid in further defining normal CSF.

References

1. ADOLPH, R.J., FUKUSUMI, H., FOWLER, M.D.: Origin of cerebrospinal fluid pulsations. Am. J. Physiol. 212, 840-946 (1967)
2. BERING, E.A., Jr.: Choroid plexus and arteriole pulsations of cerebrospinal fluid: Demonstration of the choroid plexus as a cerebrospinal fluid pump. Arch. Neurol. Psychiatry 73, 165-173 (1955)
3. BERING, E.A., Jr.: Circulation of the cerebrospinal fluid: Demonstration of the choroid plexuses as the generator of the force

flow of fluid and ventricular enlargement. J. Neurosurg. 19, 405-413 (1962)

4. BERING, E.A., Jr., INGRAM, F.D.: The arteriole pulsations of the cerebrospinal fluid - its origin, configuration and possible clinical importance. Trans. Am. Neurol. Assoc. 49, 54 (1953)

5. DARDENNE, G., DEREYMAKER, A., LACHERON, J.M.: Cerebrospinal fluid pressure and pulsatility. Eur. Neurol. 2, 193-216 (1969)

6. DAVSON, H.: Dynamic aspects of cerebrospinal fluid. Dev. Med. Child Neurol. 14 (Suppl. 27), 1 - 5 (1972)

7. DuBOULEY, G., O'CONNELL, J.: Further investigations of pulsatile movements in the cerebrospinal fluid pathways. Acta Radiol. (Diagn.) (Stockh.) 13, 496-523 (1972)

8. FOLTZ, E.L., DeFEO, D., LEDERHAUS, S.: The CSF "pulse pressure" index in hydrocephalus with clinical applications of head wrapping therapy. Scientific Program Manuscripts, Vol. 43A-43J. Am. Assoc. Neurol. Surg. 1976

9. FOLTZ, E.L.: Clinical studies in hydrocephalus. In: Cisternography and hydrocephalus: A symposium. Chapt. 16. Springfield, Ill.: Thomas 1972

10. HAKIM, S.: Biomechanics of hydrocephalus. In: Cisternography and hydrocephalus: A symposium. Chapt. 3. Springfield, Ill: Thomas 1972

11. HAKIM, S., VENEGAS, J.G., BURTON, J.D.: The physics of the cranial cavity, hydrocephalus and normal pressure hydrocephalus: Mechanical interpretation and mathematical model. Surg. Neurol. 5, 187-210 (1976)

12. KATZMAN, R., HUSSEY, F.: A simple constant infusion manometric test for measurement of CSF absorption. Neurology (Minneap.) 20, 534-544 (1970)

13. KITANO, M., OLDENDORF, W.H., CASEN, B.: The elasticity of the cranial blood pool. J. Nucl. Biol. Med. 5, 613-625 (1964)

14. LANGFITT, T.W., WEINSTEIN, J. D., KASSELL, N.E.: Compression of cerebral vessels by intracranial hypertension, I; Dural sinus pressure. Acta Neurochir. 15, 212-221 (1966)

15. LEDERHAUS, S.: Pulse pressure index (PPI) in normal and hydrocephalic dogs. Univ. Cal. Student Res. J. (1975)

16. MARMAROU, A.: A theoretical and experimental evaluation of the cerebrospinal fluid systems. Drexel University, Ph. D. Thesis, 1973

17. RYDER, H.W., ESPEY, F.E., KIMBELL, F.D.: The mechanism of change in cerebrospinal fluid pressure following an induced change in the volume of the fluid space. J. Lab. Clin. Med. 41, 423-438 (1953)

18. RYDER, H.W., ESPEY, F.E., KIMBELL, F.D.: The elasticity of the craniospinal venous bed. J. Lab. Clin. Med. 42, 944 (1953)

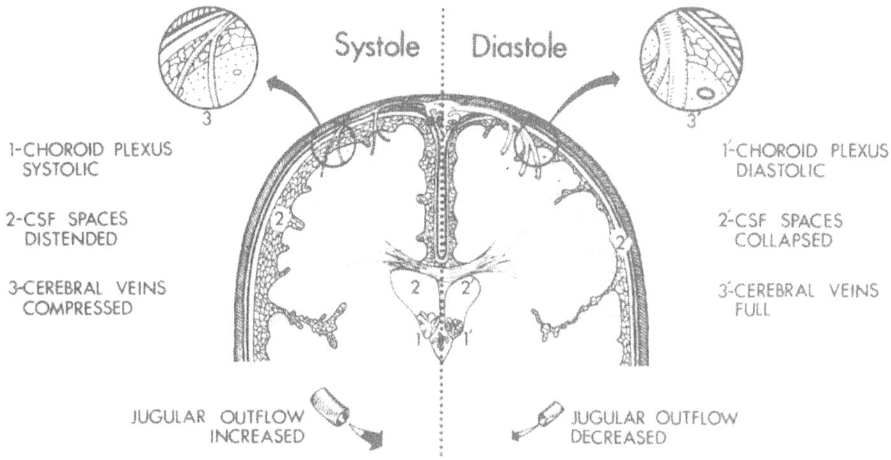

Fig. 1. Monro-Kelley doctrine of intracranial compartment compensations based on volume/pressure increase produced by choroid plexus in-thrust of arterial blood, using time base of arterial pulse itself. *Left side:* (1) systolic arterial expansion of choroid plexus (intraventricular) causing (2) CSF space distension (ventricle and subarachnoid space) which leads then to (3) compression of convexity cerebral veins and extrusion of venous blood into dural sinuses (volume venting) and a pulse of venous flow in the jugular vein. This sequence occurs during systole and immediate postsystole arterial flow. *Right side:* (1') during diastole, choroid plexus collapse/constriction within ventricle allows (2') relaxative CSF spaces (ventricles and subarachnoid spaces) with resultant (3') flood or engorgement of cerebral convexity veins and marked reduction in out-flow of dural sinus blood of jugular system. This sequence is repeated with each cardiac pulse

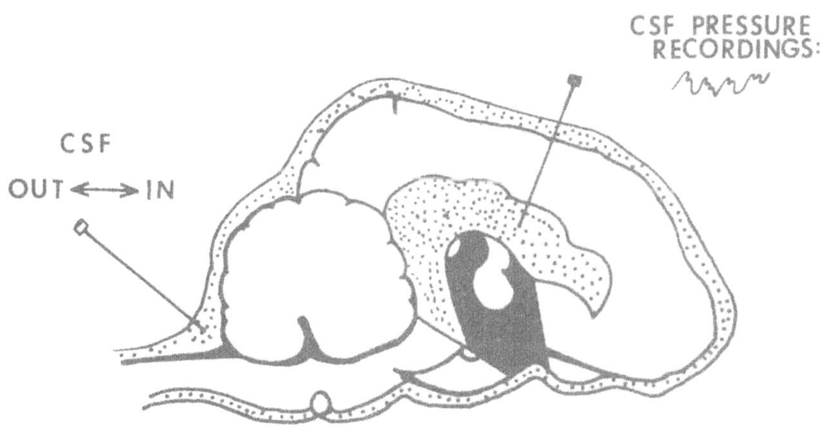

Fig. 2. Dog brain system used for measurement ventricular CSF pulse pressures during CSF volume changes induced via cisterna magna

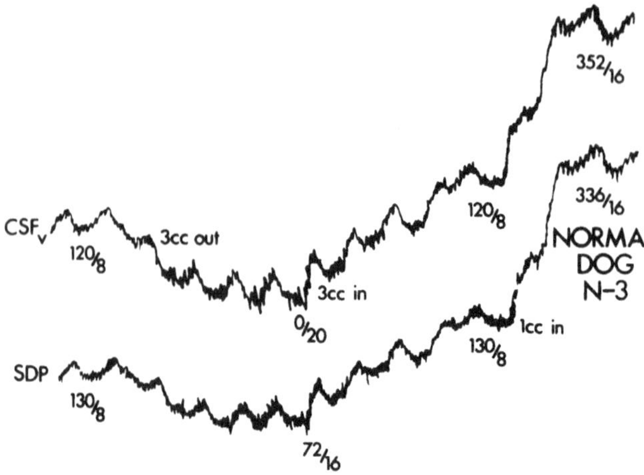

NORMAL
DOG
N-3

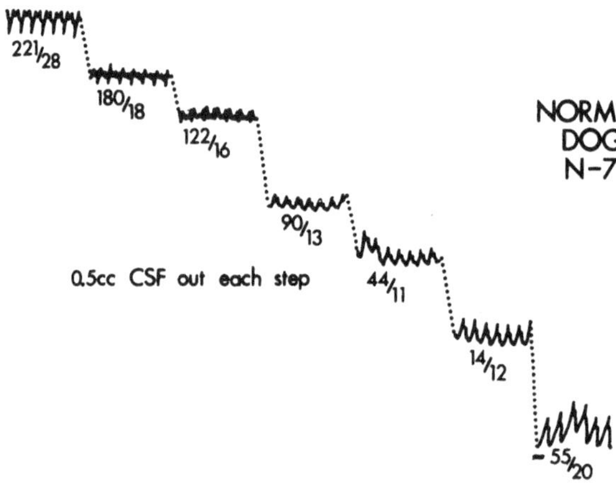

NORMAL
DOG
N-7

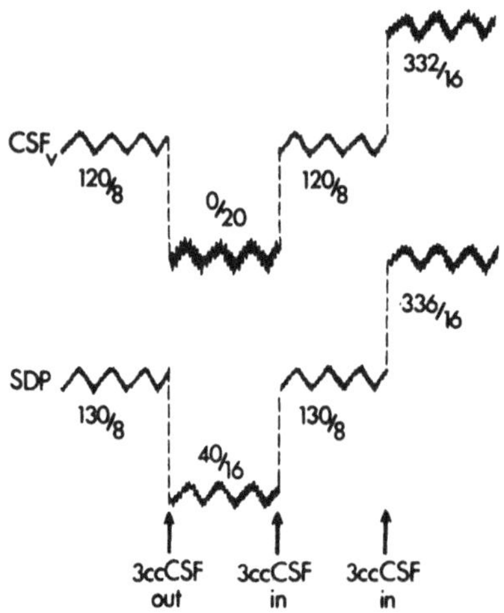

NORMAL
DOG
N-12

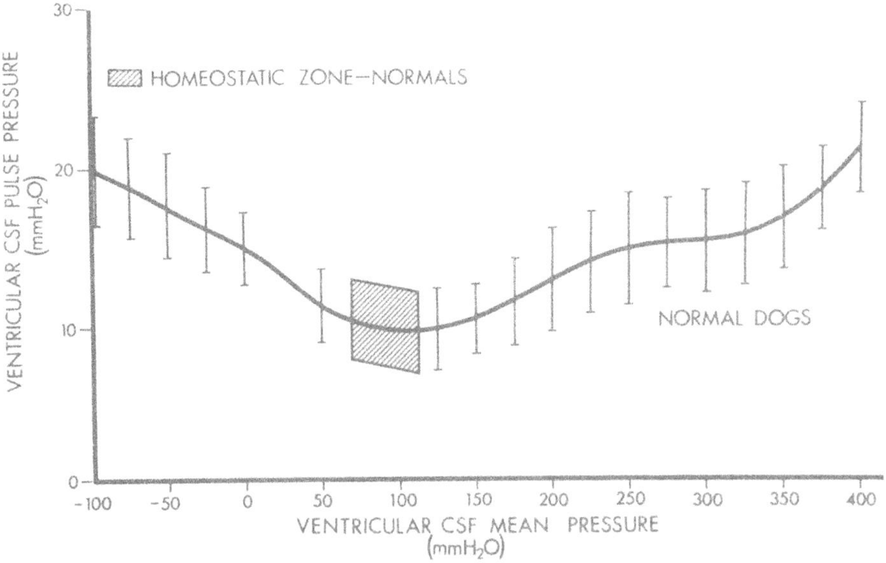

Fig. 4. Summary in 18 dogs showing mean CSF pressure (abscissa) as related to CSF ventricular pulse pressure (ordinate). Standard deviation *bars* on graph lines indicate consistent response. Pressures in mm H_2O. Homeostatic pressures (normal at start of procedure) in *diagonal line area*

◁ Fig. 3. Polygraph records of ventricular CSF mean/pulse pressures in the normal dogs. *Dog N-3*, recordings are present during homeostatic state, CSF withdrawal, CSF volume return to starting mean pressure, and CSF injection to produce high mean pressure. Pressures are recorded as mean/pulse pressure at each stage in mm H_2O (i.e., 100/10 = 100 mm H_2O mean pressure with 10 mm H_2O pulse pressure). *Note* striking *increase* in pulse pressure at *low mean* and at *high mean* CSF pressures as compared to initial, homeostatic levels. SDP = subdural pressure (paralleled CSF pressures). *Dog N-7*, record starts at high mean pressure and is reduced to a negative 55 mm H_2O mean pressure by 0.5 cc increments of CSF withdrawal. Note high pulse pressure at mean of 221 (221/28) and low pulse pressure at normal mean (44/11) with reappearance of high pulse pressure at minus 55 mean (-55/20). *Dog N-12*, record shows same type of response with 3 cc CSF removal and reinjection - i.e., normal mean (120/8); at low mean (0/20); and at high mean (332/16). These examples show change of a damped pulse pressure (amplitude) at normal mean pressure to a high amplitude undamped pulse at *both high* and *low mean pressure*

Experimental Brain Edema in Acute and Chronic Brain Abscess in Rabbits and Its Morphologic Alterations

T. WALLENFANG, J. BOHL, and G. SCHREINER

Despite advances in diagnosis, in techniques of neurosurgery, and in therapy, brain abscess remains a neurosurgical challenge. The final outcome of the brain abscess is determined by the type of abscess (acute or chronic) and by the severity of the perifocal edema due to inflammation that has not yet coalesced.

The aim of the present investigation is to examine the inflammatory brain edema in acute brain abscess and its decrease when encapsulation develops. We would like to call attention to the morphologic changes of the different tissue samples parallel to the course of edema.

Method

In the right capsula interna of 63 rabbits, 0.03 ml of a mixture of agar and bouillon with *Staphylococcus aureus* (in the ratio of 1 : 1) was inoculated under ketamine anesthesia (20-25 mg/kg body weight) (2,3,7,8). The amount injected contained between 1 and 1.5 million organisms with a low degree of pathogenicity. Beside the comparison with the contralateral hemisphere, there was a control group of 42 animals that had only received agar and bouillon injected into the right hemisphere.

The extent of the edema induced was visualized by intravenous injections of 2% Evans blue (1 ml/kg body weight) (5).

After 1, 2, 3, 5, 7, 14, 28, and 56 days, respectively, seven animals were sacrificed and the cerebral hemispheres weighed. The brain was then frozen in liquid nitrogen and sliced into four parts. One slice including half of the abscess was investigated by light microscopy. Water and electrolyte contents were determined in the following areas of the cerebral white matter: immediately around the abscess, remote from the abscess, the cortex over the abscess, and the contralateral hemisphere, which served as control.

After 2, 3, 5, 7, 14, and 28 days, both carotid arteries were cannulated, the brains were fixed by perfusion with 3.9% glutaraldehyde, embedded in epoxy resin for 1.5-µm thin sections, and samples for electron microscopy were taken from the same areas as mentioned above.

Results

Abscess formation was observed in all animals (Fig. 1). The abscess diameters were 4-7 mm and were microscopically visible up to the cortex. The abscesses showed a distinct tendency to spread in the direction of the ventricular system. The encapsulation is first seen on the 7th day. As the capsule increased in thickness in the following weeks, the edema decreased.

The maximal water accumulation around the abscess was found during the first 48 h (Fig. 2). On the 2nd day, the water content was around 5.8% higher (75.4 g/100 g wet weight) than in the contralateral hemisphere and in the control group (69.6 g/100 g wet weight) in which agar and bouillon were injected.

The water content decreased from the 2nd to the 7th day. The water content was then 70.4%. With development of encapsulation during the following weeks, the water content adjacent to the abscess was lower than in the acute phase of edema but nevertheless nearly 2% higher than normal (69.5 g/100 g wet weight).

In the areas remote from the abscess, the water content was raised only slightly less than the area around the abscess. In the acute phase, there was an increase of 4.8% (75.2 g/100 g wet weight) compared to the left hemisphere; no significant changes were seen in the control group. In the phase of encapsulation, the water content remained high up to the 14th day and returned to normal by about the 28th day. There were no significant changes in the cortex as regards the water content.

Parallel to the edema, the sodium content in the right hemisphere reached a peak in the adjacent (247 mmol/kg dry weight) and remote (250 mmol/kg dry weight) area of the acute abscess after 2 days (Fig. 3). On the 7th day, the sodium content returned to normal and then stabilized at a slightly higher level (160 mmol/kg dry weight) when encapsulation developed.

In accordance with these biochemical findings, there were striking morphologic signs of an excessive perifocal brain edema in the neighborhood of the acute abscess until the 5th day. The most predominant alterations were severe necrosis of the brain tissue in the center and focal inflammatory infiltrations at the margin of the abscess. Furthermore, there was marked degeneration of the adjacent white matter with numerous macrophages, granulocytes, and reactive astrocytic swelling. There was immense enlargement of the extracellular space, which was filled with a homogeneous plasma-like fluid, containing fragments of degenerating or necrotic cells and with erythrocytes (Fig. 4).

Some blood vessels with widened perivascular spaces in the vicinity of the abscess showed a dense fibrinoid exudation (1). This extracellular fluid seemed to reach a maximum on the 2nd day and began to spread out along the parallel arrangement of the myelinated nerve fiber bundles, especially toward the ventricular system. The cerebral cortex and the basal ganglia remained almost unaffected. From the 5th day on, there were signs of an incipient encapsulation with vascular proliferations and multiplying reactive astrocytes. By the 14th and 28th day, the abscess was already surrounded by a thick capsule and showed a marked foreign body reaction in the center. In the adjacent white matter, a reduction of myelinated nerve fibers and a reactive gliosis was noticed. In some areas an incipient status cribrosus could be observed.

While the amount of extracellular fluid gradually decreased, many astrocytes remained swollen. In all stages of the abscess formation and encapsulation, the inoculated microorganisms were encountered in the center, even after 28 days.

Summary

In the absence of therapy, brain inflammation caused by attenuated bacteria almost always led to a brain abscess. In the acute phase, there is edema formation with a tendency to spread toward the ventricular system. Whenever the edema front had reached the ventricle, the ventricular wall became stained with Evans blue and the CSF was bluish. At the same time, there was an increase in the CSF pressure, as could be proved by an experiment currently being performed. Due to disintegration of the white matter, the abscess tended to spread toward the ventricular system.

As soon as encapsulation begins, the severity of the abscess decreases and the water content disminishes. After 28 days, no organisms could be cultured. On the other hand, the disturbances of the blood-brain barrier persisted as a result of increasing size of the encapsulation. There was no complete resolution of the edema around the chronic abscess.

References

1. CERVÓS-NAVARRO, J., CHRISTMANN, U., SASAKI, S.: An ultrastructural substrate for the resolution of postirritation brain adema. In: Dynamics of Brain Edema. PAPPIUS, H.M., FEINDEL, W. (eds.), pp. 43-49. Berlin, Heidelberg, New York: Springer 1976
2. GROFF, R.A., Experimental production of abscess of brain in cats. Arch. Neurol. Psychiatry 31, 199-204 (1934)
3. HASSLER, O., FORSGREN, A.: Experimental abscess in brain and subcutis. Acta Pathol. Microbiol. Scand. 62, 59-67 (1964)
4. HIRANO, A.: The fine structure of brain edema. In: The structure and function of nervous tissue. BOURNE, G.H. (ed.), pp. 69-135. New York: Academic Press 1969
5. KLATZO, J.: Neuropathological aspects of brain edema. J. Neuropathol. Exp. Neurol. 26, 1 (1967)
6. LONG, D.M., MAXWELL, R.E., FRENCH, L.A.: The effects of glucosteroids upon cold induced brain edema. J. Neuropathol. Exp. Neurol. 30, 680-697 (1971)
7. MARKLEY, G.M.: A method for experimental production of brain abscess. Proc. Soc. Exp. Biol. Med. 47, 171-175 (1941)
8. QUARTEY, G.R., JOHNSTON, J.A., ROZDILISKY, B.: Decadron in the treatment of cerebral abscesses. J. Neurosurg. 45, 301-310 (1976)
9. REULEN, H.J.: Vasogenic brain edema. Br. J. Anaesth. 48, 741-752 (1976)
10. REULEN, H.J., TSUYUMU, M., TACK, A., FENSKE, A.R., PRIOLEAU, G.R.: Clearance of edema fluid into cerebrospinal fluid. J. Neurosurg. 48, 754-764 (1978)

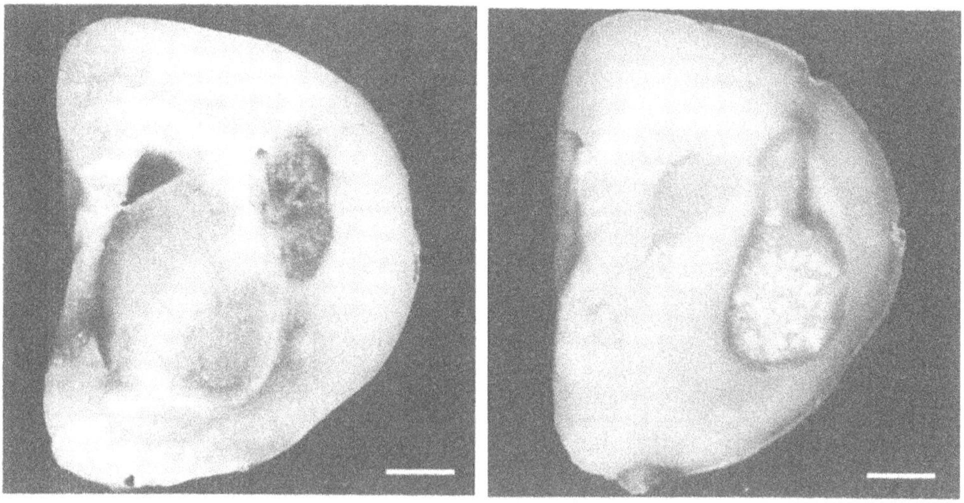

Fig. 1. *Left:* right hemisphere. Acute abscess 1 day after inoculation. x 6. *Right:* right hemisphere. Chronic abscess 56 days old with marked encapsulation. The *white line* represents 2 mm. x 6

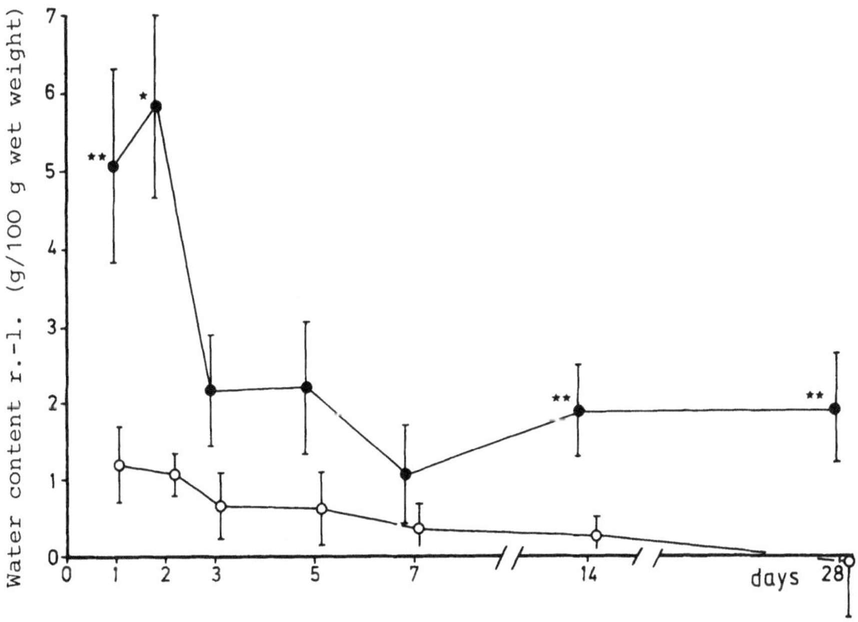

Fig. 2. Changes in water content (g/100 g wet weight) of the white matter adjacent to the acute and chronic abscess. The differences between right and left hemisphere of the abscess group (agar-bouillon-*Staphylococcus aureus*) and the control group (agar-bouillon) are compared. *, **, ***, significantly different from control; *$\underline{P}$ = 0.05; **$\underline{P}$ = 0.02; ***$\underline{P}$ = 0.01 (Wilcoxon rank sum test); ●, abscess; o, control

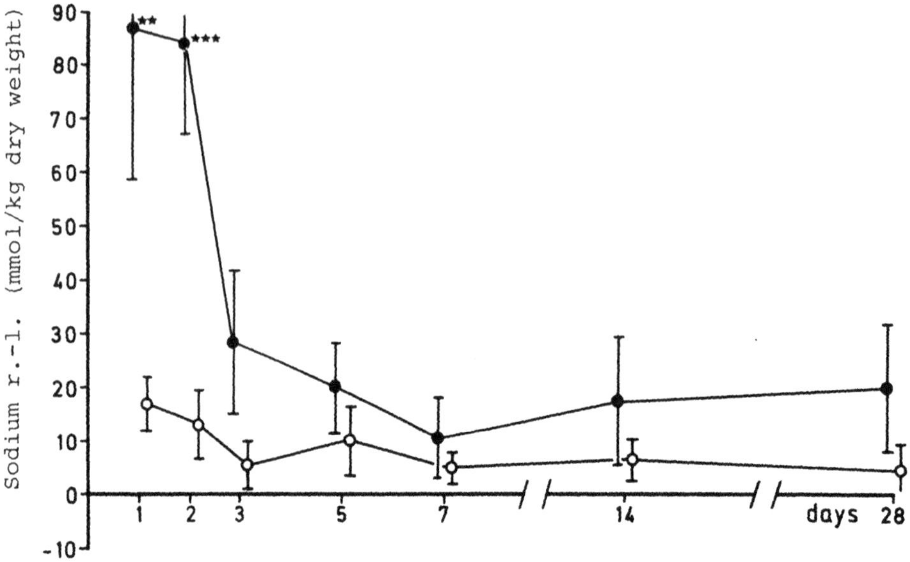

Fig. 3. Changes in sodium contents (mmol/kg dry weight) of the white matter adjacent to the acute and chronic abscess. The differences between right and left hemisphere of the abscess group (agar-bouillon-*Staphylococcus aureus*) and the control group (agar-bouillon) are compared. *, **, ***, significantly different from the control. *$\underline{P}$ = 0.5; **$\underline{P}$ = 0.02; ***$\underline{P}$ = 0.01 (Wilcoxon rank sum test); •, abscess; o, control

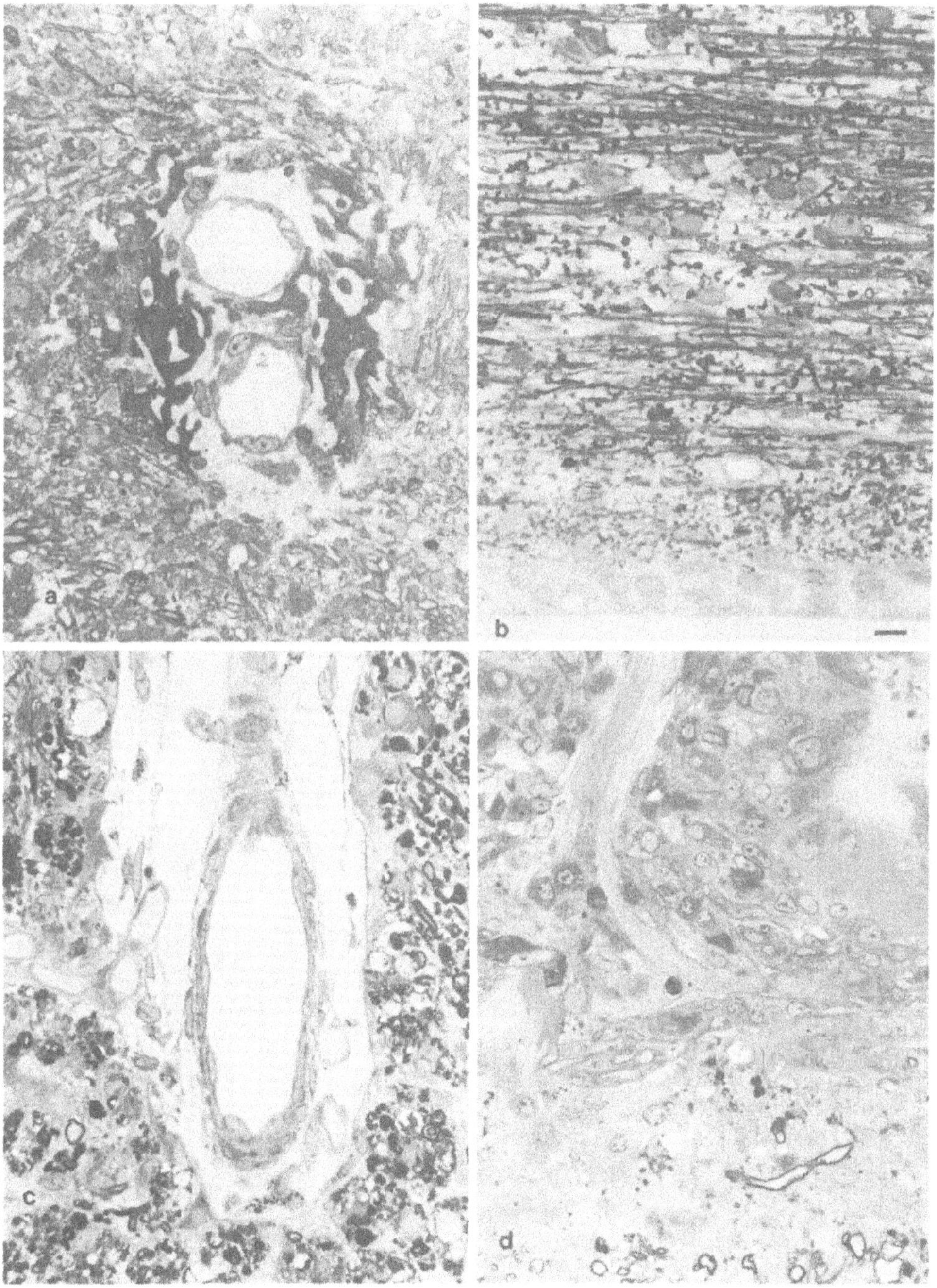

Fig.4.a Perivascular fibrinoid exudation not far from the abscess on the 2nd day. b Marked brain edema with enlargement of the extracellular space in the subependymal white matter. c Enlargement of the perivascular space of VIRCHOW ROBIN with cellular reaction on the 14th day. d Dense capsule of the abscess on the 28th day with connective tissue and glial reaction. The *black line* represents 10 μm

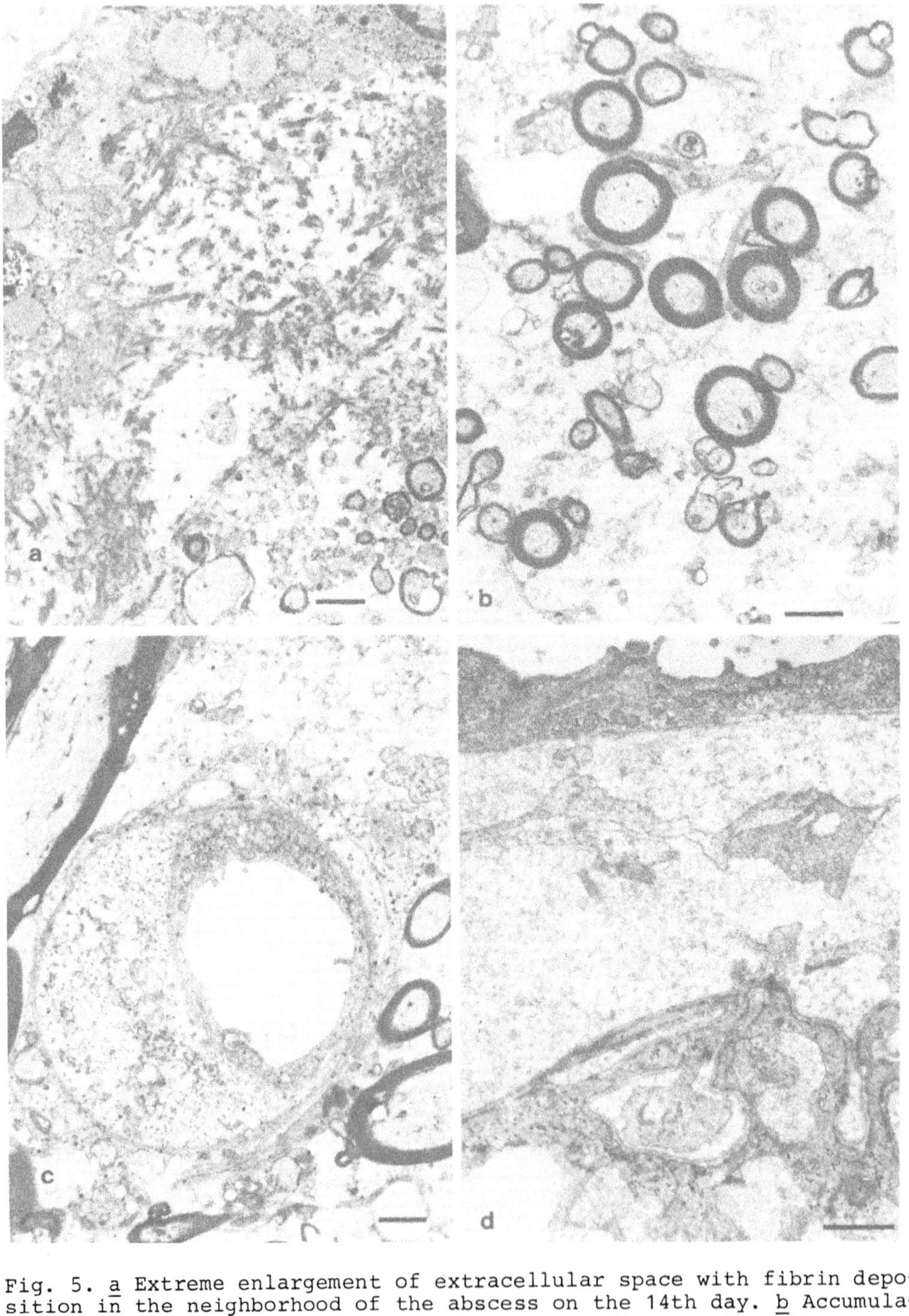

Fig. 5. a Extreme enlargement of extracellular space with fibrin deposition in the neighborhood of the abscess on the 14th day. b Accumulation of extracellular fluid even at a greater distance from the abscess on the 2nd day. c Capillary with intact endothelial cells and with swollen astrocytic processes in the vicinity on the 2nd day. d Enlargement of the perivascular space of a small cerebral vein with exudation of a plasma-like fluid on the 14th day. The *black lines* represent 1 µm

Tissue PO_2 and rCBF in Edematous Brain Cortex During Moderate and Severe Arterial Hypoxia

R. SCHUBERT, J. GROTE, and K. SCHÜRMANN

Under the conditions of normal arterial blood pressure, pronounced arterial hypoxia, caused by the reduction of arterial oxygen tension, induces a progressive increase in the total as well as in the regional cerebral blood flow (rCBF) (7,10,13). The rise in CBF seems to be one of the main mechanisms that maintains energy metabolism of the brain during arterial hypoxia. In edematous brain tissue, the blood flow regulation is disturbed, and a less pronounced blood flow increase or no increase could be observed when arterial oxygen tension was decreased below 50 mm Hg (5,16). The present experiments were performed to investigate the effect of arterial hypoxia on rCBF, tissue PO_2, and the concentrations of tissue metabolites in normal and edematous brain cortex under the conditions of arterial normocapnia and normal arterial blood pressure.

Methods

In 29 cats a local vasogenic brain edema was induced by a cryolesion to the right frontal cortex according to KLATZO (9). The edematous brain regions were stained by Evans blue intravenously injected (2% Evans blue, 1 ml/kg body weight). The animals were reanesthetized 20 - 24 h later with sodium pentobarbital (Nembutal, 30 mg/kg body weight), paralyzed with hexcarbacholinbromide (Imbretil) (1.6-2.0 mg initially and then 0.2-0.3 mg/30 min), and artificially ventilated under controlled conditions. The left femoral artery and the superior sagittal sinus were cannulated to obtain blood samples and to continuously record the arterial blood pressure and the pressure in the sinus system. Mean arterial blood pressure (MABP) and $PaCO_2$ were kept in normal ranges. After a bilateral craniotomy, the dura remained intact in 15 cats, while the dura was opened in 14 animals for the determination of tissue PO_2 in the upper layers of the brain cortex using PO_2 multiwire surface electrodes (8). rCBF was measured in both groups by means of the ^{85}Kr clearance technique. The lingual arteries were catheterized for tracer injection. Measurements were performed in the bluish stained region immediately adjacent to the lesion and in the corresponding control area of the unaffected left hemisphere during arterial normoxia as well as during moderate and severe arterial hypoxia. At the end of the experiments, the brain was instantly frozen, and water and metabolite contents were determined in the same cortical tissue areas where rCBF and tissue oxygen tension had been measured.

Results and Discussion

The mean values of tissue water content determined in the cortical area adjacent to the lesion as well as in the corresponding control region are given in Table 1. Under comparable conditions, almost

Table 1. Mean tissue water content in cortical areas of the right hemisphere immediately adjacent to a cryolesion and in the corresponding control regions of the unaffected left hemisphere under the conditions of intact and opened dura and regional brain swelling

	Control	Edema
Water content, dura intact (ml/100 g wet weight)	78.9 ± 0.3	80.2 ± 0.2
Regional brain swelling, dura intact (%)	-	7.7 ± 1.4
Water content, dura opened (ml/100 g wet weight)	78.9 ± 0.4	80.2 ± 0.4
Regional brain swelling, dura opened (%)	-	7.5 ± 1.7

identical results were obtained in both series of experiments. Regional brain swelling of the edematous tissue areas with a mean water content of 80.2 ml/100 g were calculated according to ELLIOT et al. (2) and found to be 7.5% in animals with opened dura and 7.7% in animals with intact dura.

Figure 1 summarizes the results of all blood flow measurements performed in both experimental groups under the conditions of arterial normoxia and arterial hypoxia. The upper two curves demonstrate the influence of a reduction of arterial oxygen tension on rCBF in the control regions of the unaffected hemisphere in animals with opened as well as with intact dura. During arterial normoxia and normocapnia, the mean rCBF of the control area under the opened dura was about 10% above the comparable value determined in cats with intact dura. Under both conditions, the stepwise reduction of arterial oxygen tension induced a progressive increase in rCBF of the control areas. At the same time, a considerably different blood flow behavior could be observed in the edematous cortical areas, as can be seen in the lower two curves (Fig. 1). In the two groups of experiments, rCBF of the edematous cortical areas was significantly smaller than the comparable values of the unaffected control areas; however, the blood flow reduction was less pronounced in animals with opened dura. During arterial normoxia and normocapnia in animals with intact dura, mean rCBF in cortical regions with increased water content was about 40% lower than in animals with opened dura. This observation may be of importance for the clinical treatment of a developing or existing traumatic edema. It indicates that under comparable conditions enlargement of the dura may improve regional circulation. During moderate and severe arterial hypoxia, only a slight increase in rCBF in the edematous brain areas could be determined if the dura was opened, indicating an impairment of blood flow regulation in those tissue areas with increased water content. In animals with intact dura, a similar reduction of the arterial oxygen tension had no influence on rCBF in the edematous tissue areas. This result may be explained as the consequence of a loss of regional blood flow regulation in brain tissue with increased water content. During all experiments, regional cerebral perfusion pressure was found to be the within normal range.

Since local mechanisms, such as a decrease in tissue pH (12), increase in extracellular K^+ activity, and increase in extracellular concentration of adenosine, all induced by severe tissue hypoxia, are assumed to play an important role in cerebral blood flow regulation (1,4,11), PO_2 distribution in the edematous cortical areas as well as in the uninjured control regions had to be determined under the different experimental conditions. To avoid producing additional brain injury, PO_2 surface electrodes instead of needle PO_2 electrodes were used for measuring local PO_2 in brain tissue. The electrodes employed allow the simultaneous determination of PO_2 at eight locations in a very small area (about 400 - 600 μm^2) of the upper cortical layers. The measurements were performed in the tissue areas under investigation immediately after the rCBF determination in 14 animals with opened dura. The results are summarized in Fig. 2. During arterial normoxia, similar PO_2 distributions could be found in the edematous as well as in the control area. In both regions, tissue PO_2 ranged from values near the arterial oxygen tension to values between 0 and 2 mm Hg. In spite of the fact that rCBF was significantly decreased in comparison to normal levels, the O_2 supply of the edematous brain cortex was sufficient under the conditions of arterial normoxia as indicated by the PO_2 histograms. The result can be explained by the lowered local metabolic rate of oxygen in brain cortex with increased water content as demonstrated previously (6). During moderate (PaO_2 = 54 mm Hg) and pronounced arterial hypoxia (PaO_2 = 31 mm Hg), the tissue PO_2 histograms of both compared cortical regions were shifted toward low PO_2 values. At a mean arterial PO_2 of 31 mm Hg, severe tissue hypoxia could be demonstrated in the edematous cortical areas as well as in the corresponding control areas of the unaffected left hemisphere.

In both regions, the incidence of tissue PO_2 values between 0 and 1 mm Hg increased significantly. At the same time, a pronounced increase of rCBF was observed in the control area, while in the edematous cortical tissue only small blood flow changes were found.

Pronounced arterial hypoxia induced characteristic changes of tissue metabolism in the control as well as in the edematous cortical areas. As demonstrated in Fig. 3, reduction of arterial oxygen tension from normal to about 30 mm Hg induced a significant increase in the tissue concentrations of lactate and pyruvate in both brain regions. Simultaneously, the concentration of creatine phosphate decreased, while in the mean the concentration of ATP remained unaffected. These findings indicate an enhancement of glycolysis in both cortical tissue zones.

Conclusions

Summarizing all these results, the investigations show that in cortical tissue with increased water content the normal regulation of regional cerebral blood flow during pronounced arterial hypoxia is disturbed or abolished. Although severe tissue hypoxia and a significant increase in tissue lactate could be demonstrated in the edematous cortical regions and in the control areas at a mean arterial PO_2 of about 30 mm Hg, none or, at most, a slight blood flow increase was found in the cortical regions with abnormal water content. This may be due to the increase in local tissue pressure in edematous brain regions, as shown by REULEN et al. (3,14,15), which locally counteracts changes of regional vascular resistance. Furthermore, vasoparalysis may be expected in edematous cortical areas with extremely high tissue lactate concentrations.

References

1. BETZ, E.: Cerebral blood flow: Its measurement and regulation. Physiol. Rev. 52, 595-630 (1972)
2. ELLIOT, K.A.C., JASPER, H.: Measurement of experimentally induced brain swelling and shrinakge. Am. J. Physiol. 157, 122-129 (1949)
3. FREI, H.J., WALLENFANG, Th., PÖLL, W., REULEN, H.J., SCHUBERT, R., BROCK, M.: Regional cerebral blood flow and regional metabolism in cold induced edema. Acta Neurochir. (Wien) 29, 15-28 (1973)
4. GROTE, J.: Cerebral blood flow regulation under the conditions of arterial hypoxia. In: The arterial system. BAUER, R.D., BUSSE, R. (eds.), pp. 209-215. Berlin, Heidelberg, New York: Springer 1978
5. GROTE, J., SCHUBERT, R.: Regional cerebral blood flow and oxygen supply during arterial hypoxia in normal and edematous brain tissue. In: Blood flow and metabolism in the brain. HARPER, M., HENNETT, B., MILLER, D., ROWAN, J. (eds.), pp. 926-927. Edinburgh, London, New York: Churchill Livingstone 1975
6. GROTE, J., SCHUBERT, R.: O_2 tension distribution and local O_2 consumption in normal and edematous brain cortex (in press)
7. GROTE, J., KREUSCHER, H., SCHUBERT, R., RUSS, H.J.: New studies on the influence of PaO_2 and $PaCO_2$ on regional and total cerebral blood flow. 6th Conference on Microcirculation 1970, pp. 294-297. (Aalborg). Basel: Karger 1971
8. KESSLER, M., GRUNEWALD, W.: Possibilities of measuring oxygen pressure fields in tissue by multiwire platinum electrodes. Prog. Resp. Res. 3, 147-152 (1969)
9. KLATZO, I., WISNIEWSKI, H., STEINWALL, D., STREICHER, E.: Dynamics of cold injury edema. In: Brain Edema. KLATZO, I., SEITELBERGER, F. (eds.), pp. 554-563. Wien, New York: Springer 1967
10. KOGURE, K., SCHEINBERG, P., REINMUTH, O.M., FUJISHIMA, M., BUSTO, R.: Mechanisms of cerebral vasodilatation in hypoxia. U. Appl. Physiol. 29, 223-229 (1970)
11. KUSCHINSKY, W., WAHL, M.: Local chemical and neurogenic regulation of cerebral vascular resistance. Physiol. Rev. 58, 656-689 (1978)
12. LASSEN, N.A.: Brain extracellular pH: The main factor controlling cerebral blood flow. Scand. J. Clin. Lab. Invest. 22, 247-251 (1968)
13. McDOWALL, D.G.: Interrelationships between blood oxygen tension and cerebral blood flow. In: Oxygen measurements in blood and tissues. PAYNE, J.P., HILL, D.W. (eds.), pp. 205-214. London: Churchill 1966
14. REULEN, H.J.: Vasogenic brain edema. New aspects in its formation, resolution and therapy. Br. J. Anaesth. 48, 741-752 (1976)
15. REULEN, H.J., KREYSCH, H.G.: Measurement of brain tissue pressure in cold induced cerebral edema. Acta Neurochir. (Wien) 29, 29-40 (1973)
16. SCHUBERT, R., GROTE, J.: Relationship between PaO_2 and tissue PO_2 as well as rCBF in edematous brain tissue. (in press)

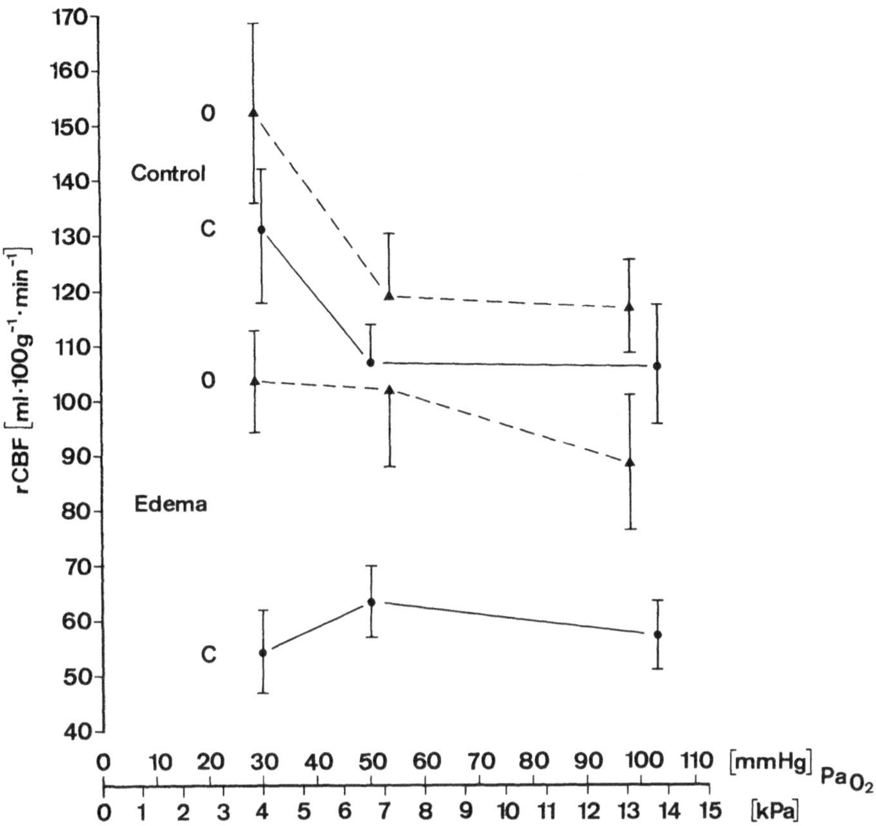

Fig. 1. Effect of the reduction in arterial PO_2 on regional blood flow in cortical areas with normal and increased water content under the conditions of opened (O) and intact dura (C) Values are mean ± SE

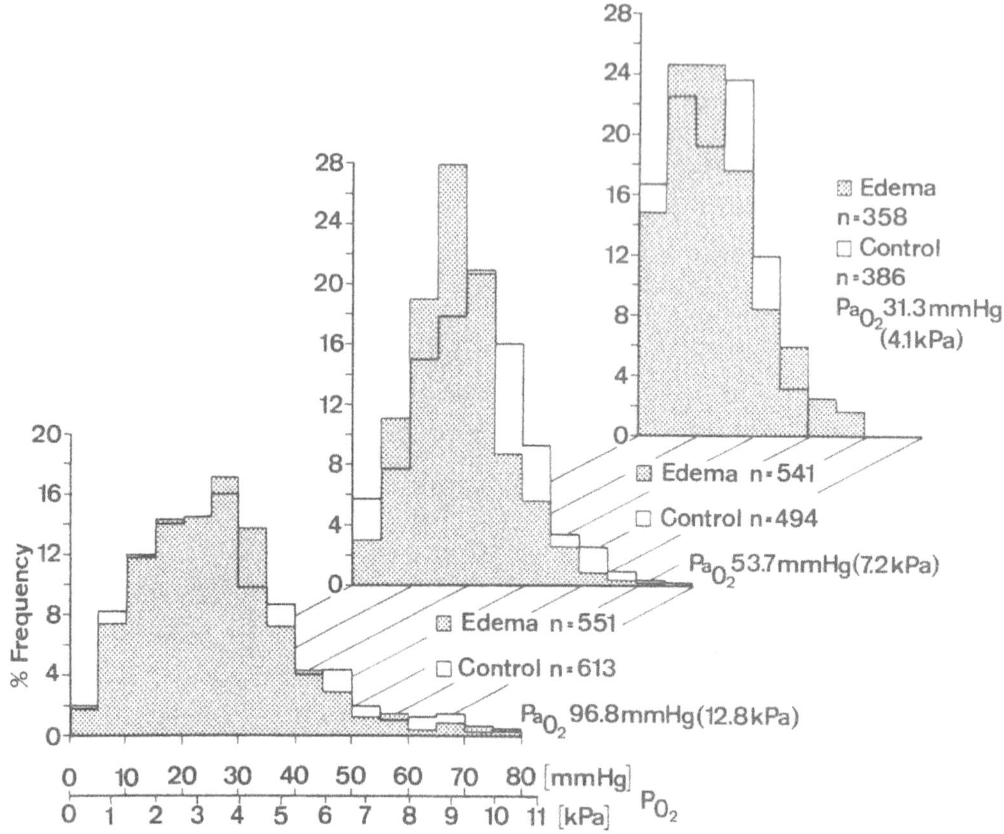

Fig. 2. Tissue PO_2 distribution in the upper layers of normal and edematous cortical areas during arterial normoxia as well as moderate and pronounced arterial hypoxia

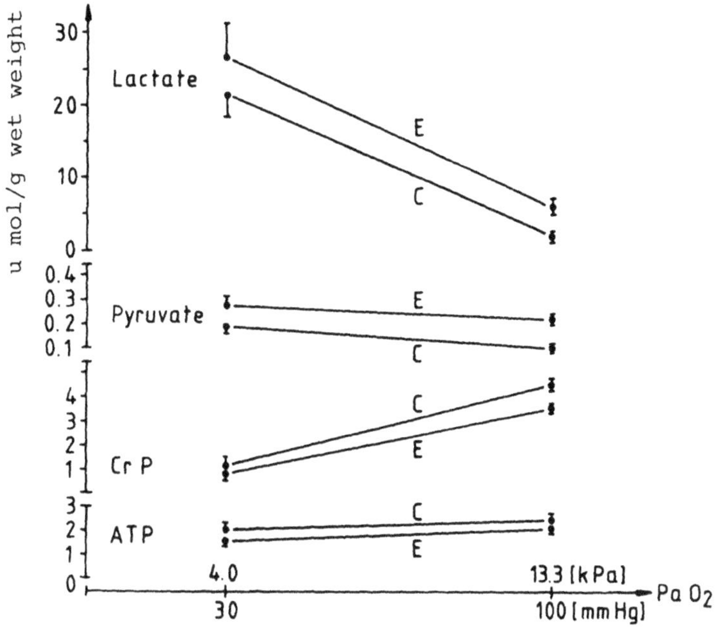

Fig. 3. Tissue metabolite concentrations in normal and edematous brain cortex during arterial normoxia and pronounced arterial hypoxia

Dysregulation of Glucose Metabolism in Patients with Brain Tumors and Injuries

E. GROTE, H. W. PIA, and W. WESEMANN

The metabolism in brain tissue depends on an uninterrupted supply of glucose. In the case of deficiency, the brain is not capable of switching to fat and protein, as other organs do. Only after several days of an inadequate glucose supply does the brain convert hydroxybutyric and acetoacetic acid into energy. Glycogen, the stored form of glucose, is not deposited in the brain but rather in the liver and muscle, which means that a constant supply of glucose to the brain is possible only through a high flow rate of cerebral blood with a sufficiently high level of glucose.

During the normal cerebral blood flow of 50 ml/100 g/min and an average glucose difference of 10 mg, the brain takes up 5 mg/100 g/min, i.e., 120 g/day, which is more than 50% of the entire glucose production of the liver and kidney. Considering the fact that the brain tissue is only 2% of the body mass, the high glucose consumption underscores the vital importance of the brain influence on the regulation of the glucose supply.

From publications in 1959 and 1962 (LAJTHA and VRBA), we know that glucose is used not only for energy but also for transamination processes in protein metabolism (Fig. 1).

Brain circulation and physiologic conditions are ensured by autoregulation. This mechanism is lost in brain edema of both cytotoxic or vasogenetic origin, and circulation becomes strongly dependent on systemic blood pressure. In the case of reduced blood flow, the glucose level must be increased to guarantee the glucose supply because the transported amount depends on its concentration and the volume of the transport medium. During normal blood flow, however, another reason for increasing the glucose level may arise. In edematous tissue, the cellular transfer of glucose may be impaired so that the supply to the cell is possible only by way of a high extra-intracellular concentration gradient.

A requirement for both mechanisms is a glucose-measuring device in a brain area from where the controlling influences originate. In 1969 OOMURA et al. (4) proved the presence of neurons in the medial and lateral hypothalamus. The activity of the neurons was glucose dependent. His concept was confirmed many times by experimentally induced hypothalamic and extradiencephalic lesions.

The blood sugar profiles of our patients with various ailments were all identical. We, therefore, assumed (Fig. 2) that deviations are not due to circadian rhythms but to regulating mechanisms. These were studied by GROTE according to tumor localization, morphology of the pathologic condition, and particularly the neurological syndrome. All patients were examined as to their reaction toward a weight-dependent glucose load.

The following groups were observed:

1) Healthy subjects without respect to age, sex, and body weight.
2) Patients with diabetes mellitus without central nervous disease.
3) All patients suffering from intracranial space-occupying lesions are summarized here. The common feature is the preoperative status without impairment of conciousness.
4) Patients with intra- and suprasellar endocrinologically inactive pituitary tumors.
5) Patients with the symptoms of global pituitary insufficiency.
6) Patients with intracranial tumors in or adjacent to the hypothalamus.
7) Patients with cortical superficial brain tumors.
8) Unconscious patients with midbrain decerebration.
9) Unconscious patients with a neurological syndrome indicating additional pontine damage.
10) Unconscious patients without regard to the level of brain stem damage.

Averaged glucose concentration determined at various times for 1 h after glucose loading gave the following results (Fig. 3). Diabetics show higher glucose concentrations than healthy subjects. Patients with preoperative tumors demonstrate a similar pattern. On the first postoperative day, a significant increase of glucose occurs, which is still present on the 7th day. The groups with pituitary tumors are not being studies further at the moment. Patients with hypothalamic tumors are characterized by an increased glucose level, which is extremely elevated on the 1st postoperative day, whereas patients with cortical superficial brain tumors show only a slightly raised postoperative value with normalization on the 7th day. All groups of unconcious patients are markedly hyperglycemic irrespective of the level of brain stem damage.

Insulin levels determed by radioimmunoassay (RIA) are low in the (Fig.4) diabetic group as expected. Patients with uncomplicated brain tumors show an elevated concentration on the 1st postoperative day with normalization on the 7th. The same phenomenon is observed in patients with intra- and suprasellar pituitary adenomas. However, postoperative hyperinsulinemia is most serious in patients with hypothalamic tumors, whereas the preoperative values are normal.

Cortical brain tumors do not differ significantly from the whole group as a standard. Midbrain decerebration leads to high insulin levels. In contrast, patients with additional lower pontine damage demonstrate the lowest insulin concentration of all groups.

All cortisol levels are elevated on the 1st and 7th postoperative days with the exception of the hypothalamic lesion group. Highest values are measured in cases of midbrain decerebration and in patients with damage to the lower brain stem as well (Fig. 5).

An abnormally high supply of glucose to the brain must affect the energy substrate in the periphery. The coordination of glucose and free fatty acid (FFA) metabolism was experimentally proved by WESTERMANN and STOCK (7). During starvation, levels of glucose and FFA react inversely. On exposure to cold, both (Fig. 6) glucose and FFA rise simultaneously to (Fig. 7) supply energy to combat cold (heat loss). After adrenalectomy and denervation, no increase is observed. The original physiologic situation is restored by administering adrenaline.

We were able to verify these findings by gas-chromatographic analysis of FFA and glucose in patients with different brain lesions. In addition we found some primary dysregulations.

The glucose supply to rat brain tissue may be quantitized and related to electric trauma at various time intervals. For this purpose animals were sacrificed 1/2, 2, 4, and 8 h after injection (Fig. 8) of glucose ^{14}C, and brain slices were prepared. Autoradiographic examination of these brain slices showed the traumatized zone to be free of ^{14}C activity. In the rest of the slice, ^{14}C activity was essentially the same regardless of time, while it decreased with time in the normal controls. Apparently, glucose metabolism is not only impaired in the traumatized area but in the entire brain as well. This finding is corroborated by experiments with glucose polymers, precursors of glucose. There is continuous washout of ^{14}C activity in the controls, whereas turnover is strongly reduced in the traumatized rat brain.

Summary

Postoperative and post-traumatic developments that are accompanied by brain lesions or midbrain lesions show a strong time-dependent correlation between hyperglycemia and injury (topography). The reason for the reactive hyperglycemia is the relative or absolute lack of glucose in brain tissue caused by edema. A therapeutic regimen has to guarantee the glucose supply to the brain by way of optimized cerebral perfusion.

References

1. GROTE, E.: Zentralnervöse Regulation und Dysregulation der Glukosehomöostase beim Menschen. Habilitationsschrift 1976
2. LAJTHA, A.: Protein metabolism of the nervous system. New York: Plenum Press 1970
3. OOMURA, Y., KIMURA, K., OOYAMA, H., MAENO, T., IKI, M., KUNIYOSHI, M.: Reciprocal activities of the ventro-medial and lateral hypothalamic areas of cats. Science 143, 484 (1964)
4. OOMURA, Y., ONO, T., OOYAMA, H., WAYNER, M.J.: Glucose and osmosensitive neurones of the rat hypothalamus. Nature 222, 282 (1969)
5. VRBA, R.: Glucose metabolism in rat brain in vivo. Nature 195, 663-665 (1962)
6. VRBA, R., GAITONDE, M.K., RICHTER, D.: The conversion of glucose carbon into protein on the brain and other organs of the rat. J. Neurochem. 9, 465-475 (1962)
7. WESTERMANN, E., STOCK, K.: The automatic nervous system and energy metabolism. J. Neuro-Visc. Rel. (Suppl. IX) 283 (1969)

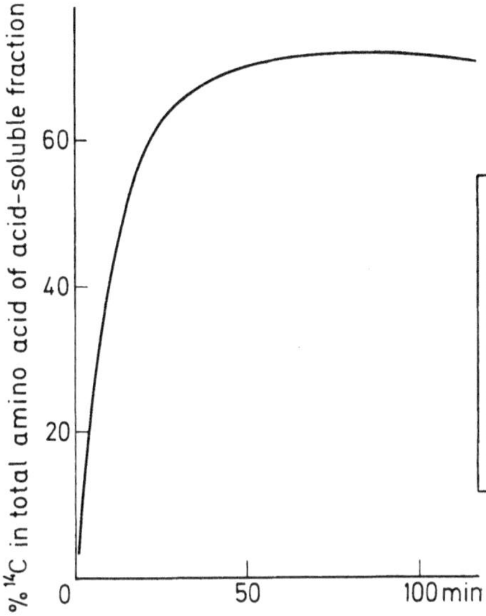

	Distribution of ^{14}C in amino acids, values in % after administration of glucose ^{14}C		
	5 min	30 min	60 min
Alanine	15	2	2
Glutamate	49	61	57
Glutamine	16	15	22
GABA	11	7	7
Aspartate	9	15	12
Serine	Traces		
Glycocoll	0.4 – 0.7		

Fig. 1. Conversion of carbohydrates into amino acids as measured by the ^{14}C content in amino acids at various times after injection of glucose ^{14}C

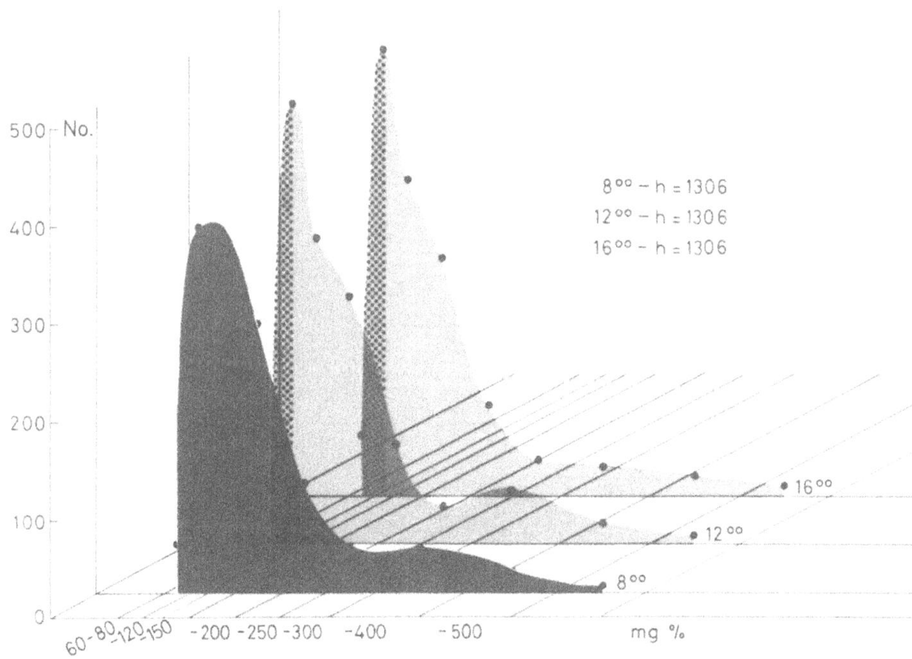

Fig. 2. Blood sugar profiles (No. = 1306) of 60 patients with brain tumors and trauma

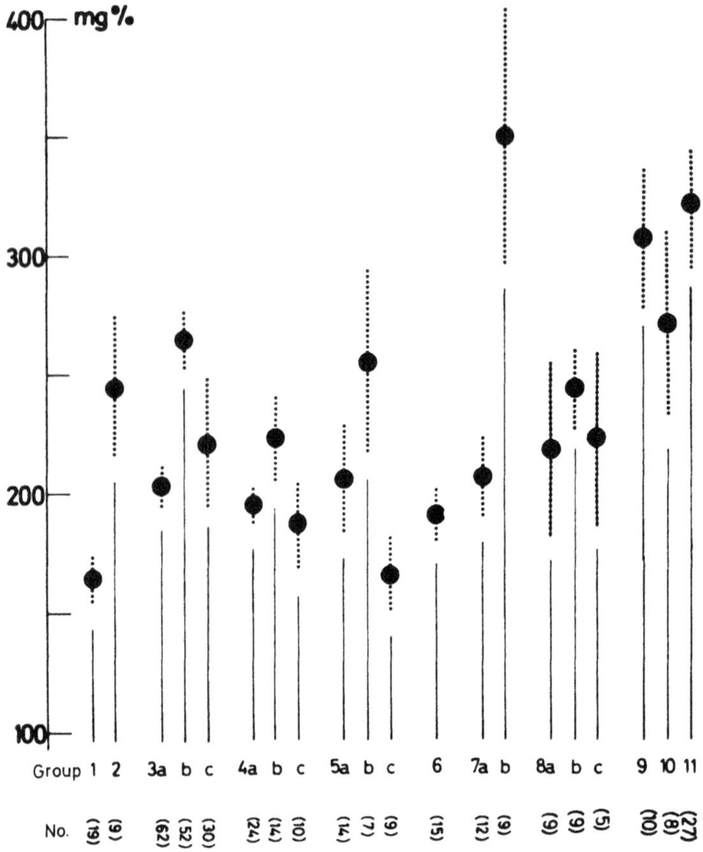

Fig. 3. Mean blood sugar concentration after a glucose tolerance test (0.33 g/kg body weight). The grouping is based on localization and symptomatologic criteria (1)

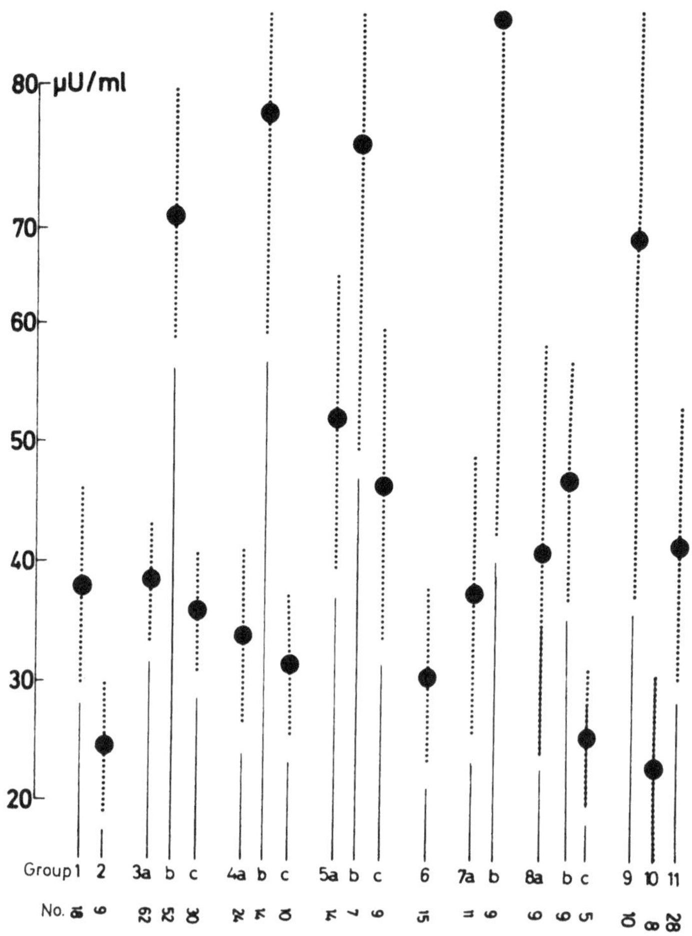

Fig. 4. Mean insulin concentrations after glucose tolerance test (0.33 g/kg body weight) (1)

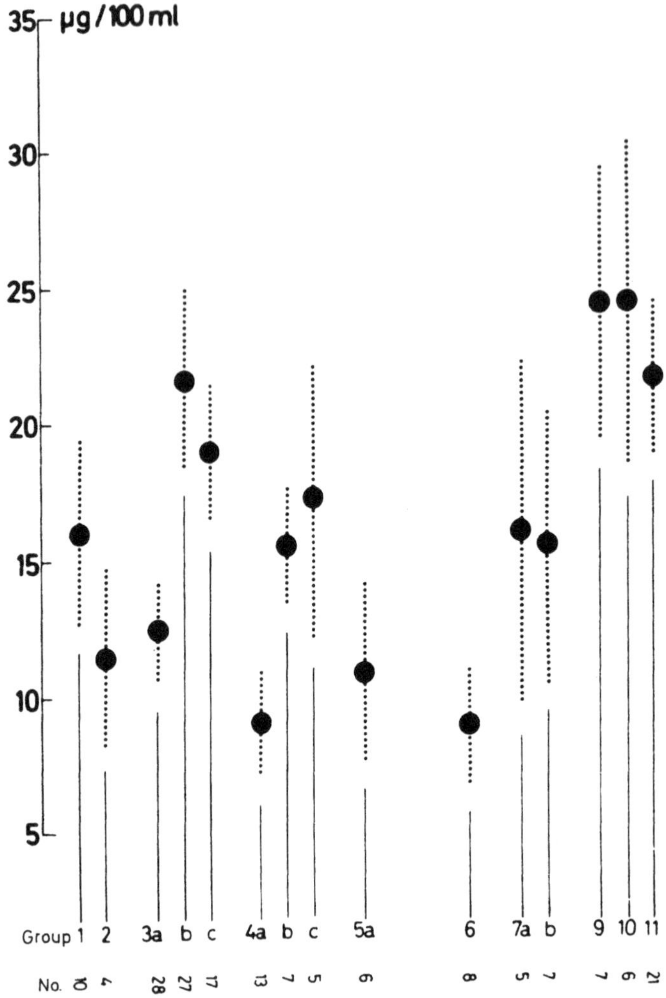

Fig. 5. Mean cortisol concentration in patients with brain tumors and trauma. The grouping is based on localization and symptomatologic criteria (1)

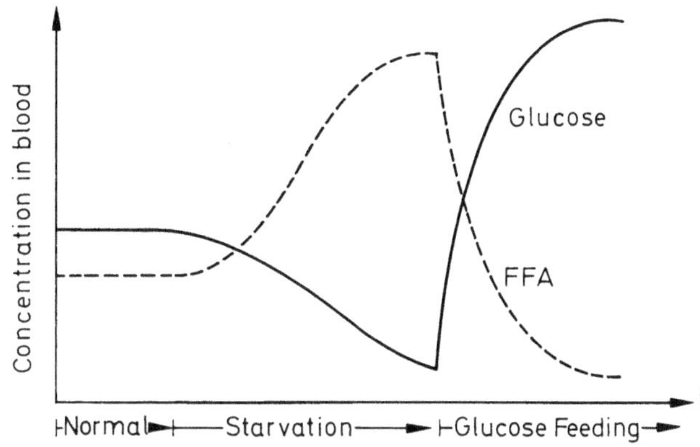

Fig. 6. The mirror image behavior of glucose and free fatty acid concentration in the blood under normal conditions, starvation, and glucose feeding (7)

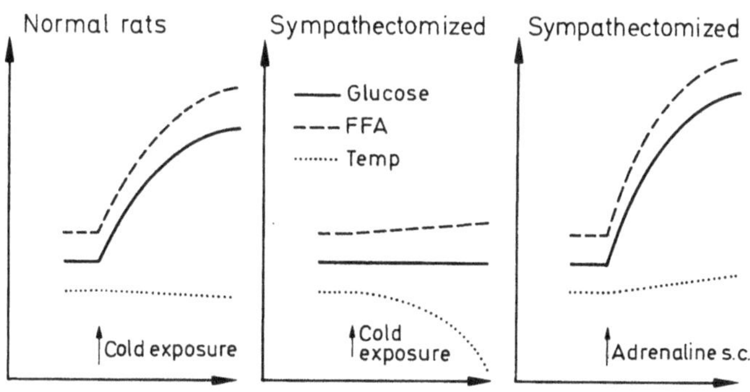

Fig. 7. Behavior of glucose and free fatty acids concentration during increased metabolic activity by cooling in normal and sympathectomized rats and during adrenaline administration of sympathectomized rats

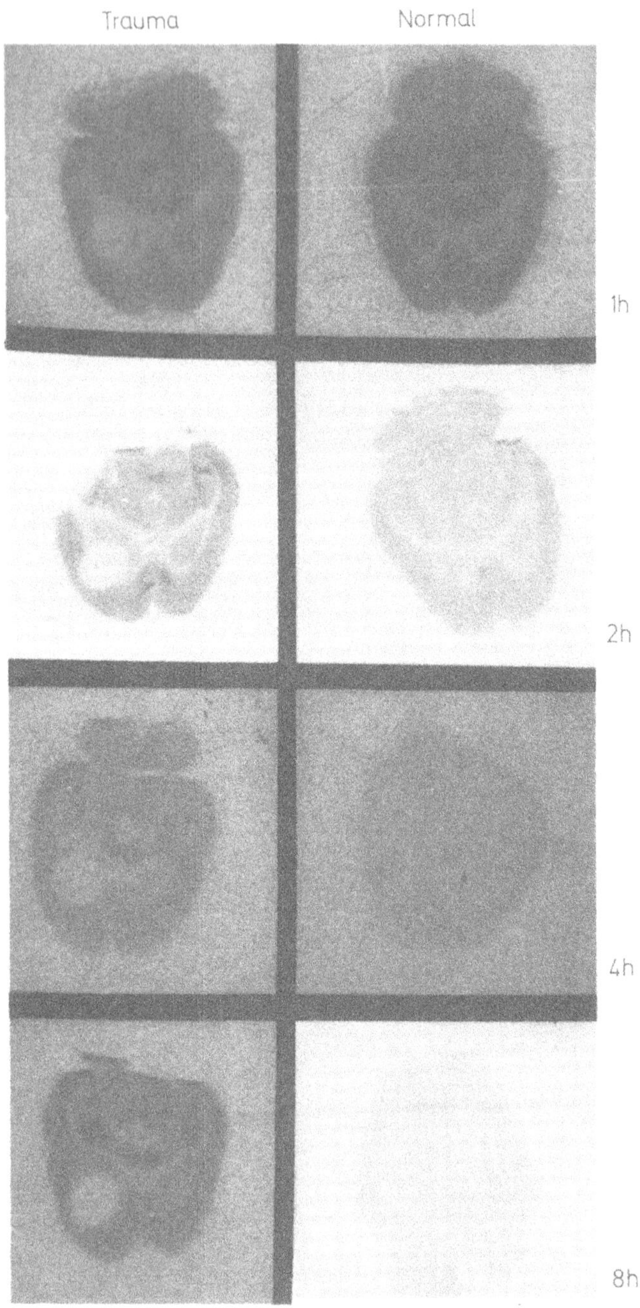

Fig. 8. Comparison of ^{14}C autoradiography of brain tissue of normal and electrotraumatized rats after 1 h, 2 h, 4 h, and 8 h

Enzymatic Activity, Electrolytes, and Osmolality in the Ventricular Fluid: the Significance of a Continuous Measurement for the Prognosis of Acute Brain Lesions

K. E. RICHARD, R. A. FROWEIN, G. HELLER, and P. ZIMMERMANN

Extent and course of an acute brain lesion with increased intracranial pressure can be recognized first of all by the degree of the neurological disturbances (20,22). Within the frame work of intensive medical care of severe brain lesions, there is an urgent need for further parameters to evaluate early prognosis of the patients.

The question of how far changes of the enzymatic activities of the blood and of the cerebrospinal fluid make it possible to assess the severity of an acute brain lesion and the prognosis was investigated experimentally and clinically by several authors, especially in cases of brain trauma (10,13,24,28,31) and of cerebrovascular disturbances (3,18). Their results, however, are exclusively based on enzymatic analyses of the *spinal* fluid.

As is well known, various authors could demonstrate that, in cases of acute brain lesion, cell enzymes from the affected areas of brain tissue enter into the ventricular fluid within 1-3 h (1,12,14,16,29). Therefore, it seems to be logical to follow the enzymatic activities in the ventricular fluid after surgery of brain tumors and intracranial hematomas.

Material and Methods

In six patients with supratentorial or infratentorial space-occupying lesions, the activities of the following enzymes were measured in blood serum and ventricular fluid for an average time of 7 days before and after surgery:

Total lactic dehydrogenase (LDH)
α-Hydroxybutyric acid dehydrogenase (α-HBDH) (i.e., isoenzyme 1 and 2 of LDH)
Aspartate aminotransferase (GOT)
Creatine kinase (CK)

The upper limits for serum and cerebrospinal fluid are taken from the literature (4,7,9,12,14,30,32).

Furthermore, the following substances were regularly examined: in the ventricular fluid lactate, sodium, and chloride ions including osmolality, protein, and urea. The mean *ventricular fluid pressure* (VFPmx) during periods of ventricular 12 h were calculated from the continuous pressure curves (20).

The *electric conductivity* of the ventricular fluid was measured by a "flowthrough measuring cell" type LDM-S (RTW Company, Weilheim, West-Germany) (cell factor K = 10 · cm^{-1}), at a constant temperature of of 25° C. The *specific conductivity* of VF was calculated from the product of the VF conductivity and the cell factor.

Concerning *neurological functions*, the state of consciousness, responsiveness, pupillary reaction, motor function, tonus, and respiratory function assessed (20,22). Using a numerically calculated index, the following grades of neurological deficites were differentiated:

No deficit (index 6)
Slight to moderate deficit (index 7-11)
Severe deficit (index 12-17)
Very severe deficit (index 18-24) (see RICHARD and FROWEIN 1978).

Results

Case 1

A 71-year-old woman (F.H., 1084/78) (Fig. 1): on the 1st day after extirpation of a large cerebellopontine neurinoma, the VF activities of LDH and α-HBDH were significantly elevated, while coma with severe neurological disturbances (coma 2) persisted. CK activity was slightly increased; GOT was normal. On the 3rd day neurological functions began to recover. Simultaneously with an augmented blood content of VF, the VF-LDH was increased. The other enzymes rapidly declined to normal activities. At the same time, the VF lactate initially elevated up to 3.2 mmol/liter began to normalize. VF Na^+ and Cl^- remained constantly in the normal range. VF osmolality and VF urea rose due to a renal failure with retention of BUN. The electric conductivity left the normal range of 12.000 to 13.500 μS only for a short time. Until the 7th postoperative day, we measured only slight VFP increases up to 30 mm Hg. In the further course, the patient slowly recovered. On the 18th postoperative day, there still was a slight neurological global dysfunction with complete normalization of the VF enzymes.

Case 2

A 38-year-old woman (F.F., 1017/78) (Fig. 2): after acute onset of headache and nausea on admission, coma grade 3. CT diagnosis of a hemorrhage into the right cerebellar hemisphere. The preoperative analysis of enzymes showed strikingly high values of CK in VF and serum. LDH and α-HBDH were also highly elevated. GOT, however, was not elevated. After removal of the hematoma, significant lower activities of VF enzymes. On the 2nd postoperative day, again slight increase of LDH and CK parallel to a small rise of lactate up to 3.2 mmol/liter. VF conductivity, osmolality, and VFP were normal. Full recovery.

Case 3

A 55-year-old woman (W.T., 640/78) (Fig. 3): recurrency of an ependymoma of the fourth ventricle. Postoperatively high enzymatic activities in the VF in connection with an increase of lactate up to 4.5 mmol/liter. Despite continuing semiconsciousness with severe neurological deficit, only the CK and the GOT declined to normal values on the 4th postoperative day. On the 6th day, removal of the pressure-controlled external drainage. A few hours later, acute respiratory arrest with dilated and fixed pupils and isoelectric EEG. VFP rose to high levels. In spite of continued external drainage, no recovery. VF lactate rose up to 4.5 mmol/liter. Strikingly large fluctuations of Na^+ and Cl^- ion concentration as well as of the osmolality and the VF conductivitiy.

Case 4

A 50-year-old man (R.H., 1148/78) (Fig. 4): metastasis in the left lateral ventricle. Preoperatively the total LDH and the α-HBDH and the CK in the VF were distinctly above the upper normal limits. After decrease of enzymatic activity on the 2nd postoperative day, once more steep increase of the LDH and the α-HBDH in connection with an extreme increase of lactate concentration, which was only slightly elevated before. Absence of an increase of VF CK and VF GOT.

In the evening of the third postoperative day, coma 3. Diagnosis of a bacterial contamination of the VF. Under antibiotic treatment, only temporarily slight improvement of the values. Fatal outcome on the 13th postoperative day.

Case 5

A 55-year-old woman (G.A., 1173/78) (Fig. 5): 1 day after subtotal extirpation of a bifrontal malignant astrocytoma, acute development of coma 3. In addition to a severe shift of the midline, CT showed blood clots in both lateral ventricles. The analyses of the distinctly bloody VF (Hb 0.28 g%), VF demonstrated high values of lactate, total LDH, α-HBDH, and CK. In the further course, only transitory decrease of the enzymatic activities and the lactate of the VF. On the 6th day, acute circulatory collapse with coma 3. The activities of LDH and α-HBDH rose once more. At the same time as a progressive renal failure, an increase of VF urea was measured, corresponding to an increasing VF osmolality and electric conductivity in spite of a high protein content.

Case 6

A 16-year-old girl (J.I., 1142/48) (Fig. 6): acute traumatic hematoma and contusion of chest. In the posttraumatic course up to the 5th day continuous increases of LDH, α-HBDH, and CK in the VF were measured. After that, despite lasting high serum activities, gradual fall of VF enzymes. On the 16th day, change from coma to stupor. Transition to an apallic state. Contrary to the VF lactate concentration, the enzymatic VF activities were not yet normalized.

Conclusion

All patients examined during the early postoperative period of the first 3 days were comatous with severe neurological deficits as an expression of a serious brain lesion. Therefore, we cannot arrive at any conclusion as to how these parameters are affected in less serious cases of brain lesions. However, how far could we get at a statement about the severity of brain dysfunction and the prognosis on the basis of these findings?

1) The *enzymatic activities* of the *blood serum* were only slightly elevated above the upper normal limits and fell again in favorable

courses. Continuously high or increasing CK activities are probably due to tissue lesions in other organs, e.g., the heart muscle (case 6).

2) All *VF enzymes* were highly elevated, with the exception of GOT, during the first days. The activity of *CK*, which is normally very low in the VF, was always distinctly and continuously elevated, surprisingly to the same extent both in survivors and in the patients with fatal outcome (Fig. 7). Although this enzyme does not originate from red cells of the bloody VF or from the tumor tissue but from the damaged brain tissue areas (4), its augmentation allows no reliable conclusion as to the extent of brain lesion or to prognosis. This is in contradiction to the opinion of several authors (9,10,12, 14,28,31). Likewise, the *total LDH* and its isoenzymes 1 and 2, the α-HBDH, showed pathologically elevated activities independent from the outcome. A main source of these enzymes are the red and white cells in the ventricular fluid blood stained postoperatively (2,11, 14,27). Secondary increments also lead one to suspect a pleocytosis or an infection of the CSF (13). A continuous and rapid decrease, however, correlated well with an improvement of the neurological condition. The most reliable parameter for an assessment of the postoperative course, in our experience, is represented by the *lactate concentration* of the ventricular fluid. In three survivors, the lactate levels were only slight elevated. In contrast, the VF lactate concentrations of the three patients with an unfavorable outcome were distinctly higher, without a tendency toward normalization. This is in agreement with our previous findings (21). Among 39 patients with infratentorial space-occupying lesions, the lactate level fell progressively in those who survived but remained high in those with an unfavorable outcome.

3) Until now the *electric conductivity* of the VF proved to be a relatively constant parameter in the range of 12.000 - 13.000 μS (26). With constant temperature, this parameter increases by the number of moveable carriers of an electric potential, i.e., sodium, chloride, lactate, and possibly urea ions in the ventricular fluid (8,15). On the other hand, it decreases with diminution of these ions or with increasing VF protein content. Therefore, it is understandable from the hitherto existing data that there is no simple parallelism of electric conductivity and the osmolality (17) of the ventricular fluid, as various authors assumed (6,8).

Summary

In six patients the following parameters were continuously measured over a period of 7 days before and after surgery of space-occupying lesions: activities of enzymes in blood serum and ventricular fluid (LDH, α-HBDH, CK, GOT), lactate in the VF, Na^+ and Cl^- ions in the VF, osmolality, protein, urea, and electric conductivity in the VF. The neurological condition was continuously recorded.

Blood enzymes were slightly elevated and fell again in favorable courses. VF, LDH, α-HBDH, and CK were highly elevated. However, their augmentation allowed no conclusion as to the extent of brain lesion or to prognosis. The most reliable parameter for an assessment of the postoperative course seems to be the VF lactate concentration. The relatively constant electric conductivity of VF shows no simple parallelism to VF osmolality.

References

1. AKASHI, K.S.: Studies on the changes in GOT, GPT and LDH of the cerebrospinal fluid in experimental head injuries. J. Med. Soc. Tokio Univ. 13, 1-18 (1966)
2. DELANK, H.W., ENGELMANN, G.: Die Laktatdehydrogenase und deren Isoenzyme im Liquor cerebrospinalis. Dtsch. Z. Nervenheilkd. 187, 256-264 (1965)
3. DENHAM, H.J., HODKINSON, H.M.: Serum enzymes and prognosis in cerebral infarction. Age Ageing 2, 86-91 (1973)
4. FRICK, E.: Über die Kreatinkinase im Liquor cerebrospinalis. Klin. Wschr. 45, 973-977 (1967)
5. FROWEIN, R.A., STEINMANN, H.W., AUF DER HAAR, K., TERHAAG, D.: Grenzen der Klassifikation und Prognose schwerer Hirntraumen. Adv. Neurosurg. 5 (1978)
6. HELLER, H., JAEHRIG, K.: Konduktometrische Untersuchungen zur renalen Elektrolytausscheidung bei untergewichtigen Neugeborenen. Kinderaerztl. Prax. 41, 438-447 (1973)
7. HELLER, W., OLDENKOTT, P.: Klinisch-chemische Diagnostik bei Hirntumoren und Hirnverletzungen. Dtsch. Med. Wochenschr. 96, 1222-1224 (1971)
8. JAEHRIG, K., BOGUN, K.R., GRIMMER, J.: Die Konduktometrie zur orientierenden Messung der Harnelektrolytkonzentration. Urologe (A) 16, 204-207 (1977)
9. KALTIALA, E.R., HEIKKINEN, E.S., KAERKI, N.T., LARMI, T.K.: Cerebrospinal fluid and serum transaminases and lactic dehydrogenase after head injury. Acta Neurol. Scand. 44, 124-129 (1968)
10. KLUN, B.: Spinal fluid and blood serum enzyme activity in brain injuries. J. Neurosurg. 41, 224-228 (1974)
11. LANG, G., SCHURICHT, G., REICHEL, F.: Die Liquoruntersuchung unter besonderer Berücksichtigung der Liquorenzyme beim Schädelhirntrauma. Z. Aerztl. Fortbild. (Jena) 70, 678-679 (1976)
12. MAAS, A.J.R.: Cerebrospinal fluid enzymes in acute brain injury. J. Neurol. Neurosurg. Psychiatry 40, 655-674 (1977)
13. NELSON, P.V., CAREY, W.F., POLLARD, A.C.: Diagnostic significance and source of lactate dehydrogenase and its isoenzymes in cerebrospinal fluid of children with a variety of neurological disorders. J. Clin. Pathol. 28, 828-833 (1975)
14. NORDBY, H.K., TVEIT, B., RUUD, I.: Creatine kinase and lactate dehydrogenase in the cerebrospinal fluid in patients with head injuries. Acta Neurochir. (Wien) 32, 209-217 (1975)
15. PAPIERKOWSKI, A.: Der elektrische Widerstand des Liquor cerebrospinalis bei entzündlichen Erkrankungen des Zentralnervensystems bei Kindern. Paediatr. Paedol. 10, 336-341 (1975)
16. PATBERG, W.R., GO, K.G., TEELKEN, A.W.: Isolation of edema fluid in cold-induced cerebral edema for the study of colloid osmotic pressure, lactate dehydrogenase activity, and electrolytes. Exp. Neurol. 54, 141-147 (1977)
17. QUINCKE, H.: Die diagnostische und therapeutische Bedeutung der Lumbalpunktion. Dtsch. Med. Wochenschr. 46, 1825-1829 (1905)

18. RABOW, L., TIBBLING, G.: Serum enzyme activity of hydroxybutyric dehydrogenase (HBD) and heat inactivated lactate dehydrogenase (LD) after operations on intracranial aneurysms. Acta Neurochir. (Wien) 32, 199-207 (1975)

19. RICHARD, K.E.: Ventricular fluid pressure measurement by micro-catheter and pressure-controlled external fluid drainage. Acta Neurochir. (Wien) 38, 73-87 (1977)

20. RICHARD, K.E.: Langzeitmessung des Ventrikelliquordruckes bei intrakraniellen raumfordernden Prozessen und akuten Hirnschädigungen. Ph. D. Dissertation, University of Cologne (1978)

21. RICHARD, K.E.: Longterm measurement of ventricular fluid pressure in tumors of fossa posterior. Adv. Neurosurg. 5, (1978, in press)

22. RICHARD, K.E., FROWEIN, R.A.: The relationship between intracranial pressure, disturbances of brain function and prognosis. Neurosurg. Rev. 1/2, 25-36 (1978)

23. RICHARD, K.E., FROWEIN, R.A., VANNER, G.K.: Ventricular fluid pressure in posterior fossa tumors of childhood. Mod. Probl. Paediatr. 18, 35-39 (1977)

24. SCHLAG, G.: Schädelhirntrauma-enzymatische und biochemische Liquoruntersuchungen. Monatsschr. Unfallheilkd. 73, 1-12 (1970)

25. SMITH, S.E., CAMMOCK, C.V., DODDS, M.E., CURRY, H.J.: Glutamic oxalacetic transaminase in the evaluation of acute injury to the head. Am. J. Surg. 99, 713-716 (1960)

26. TASZEW, T., IWANOWA, D.: I-sledowanija ob elektrowodimosti likwora. Folia Med. (Plovdiv) 3, 9-14 (1961)

27. VARA-LOPEZ, R., VARA-THORBECK, R.: Modification in the activity of some enzymes of the cerebrospinal fluid in patients with intracranial tumors. J. Neurosurg. 34, 749-752 (1971)

28. VILLAR, J.L. del, NAVARRO, I.R., RAMOS, G., GONZALEZ, F.M.J.: (CPK of CSF in head trauma: its prognostic value). CPK del LCR en traumatismos de craneo: su valor prognostico. Rev. Clin. Esp. 129, 487-488 (1973)

29. WEIDNER, A., STOLKE, D., DIETZ, H.: Effects of a local cryogenic lesion on enzyme activities in cat brain. Adv. in Neurosurg. 4, 212-216 (1977)

30. WILKINSON, J.H.: The principles and practice of diagnostic enzymology. London: Arnold 1976

31. WOLFF, H., ZERNA, M.: Das Verhalten der Malatdehydrogenase und Laktatdehydrogenase im Liquor nach Schädelhirntraumen. Zentralbl. Chir. 90, 701-705 (1965)

32. WOLINTZ, A.H., JACOBS, L.D., CHRISTOFF, N., SOLOMON, M., CHERNIK, N.: Serum and cerebrospinal fluid enzyms in cerebrovascular disease. Arch. Neurol. 20, 54-61 (1969)

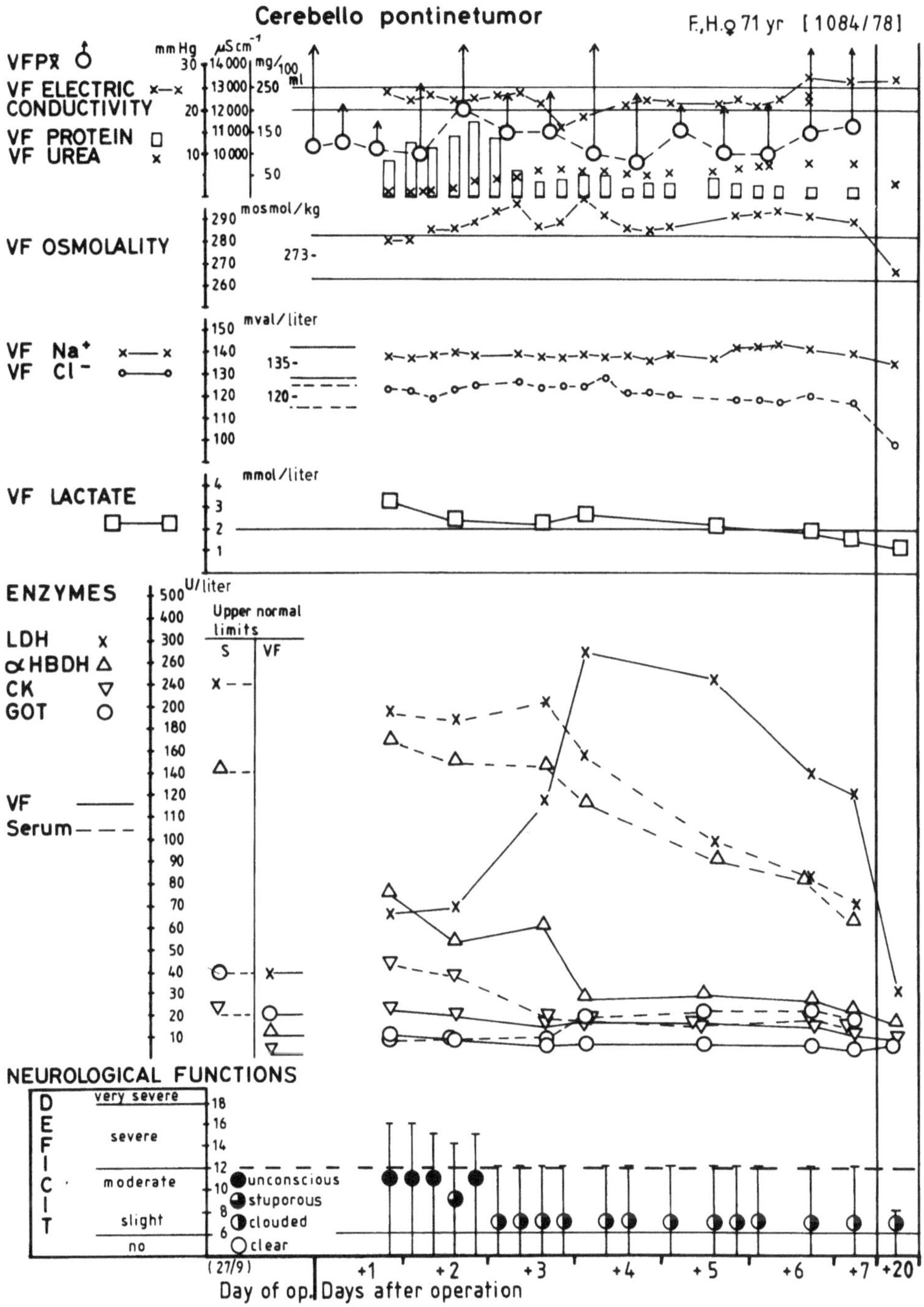

Fig. 1. Example of a favorable course

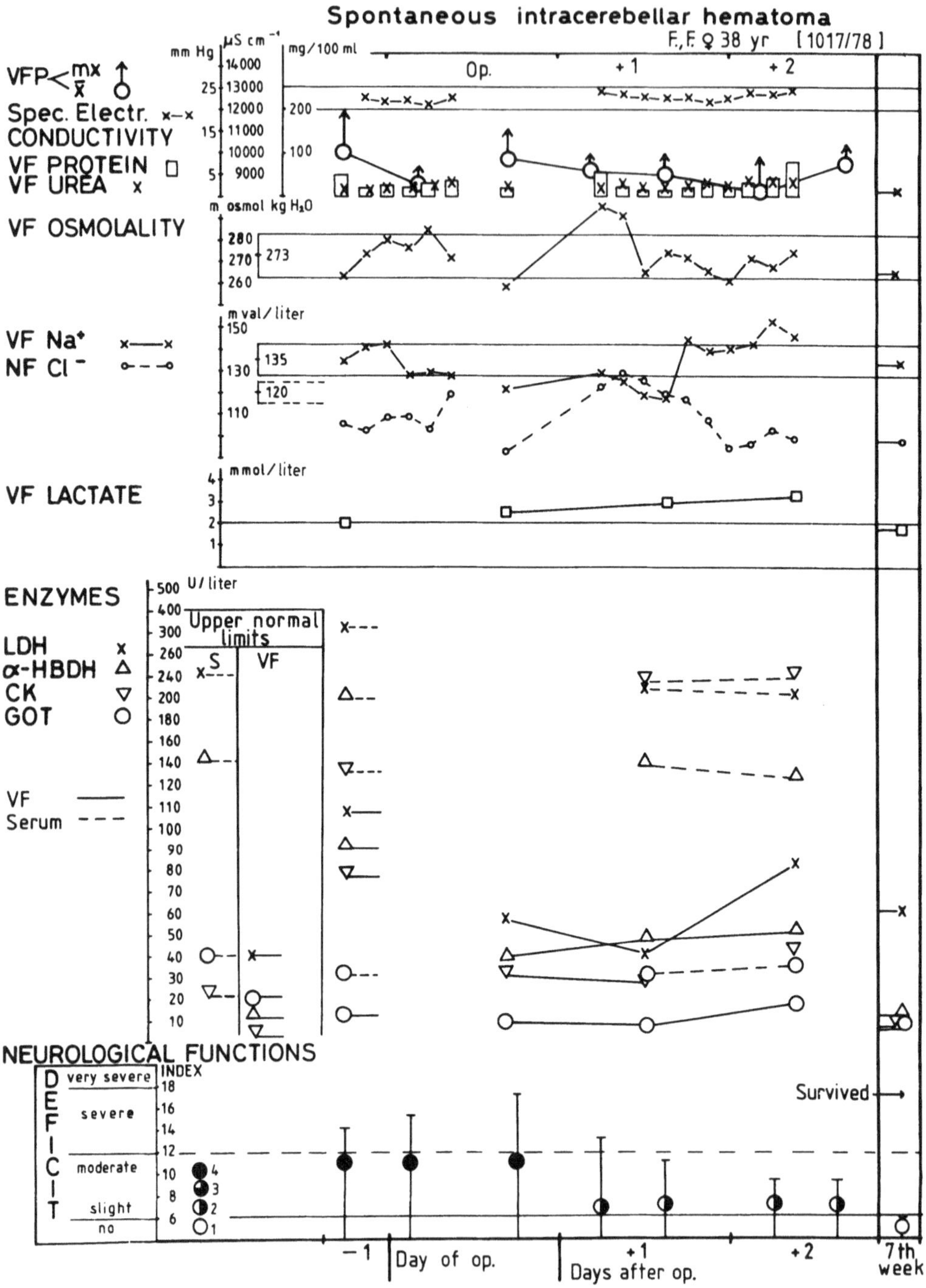

Fig. 2. Example of a favorable course

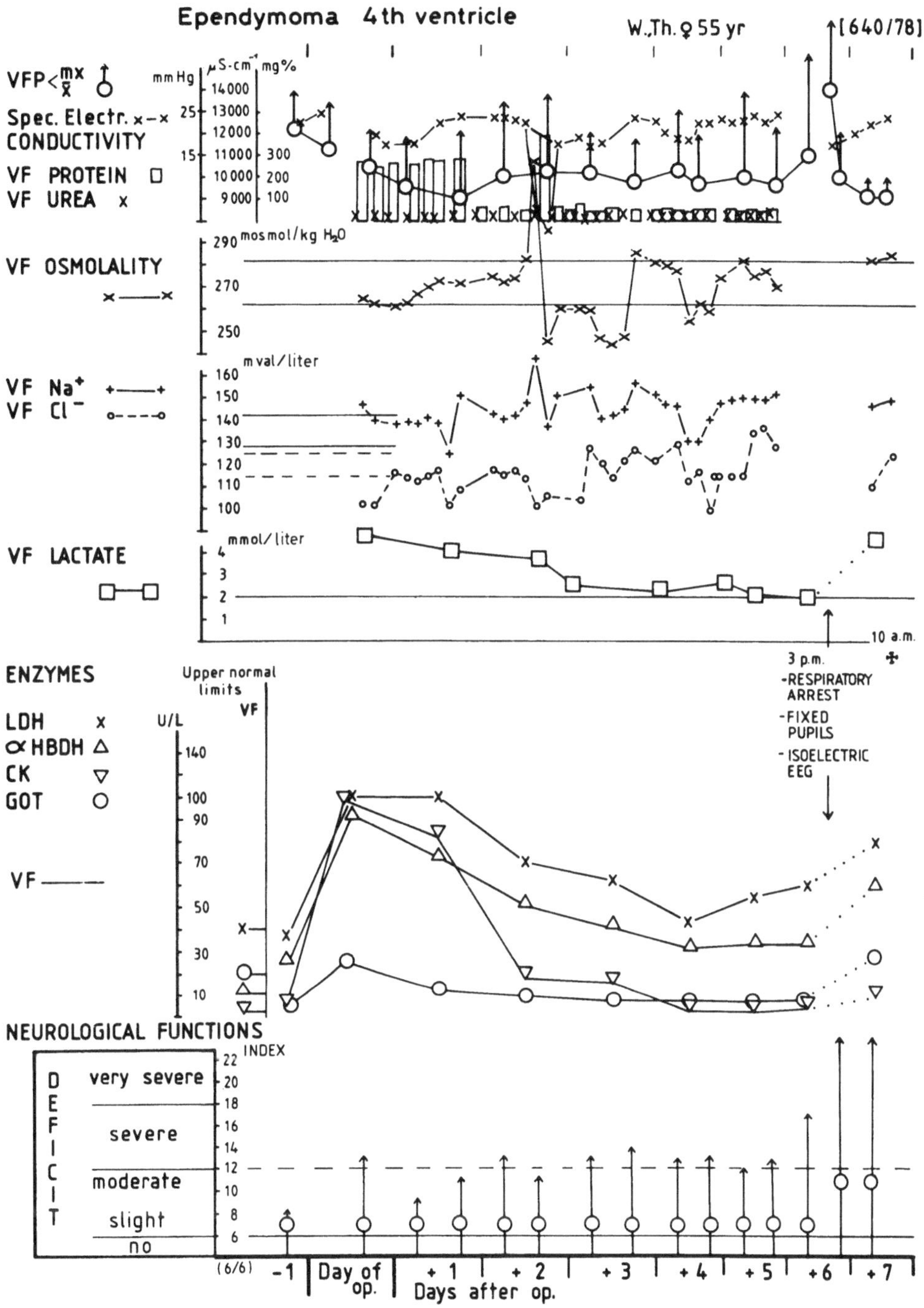

Fig. 3. Example of an unfavorable course

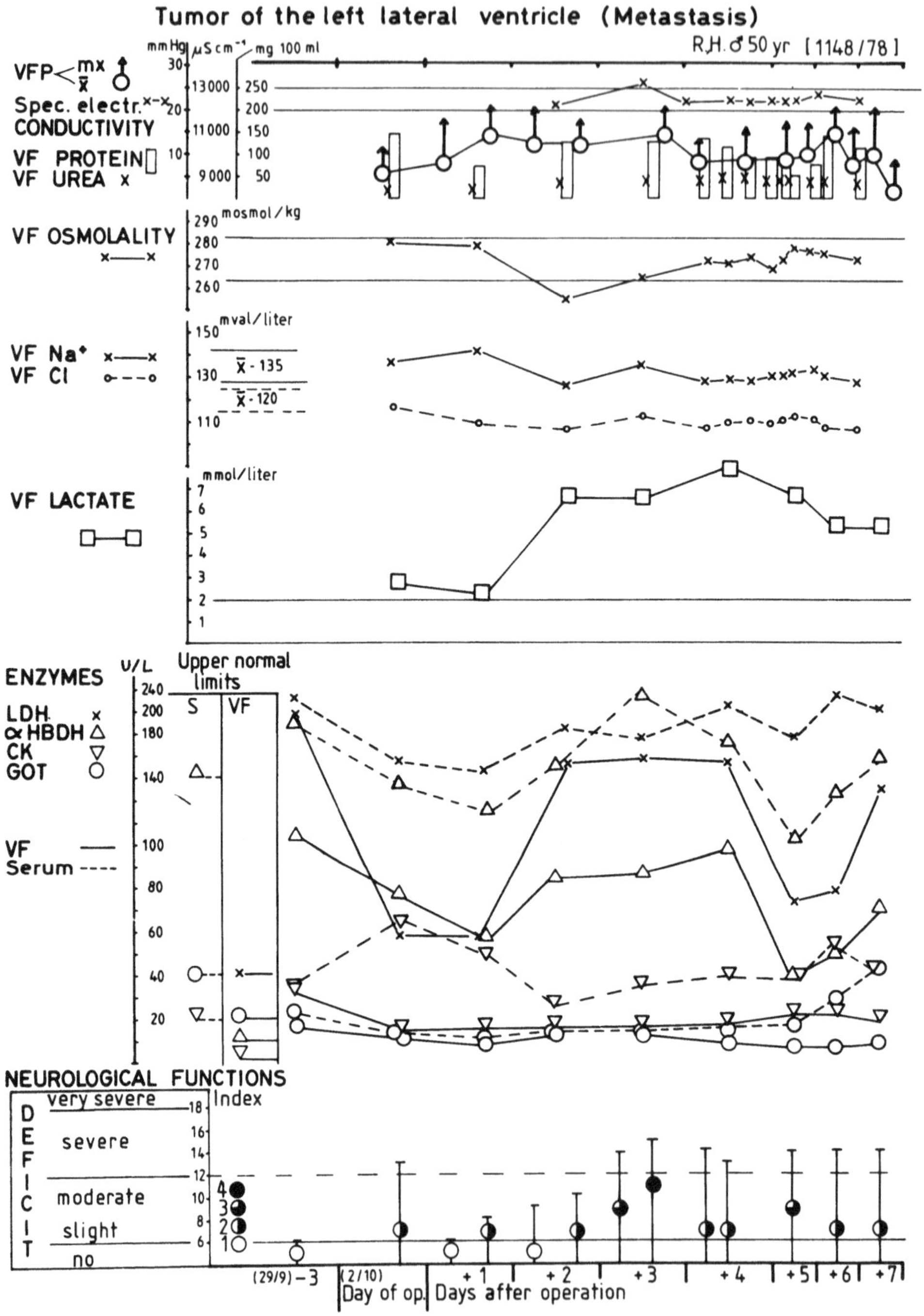

Fig. 4. Example of a complication by CSF infection

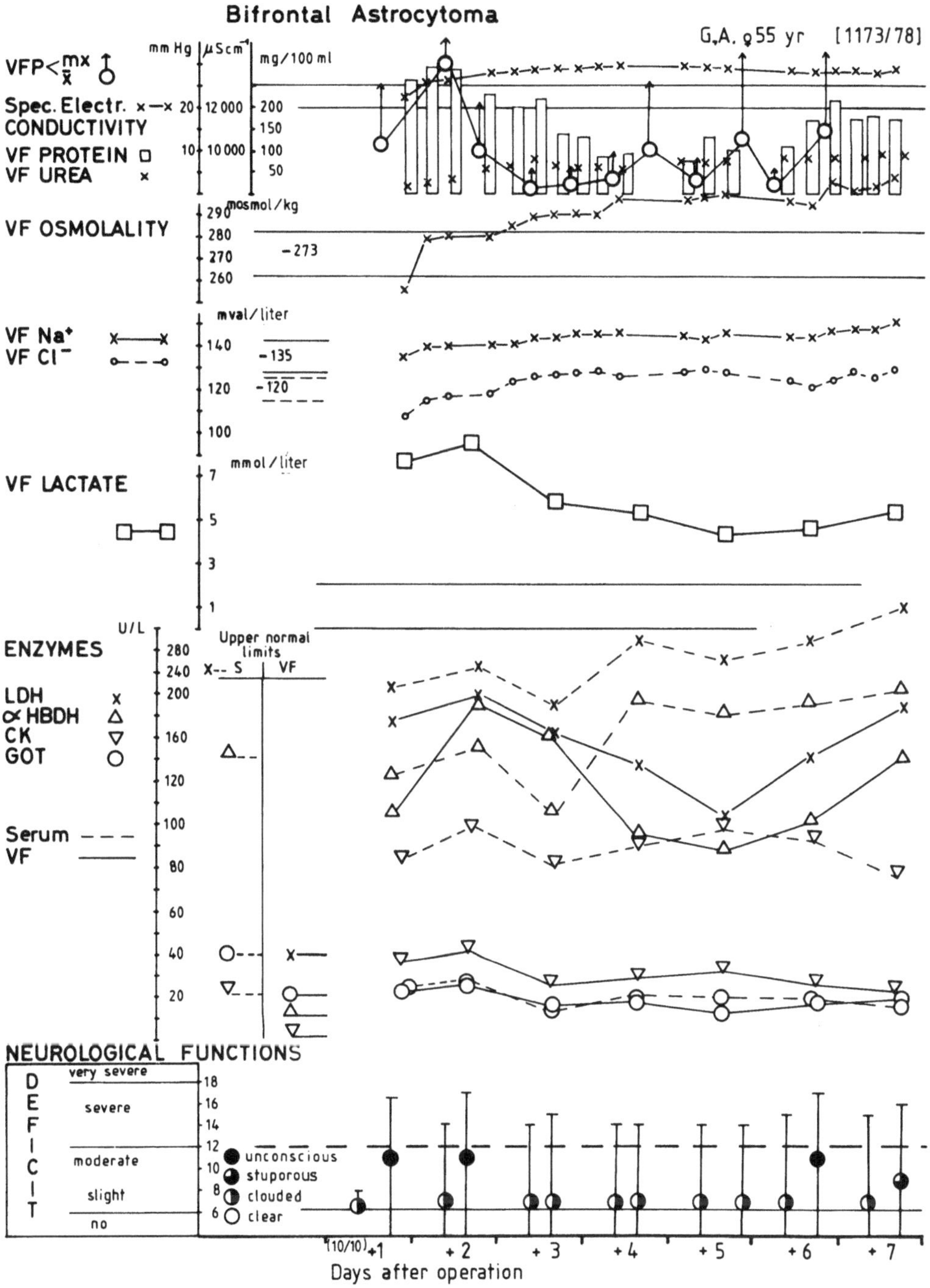

Fig. 5. Example of an unfavorable course

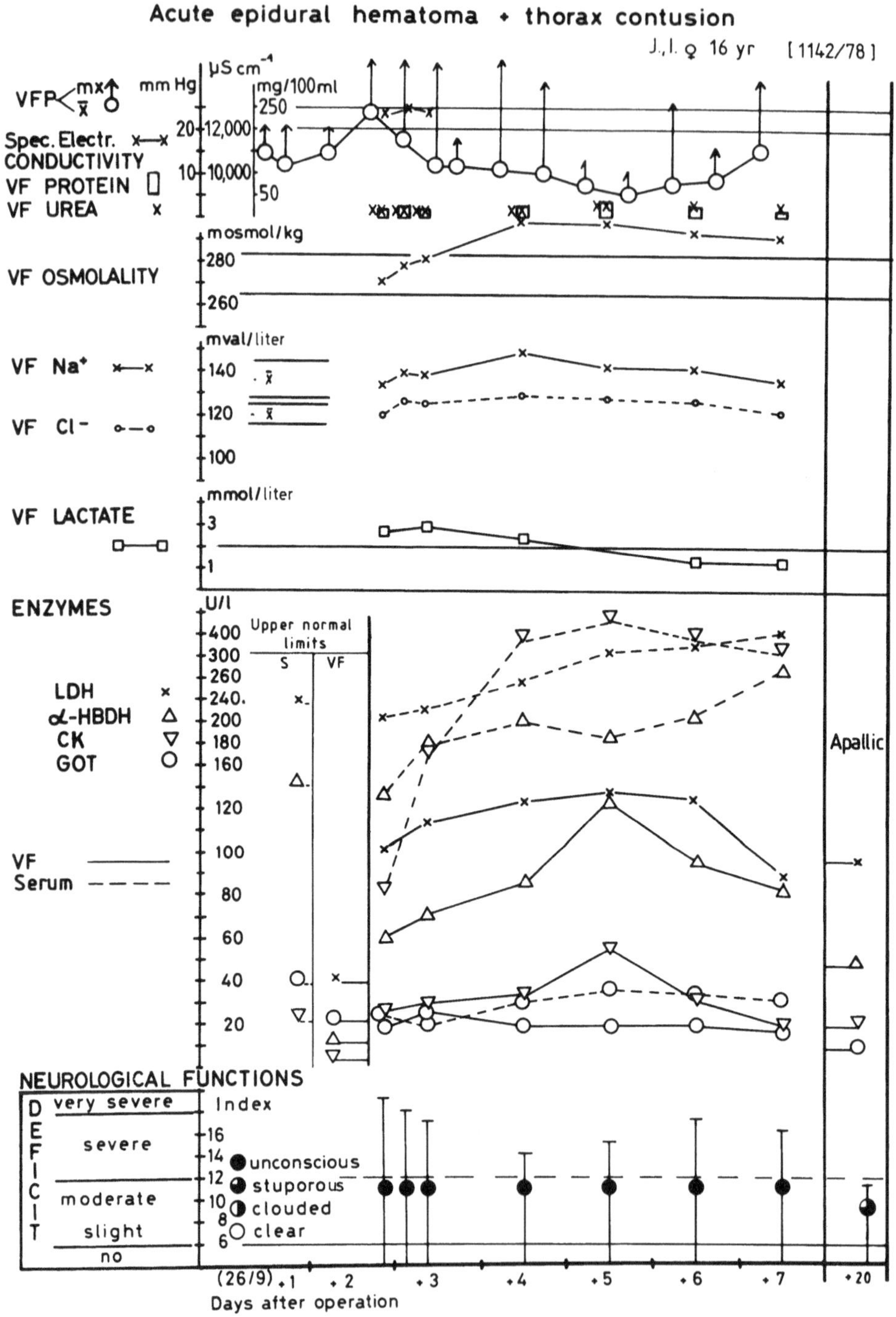

Fig. 6. Example of a combined trauma of brain and chest with development of an appallic state

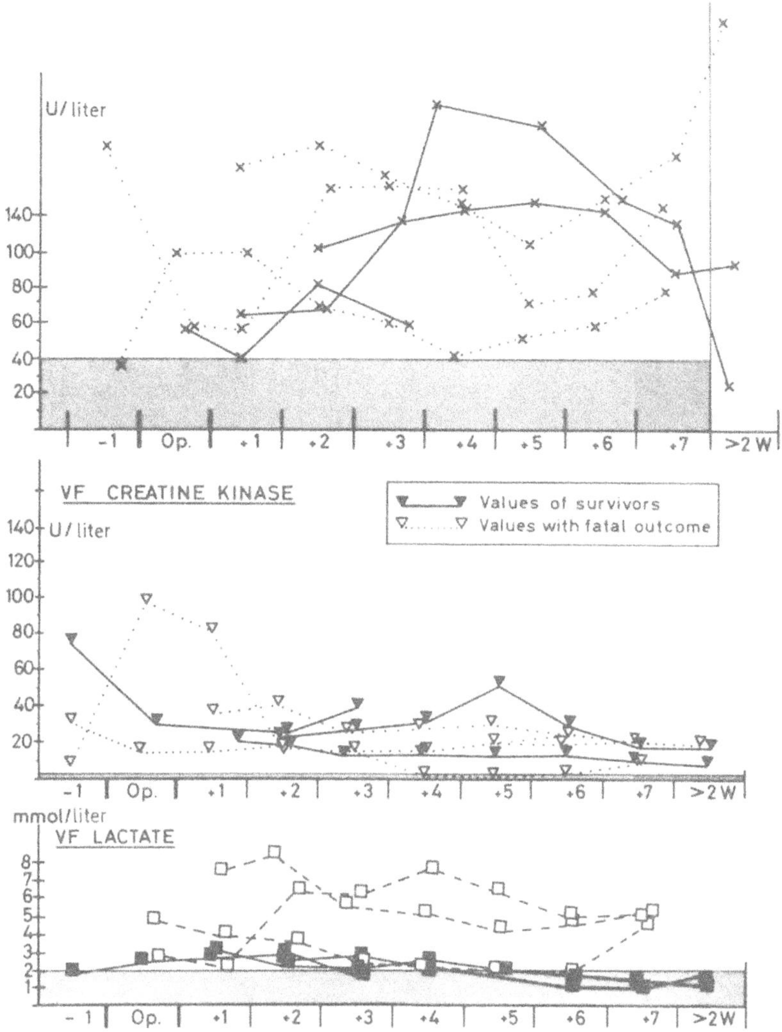

Fig. 7. Comparison of VF dehydrogenase, VF creatine kinase, and VF lactate in the postoperative course after severe brain lesions

Prognostic Value of Somatosensory-Evoked Potential Patterns and Neurosecretory Findings in Severe Brain Injury[1]

F. O. MILTNER, E. HALVES, and E. MAY

Introduction

Cerebral somatosensory-evoked responses (SEP) triggered by stimulation of peripheral nerves are widely accepted as diagnostic indices of conductive properties of the human somatosensory system (2,3,4,7,9). Although SEPs are at least indicators of neuronal population responses, when generated in relevant areas, they provide, in addition, clues to some of the neuronal processes mediating the function of those areas (5,6,8,14,18,19).

In normal subjects, wave forms, amplitudes, and latencies show variations with age, vigilance levels, stimulation parameters, and location of electrodes (2,16). In patients suffering from neurological disorders, either structural lesions or/and functional disturbances, the SEP may be affected by disturbances of the cortex, brain stem, spinal cord, and peripheral nerves. Especially in cases of severely brain-injured patients, very complex lesion patterns are observed, often including dysfunctions at multiple levels of the neuraxis. Therefore, localization of the lesion sites only by neurophysiologic methods (EEG, multimodal-evoked potentials TMEP), and contingent negative variation (CNV)) is thought to be impossible (14,22). In practice, during the early phases of neurosurgical intensive care, the examination of a patient's present state needs the documentation of structural lesions by computer axial tomography (CAT) and the recording of the development of the neurological condition (11,15). Some workers have suggested, in spite of all difficulties, that coma level and focal neurological defects are reflected by multimodal-evoked potential studies (11). From a clinical point of view, the present investigation has been planned with the following aims:

1) To study the general characteristics of the early and later SEP components in relation to coma level and lesion site
2) To select SEP patterns and variations, which could be used in clinical assessment
3) To cast some light upon the interrelationship of EEG patterns and dysfunctions of the hypothalamic-pituitary axis

Methods

Observations were made on patients with severe brain injury in extensive serial studies. These patients were divided into three groups (No. = 163):

1 Supported by the "Deutsche Forschungsgemeinschaft" SFB 33 (Arbeitsgruppe A3).

Group 1: comatose patients with neocortical lesions

Group 2: patients with brain stem lesions

Group 3: patients after brain death

The pathology of these cases was verified on the basis of all informations available: clinical course, computer axial tomography, and postmortem pathologic examination.

Somatosensory-evoked potentials (SEP) were recorded from the points F3-C3, F4-C4, nuchal and tympanal of the 10/20 system. For stable recordings over longer periods, we used needle electrodes. The bioelectric signals were amplified with a conventional six-channel EEG machine and fed into a four-channel averaging computer (Nicolet 1072). The recording system had a band pass ranging from the time constant 0.3 to 2 kc within 3 dB. Routinely, 128 responses to median nerve stimulation were averaged. Occasionally we summed up to 500 times.

The stimulating needle electrodes were inserted subdermally bilateral over the median nerves proximal to the wrist with the cathode 3 cm proximal to the anode. Electric stimuli were applied at a rate of 1/s, pulse duration of 0.1 ms, and supralimitary, constant intensity. Sequentially, both median nerves were stimulated and the SEPs plotted. Sweep durations were varied from 40 ms to 200 ms.

Results

With the use of our mobile equipment, it was possible to record SEPs in comatose patients under the demands of the intensive care unit. The evoked potential patterns were correlated with the clinical neurological course, computer axial tomography, operative or postmortem findings. The electroclinical data allowed differentiation of our findings into three categories:

1) Hemisyndromes and lesion patterns with more or less predominant hemispheric, neocortical lesioning
2) Brain stem syndromes, which were classified as
   - Upper brain stem syndrome (Mittelhirnsyndrom)
   - Lower brain stem syndrome (Bulbärhirnsyndrom)
   - More or less pronounced unilateral, incomplete brain stem lesioning at different structural levels
3) Brain death

1) SEP Patterns in Extended Neocortical Lesions

In patients with neurological hemisyndromes and radiologically verified extended lesions restricted to one cortical hemisphere, we observed SEP patterns as shown in Fig. 1. After comparison of the SEPs resulting from bilateral, symmetric stimulation of both median nerves, it is now evident that the injured somatosensory cortex did not respond, in contrast to the well-formed primary response of the less desintegrated hemisphere.

2) SEP Patterns in Brain Stem Syndromes

Thalamic or pretegmental lesions located in the midline structures often cause the clinical picture of the so-called upper brain stem (Mittelhirnsyndrom). The characteristic SEP pattern, which often persisted even until the reintegration during the apallic syndrome, is shown in Fig. 2. Marked differences in amplitudes of the primary responses, with its maximum at the contralateral side are recorded. As a rule, a close correlation was found in such patients between the duration of the evoked response and the degree of reintegration of sensorimotor functions.

Lesions of the midline structures at the pontine and prepontine level caused a so-called lower brain stem syndrome (Bulbärhirnsyndrom). If this syndrome was fully developed, no SEPs were picked up from the scalp electrodes; only at the nuchal level was a typical response obtained (Fig. 3).

More or less pronounced unilateral, incomplete traumatic brain stem lesions are responsible for more complex SEP patterns. Figure 4 shows the characteristic responses of an incomplete pretectal lesion including one cerebral peduncle. In Fig. 5 the response pattern of an incomplete lesion at the pontine level is documented.

3) Brain Death

When brain death was evident following severe brain injury, no SEPs were observed at the cortical or nuchal level. Transitional stages, especially in patients under controlled respiration, were well distinguished by the far field response technique both after stimulation of median nerves and stimulation of the trigeminal afferents.

4) Neuroendocrine Technique

In addition to our electroclinical approach, described above, we employed neuroendocrine techniques to study the functional relationship of the hypothalamic-pituitary system under the conditions of acute disintegration of cerebral function following severe brain injury.

In general, we measured a marked increase in serum concentrations of cortisol, human growth hormone (HGH), and prolactin (PRL) during the acute post-traumatic hospital course. In detail, however, our findings show a pronounced variability so that, at present, only selected cases can be demonstrated. Figure 6 shows the spontaneous serum concentrations and response characteristics of pituitary hormones in two cases with lower brain stem syndrome (K.H.E. and R.R.) and in a patient following brain death (W.S.). Notice the high concentrations of corticotropin-releasing factor (CRF) and prolactin release inhibiting factor (PIF), as well as the dissociative effect of thyrotropin-releasing hormone (TRH) stimulation, with a normal rise of thyroid-stimulating hormone (TSH) but a subnormal PRL response. In brain death we did not observe HGH response to arginine stimulation, which supports the opinion that arginine may act as a false releasing hormone. Figure 7 illustrates the response patterns of a case of brain death in contrast to the characteristics of a case with limbic seizures and its more functional hypothalamic disturbances.

Discussion

Our present findings support the concept that event-related bioelectric signals may serve as a diagnostic index of the cerebrospinal structures (1,4,8,19). The data presented agree with the previously published facts from animal models and studies on patients suffering from degenerative diseases or from neurological defects of other causes (10,15). A few workers have investigated patients with neurological disorders following brain and spinal trauma (7,8,9,11,13,17,18,19). We agree partially with the concept that vigilance variations are reflected by changes of the late components of the SEP. Our investigation, however, focused on the earlier components of the SEPs for several reasons:

1) Late SEP components are less constantly reproducible, even in healthy subjects.
2) The early parts of the SEPs are well investigated with respect to their origin and spatiotemporal distribution.
3) The far field response technique was applied only occasionally in addition ot the conventional SEPs due to the presence of artifacts.

The comparative study of bioelectric and neuroendocrine data showed only a poor correlation in brain death and lower brain stem syndrome. This may be due to the widely independent organization of the somatosensory system from the homeostatic regulation of the "milieu interne". SEP patterns, especially in the upper brain stem syndrome and in transitional stages, need further investigation. We suppose that the marked differences in amplitudes of the primary response may be explained as a lack of amplifier function of the midbrain reticular formation.

Summary

Somatosensory-evoked potentials were recorded bipolarly from the points F3-C3, F4-C4, nuchal and tympanal points of the 10/20 system. The results obtained from stimulation of both median nerves alternately were compared. In patients showing a fully developed brain death, no bioelectric responses were recorded. The lower brain stem syndrome was characterized by altered somato-sensory-nuchal potentials and a lack of cortical SEPs. In the upper brain stem syndrome, a very typical SEP pattern was recorded, which shows severe variations concerning the second part of the response and obvious difference in the amplitudes of the primary response. Transitional stages were isolated. It remains open to discussion whether this pattern depends on disturbed thalamocortical interactions or is due to a disintegrated function of the mesencephalic reticular formation (MRF).

Prolactin effects of TRH stimulation of the pituitary gland were compared to the increase in prolactin secretion following chlorpromazine block of PIF secretion. Neurosecretion was tested in brain death and decerebration syndromes. Neuroendocrine data were correlated to the bioelectric findings.

References

1. BRICOLO, A., TURAZZI, S., FACCIOLI, F., ODORIZZI, F., SCIARRETTA, G., ERCULIANI, P.: Clinical application of compressed spectral array in long-term EEG monitoring of comatose patients. Electroencephalogr. Clin. Neurophysiol. 45, 211-224 (1978)

2. CALLAWAY, E., HALLIDAY, R.A.: Evoked potential variability: Effects of age, amplitude and methods of measurement. Electroencephalogr. Clin. Neurophysiol. 34, 125-133 (1973)

3. COHN, R.: Bilateral simultaneous summated cortical responses to delayed bilateral and single median nerve stimulation. Electroencephalogr. Clin. Neurophysiol. 29, 612-615 (1970)

4. CRACCO, R.A.: The initial positive potential of the human scalp-recorded somatosensory evoked response. Electroencephalogr. Clin. Neurophysiol. 32, 623-629 (1972)

5. CRACCO, R.A., BICKFORD, R.G.: Rochester, Minn. Somatomotor and somatosensory evoked responses. Arch. Neurol. 18, 52-68 (1968)

6. DESMEDT, J.E., BRUNKO, E., DEBECKER, J., CARMELIET, J.: The system bandpass required to avoid distortion of early components when averaging somatosensory evoked potentials. Electroencephalogr. Clin. Neurophysiol. 37, 407-410 (1974)

7. DOLCE, G., FROMM, H., IONESCU, A.: Reaktionspotentiale beim Apallischen Syndrom. EEG EMG 2, 95-99 (1972)

8. ERTEKIN, C.: Comparison of the human evoked Electrospinogram recorded from the intrathecal, epidural and cutaneous levels. Electroencephalogr. Clin. Neurophysiol. 44, 683-690 (1978)

9. FEINSOD, M.M.D.: Electrophysiological correlates of traumatic visual damage. In: Head injuries. Proceedings of the second Chicago Symposium on Neural Trauma. McLAURIN, R.L. (ed.), pp. 95-100. New York, San Francisco, London: Grune & Stratton 1976

10. GÖTTE, J., KUBICKI, St., KÜHN, K., STÖLZEL, R.: Klinische Anwendung somato-sensorisch evozierter kortikaler Potentiale. EEG EMG 4, 86-96 (1973)

11. GREENBERG, R.P., MAYER, D.J., BECKER, D.P.: The prognostic value of evoked potentials in human mechanical head injury. In: Head injuries. Proceedings of The Second Chicago Symposium on Neural Trauma. McLAURIN, R.L. (ed.), pp. 81-88. New York, San Francisco, London: Grune & Stratton 1976

12. GROTE, E.H.: Neuroendocrinological differential diagnosis of cerebral death. 6th Int. Congr. Neurol. Surg., Abstr. 664 p. 253. Sao Paulo 1977

13. HUME, A.L., CANT, B.R.: Conduction time in central somatosensory pathways in man. Electroencephalogr. Clin. Neurophysiol. 45 (3), 361-374 (1978)

14. HUTCHINSON, J.W., KUSSKE, J.A., VERZEANO, M.: Cortical and thalamic activity in the late phases of somatosensory evoked potentials. Electroencephalogr. Clin. Neurophysiol. 45 (1), 45-51 (1978)

15. JÖRG, J.: Die elektrosensible Diagnostik in der Neurologie. Schriftenreihe Neurologie-Neurology Series. Berlin, Heidelberg, New York: Springer 1977

16. KATZ, S., MARTIN, H.F., BLACKBURN, J.G.: The effects of interaction between large and small diameter fiber systems on the somatosensory evoked potential. Electroencephalogr. Clin. Neurophysiol. 45 (1), 45-51 (1978)

17. NAKANISHI, T., SHIMADA, Y., SAKUTA, M., TOYOKURA, Y.: The initial positive component of the scalp-recorded somatosensory evoked potential in normal subjects and in patients with neurological disorders. Electroencephalogr. Clin. Neurophysiol. 45 (1), 26-33 (1978)

18. OMMAYA, A.K., GENNARELLI, Th.A.: A physiopathologic basis for noninvasive diagnosis and prognosis of head injury severity. In: Head injuries. Proceedings of the Second Chicago Symposium on Neural Trauma. McLAURIN, R.L. (ed.), pp. 49-73. New York, San Francisco, London: Grune & Stratton 1976

19. PEROT PHANOR, L.: Evoked potentials assessment of patients with neural trauma. In: Head injuries. Proceedings of the Second Chicago Symposium on Neural Trauma. McLAURIN, R.L. (ed.), pp. 77-79. New York, San Francisco, London: Grune & Stratton 1976

20. RUDMAN, D., FLEISCHER, A.S., KUTNER, H., RAGGIO, J.F.: Suprahypophyseal hypogonadism and hypothyroidism during prolonged coma after head trauma. J. Clin. Endocrinol. Metab. 45, 747-754 (1977)

21. SCHWINN, G., von zur MÜHLEN, A., KÖBBERLING, J., HALVES, E., WENZEL, K.W., MEINHOLD, H.: Plasma prolactin levels after TRH and chlorpromazine in normal subjects and patients with impaired pituitary function. Acta Endocrinol. (Kbh.) 79, 663-676 (1975)

22. WICKBOLDT, J., MILTNER, F.: Effects of anti-Parkinsonian drugs on behavior and EEG of comatose patients. In: Head injuries. Proceedings of the 28th Annual Meeting of the Deutsche Gesellschaft für Neurochirurgie. FROWEIN, R.A., WILCKE, O., KARIMI-NEJAD, A., BROCK, M., KLINGER, M. (eds.), pp. 83-87. Berlin, Heidelberg, New York: Springer 1978

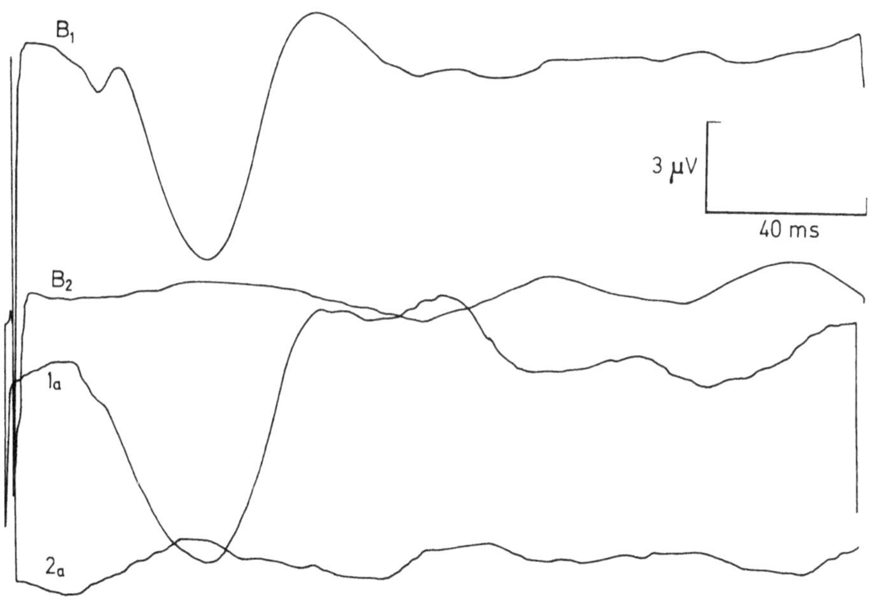

Fig. 1. Somatosensory-evoked responses picked up at the scalp points F3-C3 *(trace 1)* and F4-C4 *(trace 2)* after sequential stimulation of the right median nerve *(upper traces)* and left median nerve *(lower traces)*. Note the Early SEP components only over the *left* hemisphere

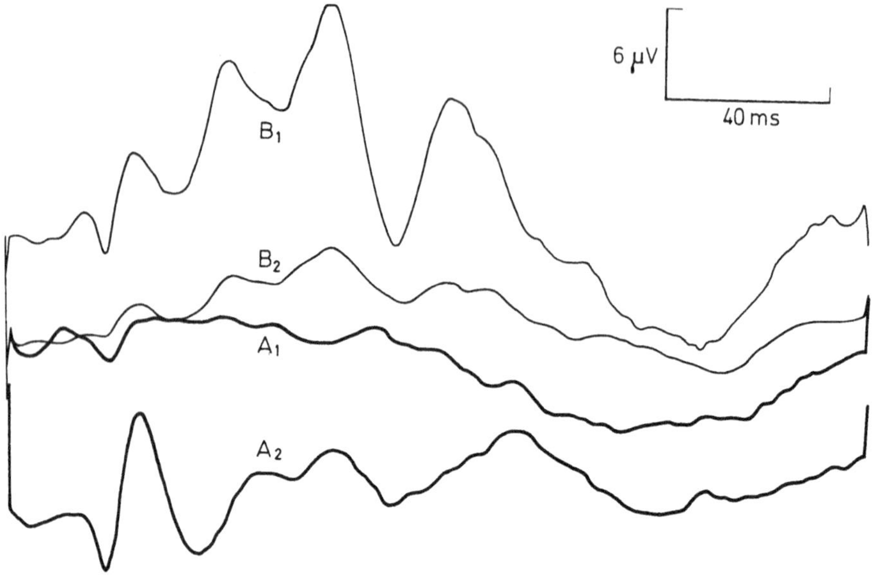

Fig. 2. SEP pattern of case with a so-called upper brain stem syndrome (Mittelhirnsyndrom). *Trace 1*, F3-C3; *trace 2*, F4-C4. *B*, stimulation of right median nerve; *A*, stimulation of left median nerve. Note the marked differences in amplitude and maximal response contralateral to the stimulation site

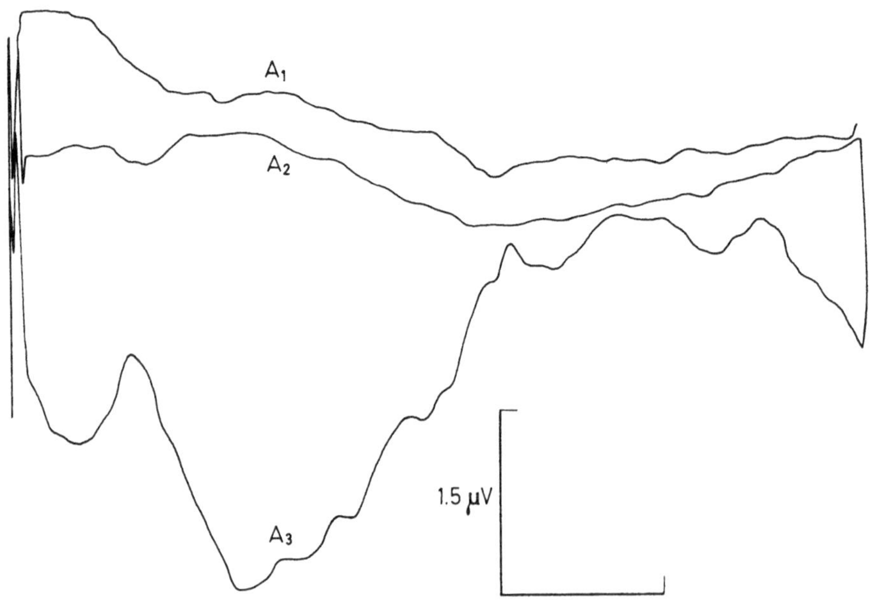

Fig. 3. Early components of SEP after left median nerve stimulation. *Trace 1*, F3-C3; *trace 2*, F4-C4; *trace 3*, nuchal-suboccipital. The cortical *traces* record only volume conducted potentials

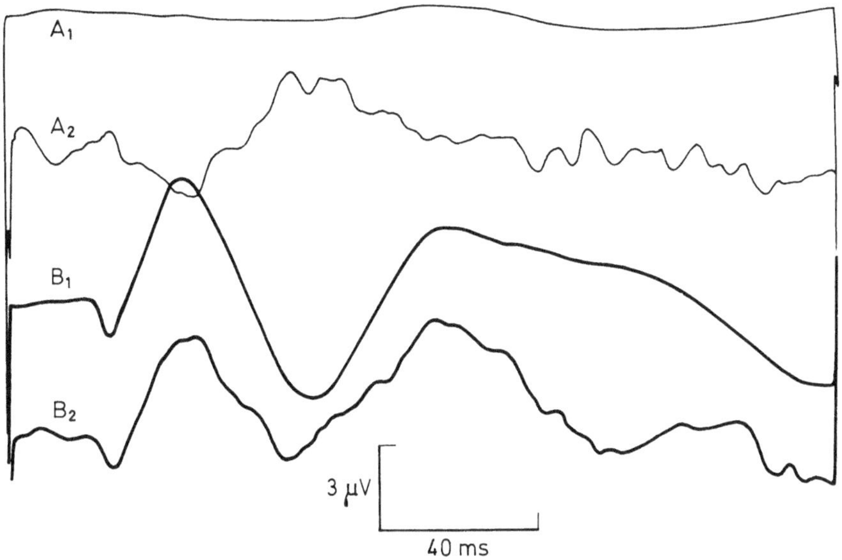

Fig. 4. Cortical responses after sequential median nerves stimulation. *A*, left median nerve; *B*, right median nerve. Unilateral incomplete lesion at the pretectal-cerebral peduncle level. *Trace 1*, F3-C3; *trace 2*, F4-C4

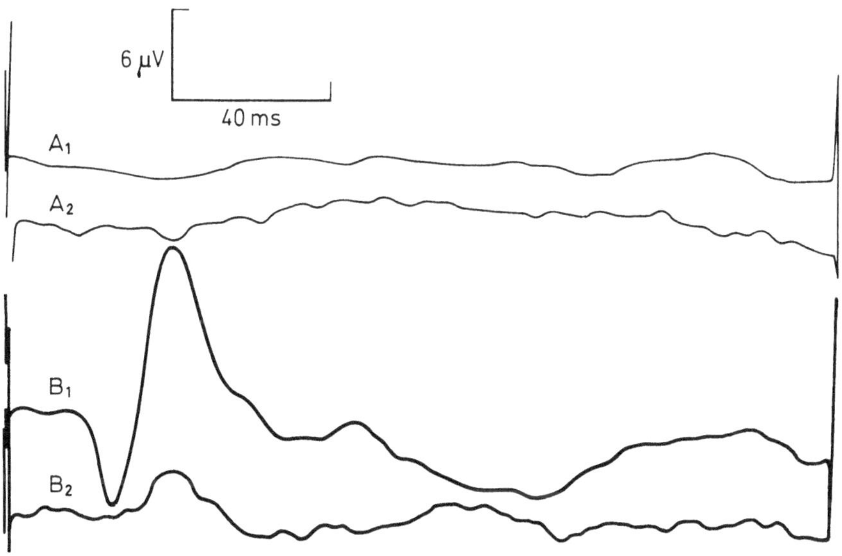

Fig. 5. SEP pattern, typical for incomplete, unilateral lesion at the pontien level. *A*, stimulation of the right median nerve. *Trace 1*, F3-C3; *trace 2*, F4-C4. Early response of noticeable amplitude only in B_1

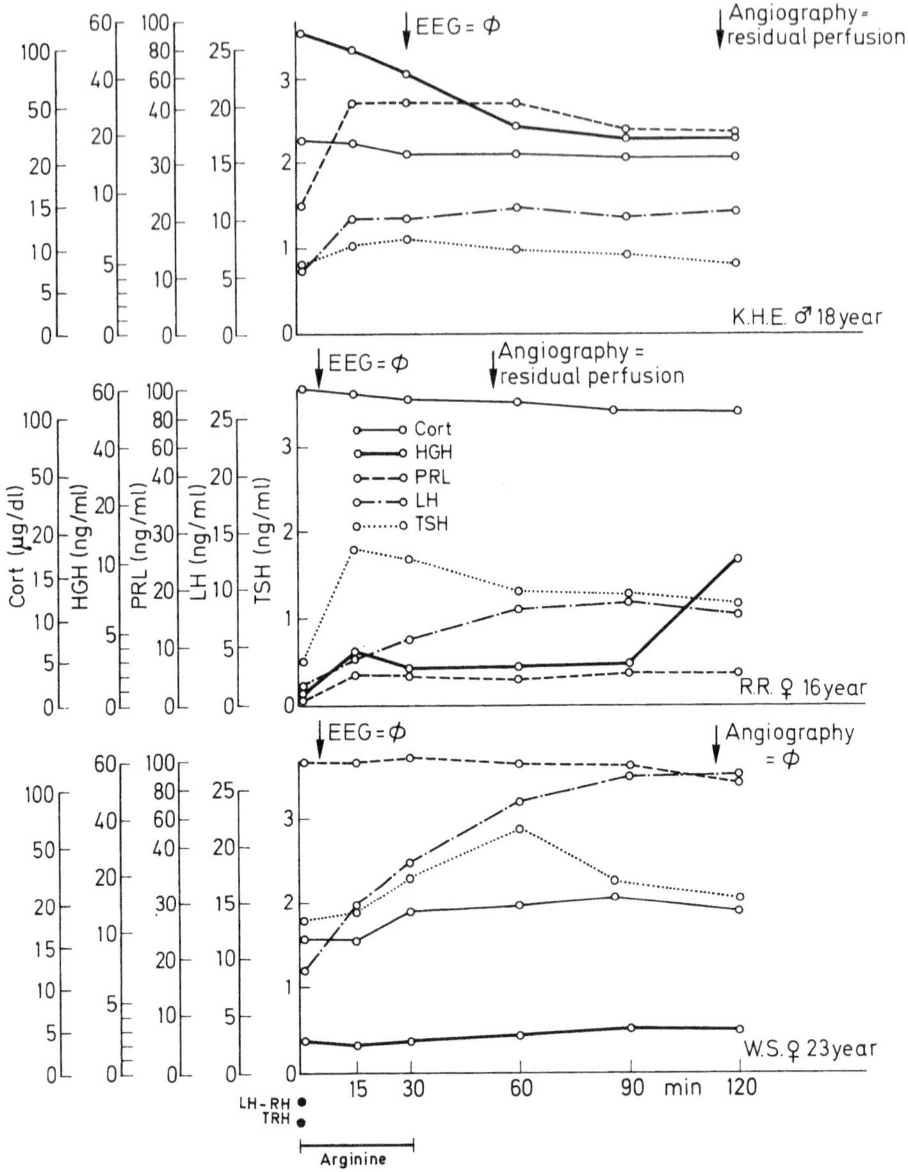

Fig. 6. Spontaneous serum concentrations of hormones of the hypothalamic-hypophyseal system and response characteristics in lower brain stem syndrome (K.H.E. and R.R.) and brain death (W.S.)

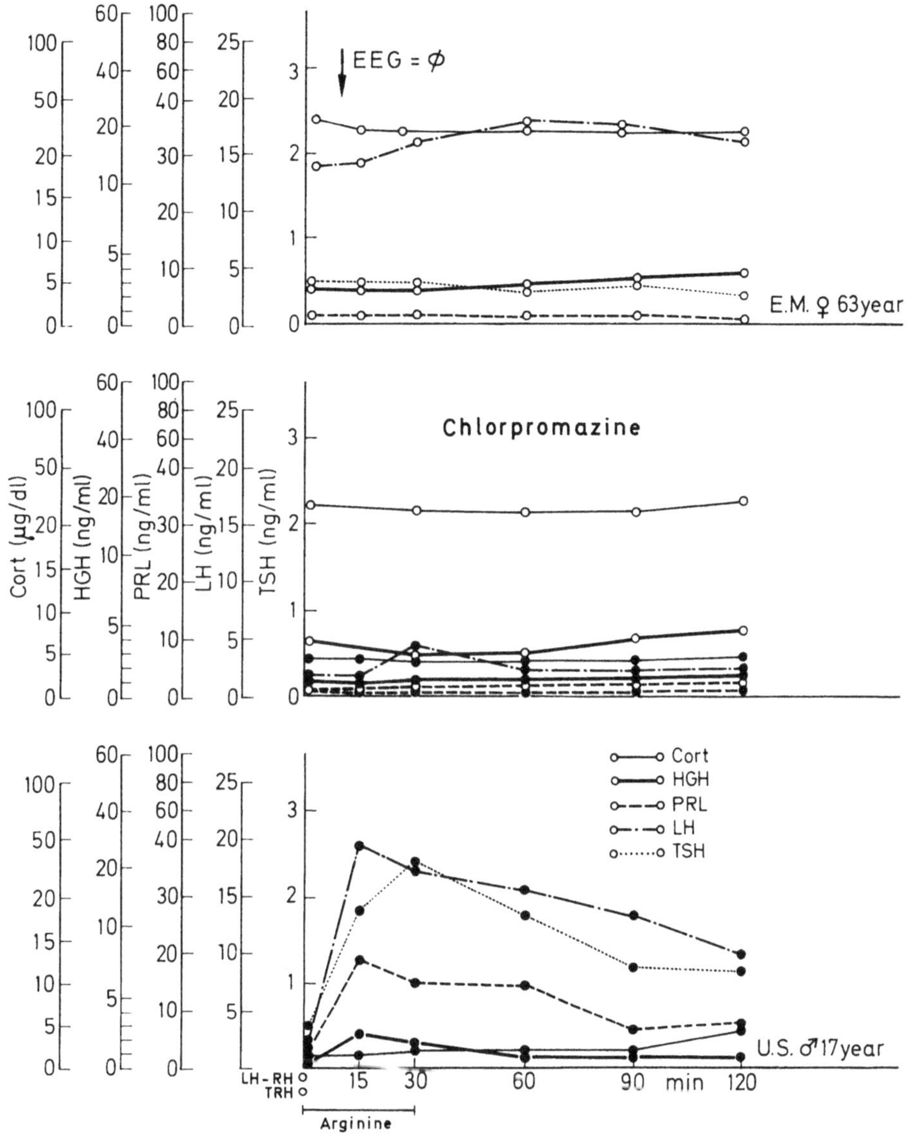

Fig. 7. Spontaneous levels and response pattern of hypothalamic-hypophyseal hormones in brain death (E.M.) in contrast to the functional disturbances caused by limbic seizures (U.S.)

Use of CT Cisternography, RISA Cisternography, and the Infusion Test for Predicting Shunting Results in Normal Pressure Hydrocephalus (NPH)

CH. SPRUNG and TH. GRUMME

After the simultaneous development of CT scanning (1,14) and of the safe water-soluble contrast medium Metrizamide (8,9,10,21) in 1973, a new method was available for the evaluation of CSF dynamics in patients with NPH, first described by GREITZ and HINDMARSH in 1974 (11). Since then, various authors (2,3,4,5,7,12,13,18,19,20,22) have used CT cisternography with Metrizamide to increase our knowledge of normal CSF dynamics and disturbed CSF flow patterns in patients with NPH.

JACOBS and KINKEL (15) demonstrated the superiority of the CT scan over pneumoencephalography in the diagnosis of NPH. Similarly, it has been claimed that CT cisternography has some advantages over RISA cisternography and may even replace the latter method (3). Until now, the correlation between normal or abnormal CSF flow patterns and the impact on surgery has not been evaluated. The purpose of the present communication is to compare the three most important diagnostic tests applied to patients with suspected NPH and to assess the value of these procedures in the prediction of the surgical outcome.

Methods

Of 69 patients admitted to our hospital since 1974 with typical signs and symptoms of NPH, 19 underwent CT cisternography performed according to the method described by GREITZ and HINDMARSH (11,12,13). In nearly all cases, the lumbar introduction of Metrizamide was performed immediately after the lumbar infusion test described by KATZMAN and HUSSEY (17). We used 10 ml of a solution containing 170 mg Metrizamide per milliliter, equivalent to 1.7 g iodine. The amount of our isotonic solution of Metrizamide is relatively low in comparison to that used by other authors (Table 1). All patients were sedated with 100 mg of phenobarbital.

After removal of the spinal needle, the patient was placed in the supine position, a firm pillow was placed under the head, and the foot end of the bed was raised about 15° for 24 h after the injection to bring the bolus of contrast medium up to the cervicodorsal junction (Fig. 1).

Intrathecal Metrizamide with cranial CT represents an important alternative method for evaluating CSF kinetics, especially in patients with suspected NPH. CT scans using a MARK-1 and 1010 EMI scanner were performed before and 3, 6, 24, 48, and - occasionally - 72 h after the lumbar injection of Metrizamide. Eleven of these patients were also studied with RISA cisternography. The procedure was performed at least 2 weeks before or after the other diagnostic procedures to prevent leakage from the spinal tap. A control group of six volunteers with normal CSF pathways was studied with CT cisternography after routine lumbar myelography with Metrizamide.

Table 1. Volume and concentration of metrizamide used by different authors to evaluate CSF kinetics. The considerable differences render comparison difficult

Authors	Year	No. of patients (hydroc.)	Volume (ml)	Concentration (mg I/ml)	Iodine (g)
GREITZ and HINDMARSH	1974	9 (1)	8-18	170-300	2.75
HINDMARSH	1975	15 (10)	18-36	85-170	1.7 -3.4
HINDMARSH	1977	48 (39)	10-36	85-170	1.7 -1.85
DRAYER and ROSENBAUM	1977	25 (17)	6- 7	190	1.14-1.33
ROSENBAUM and DRAYER	1977	47 (40)	6	190	1.14
SACKETT	1977	21 (5)	19	170	6.75
ENZMANN	1977	13 (9)	12	170	2.04
DRAYER	1978	11 (11)	2- 5.5	190	0.38-1.05
SPRUNG and GRUMME	1978	25 (19)	10	170	1.7

Results

Classification of the lumbar infusion test to determine normal and abnormal curves was carried out following the criteria established by KATZMAN and HUSSEY (4) and demonstrated in detail in a previous paper (23). The results of RISA cisternography were evaluated according to standards proposed by TATOR et al. (26).

CT cisternography was only classified as normal or negative when no reflux into the lateral ventricles occurred or when CSF attenuation was minimal after 6 h and baseline after 24 h.

Figure 2 represents a normal test result of CT cisternography performed in a hydrocephalic patient with neurological symptoms of NPH. Only 4 of the 19 patients showed such patterns, while all volunteers except two in the control group had such findings. The basal cisterns and the fourth ventricle were filled in all normal subjects after 3 h. The highest attenuation coefficients in this region were reached 6 h after injection of the contrast medium and decreased after 24 h when passage of Metrizamide to the lateral convexity and parasagittal region took place. As DRAYER et al. (2,3) also observed, we found that nearly all patients with normal CSF kinetics showed more parasagittal "blush" than did the group with apparently disturbed CSF dynamics. At 48 h the appearance of the CT scans was baseline in all patients of this group.

We considered significant reflux into the lateral ventricles and stasis lasting up to 48 h or more as a pathologic or positive CT cisternography (Fig. 3a and b). Thirteen patients demonstrated both significant reflux with CSF attenuation values above those of the surrounding brain tissue and stasis lasting up to 48 h or more, while 2 patients showed isodense CSF attenuation after 24 h. This represents 15 positive or pathologic test results.

Criteria of preoperative reliability and prognostic value of our various tests were developed on the basis of results of the shunting operation in 15 surgical patients and the clinical follow-up in the nonoperative group. The CT follow-up and an improved or unchanged clinical course in four patients not operated on confirmed a posteriori our decision to avoid unnecessary draining procedures in these patients. Table 2 lists the results of all tests performed in patients with suspected NPH, the surgical outcome, and the cases with incongruent test results.

Table 2. Comparison between the prediction of the individual tests and the surgical outcome

Case No.	Inf. test[a]	CT cist.[a]	RISA cist.	Results after shunting	Discrepancy
1) E.W.	-	+	+	Ø[b]	Inf./CT cist.
2) M.S.	+	+	+	Good	
3) H.S.	+	+	(-)	Poor	CT cist./RISA
4) H.P.	(+)	+	Ø	Excellent	
5) K.P.	+	+	+	Excellent	
6) W.T.	+	-	-	Excellent	Inf./CT cist.
7) K.V.	+	+	Ø	Excellent	
8) U.M.	(+)	(-)	Ø	Good	Inf./CT cist.
9) H.K.	(+)	+	+	Good	
10)	+	(-)	+	Ø	Inf./CT cist.
11) G.H.	(-)	(+)	(+)	Ø	Inf./CT cist.
12) H.G.	+	+	Ø	Excellent	
13) W.R.	+	+	Ø	Good	
14) S.B.	+	+	+	Excellent	
15) K.S.	(+)	(-)	-	Excellent	Inf./CT cist.
16) E.M.	-	-	Ø	Ø	
17) B.P.	(+)	+	Ø	Excellent	
18) C.B.	+	+	+	Poor	
19) M.B.	+	+	Ø	Good	

a Key to prediction of surgical outcome:
+ indicates that test predicts excellent surgical results;
(+) indicates that test predicts good surgical results;
(-) indicates that test predicts poor surgical results;
- indicates that test predicts no improvement.
b Ø indicates that test or operation was not performed.

As documented in Table 3, prediction on the basis of a single test, taken as a sole criterion for operation, is hazardous. A prediction is considered correct positive when a test result favoring operation is followed by improvement after surgery. We defined failure to improve from surgery after a single negative test as a correct negative prediction. False prediction was defined as a discrepancy between test results and surgical outcome.

Table 3. Reliability of individual tests for the prediction of treatment results

	Inf. test[a]	CT cist.[a]	RISA cist.[a]
Correct positive	13	10	4
Correct negative	3 (3)	2 (2)	1
False positive	3 (1)	4 (2)	4 (3)
False negative	0	3	2
Total	19 (4)	19 (4)	11 (3)

a The numbers in parentheses indicate patients treated with conservative measures.

Our statistics are the first to demonstrate that CT cisternography is not superior to other tests as a sole predictor of successful surgical shunting. Note the tendency of all tests to predict a successful surgical outcome without demonstrating corresponding results in follow-up studies.

Discussion

The plain CT scan was considered superior to pneumencephalography (15) and complementary to isotope cisternography (6) for differentiating patients with primary cerebral atrophy from those with NPH. HINDMARSH (12,13) observed that findings in CT cisternography were entirely in agreement with the results of isotope cisternography when simultaneous injection of both media was performed.

CT cisternography has proved a valuable indicator of CSF flow patterns. The advantages of CT cisternography over RISA cisternography are high resolution and low radiation dose, providing better anatomic and physiologic insights into the nature of CSF transport disorders (2-5, 7,12,13,18-20,22).

It has been claimed that CT cisternography would supersede other diagnostic tests in the diagnosis of NPH (2,3). However, it is hazardous to define a test result as pathologic, thus giving a reliable prediction for surgical outcome, without correlating these findings with the further clinical course or the results of surgical therapy. This was well-documented for isotope cisternography by JACOBS et al. (16) and for the infusion test (24). Our statistics are the first to demonstrate that CT cisternography is not superior to other tests as a sole predictor of successful surgical shunting. As stated before (23), one must take into account all three tests in addition to the history and neurological signs and symptoms to avoid useless operations.

In our opinion, contrary to HINDMARSH (12) and in agreement with SACKETT and STROTHER (20), the result of CT cisternography depends strongly on 1. the concentration and volume of Metrizamide, 2. the site of injection, and 3. the patient's position (Figs. 4 and 5). Improved standardization of CT cisternography is necessary to gain comparable results and to improve the prognostic value where shunting procedures are concerned.

The main drawback, as compared to both other tests, seems to be a comparatively high incidence of side-effects - mainly nausea, vomiting, and headaches - that occurred in about 40% of our patients. Furthermore, the adverse reactions correlate well with the amount of Metrizamide entering the ventricles.

Summary

A comparative analysis of three different diagnostic tests performed in 19 patients is presented. Results in CT cisternography were shown to depend strongly on the position of the patient and especially upon the volume and concentration of Metrizamide. We want to emphasize the necessity of standardization. Adverse reactions increase with the amount of intraventricular reflux. CT cisternography is not superior to other tests as a sole predictor of successful surgical shunting.

References

1. AMBROSE, J.: Computerized transverse axial scanning (tomography). Part 2. Clinical application. Br. J. Radiol. 46, 1023 (1973)
2. DRAYER, B.P., ROSENBAUM, A.E., HIGMAN, H.B.: Cerebrospinal fluid imaging using serial metrizamide. CT cisternography. Neuroradiology 13, 7-17 (1977)
3. DRAYER, B.P., ROSENBAUM, A.E.: Metrizamide brain penetrance. Acta Radiol. (Suppl.) (Stockh.) 355, 280 (1977)
4. DRAYER, B.P., ROSENBAUM, A.E.: Pediatric metrizamide CT cisternography: Cerebrospinal fluid circulation and hydrocephalus. Neurology (Minneap.) 28, 71-77 (1978)
5. ENZMANN, D.R., NORMAN, D., NEWTON, T.H.: Computer tomography in cisternography with metrizamide. Acta Radiol. (Suppl.) (Stockh.) 355, 294 (1977)
6. GADO, M.H., COLEMAN, R.E., LEE, K.S.: Correlation between computerized transaxial tomography and radionuclide cisternography in dementia. Neurology (Minneap.) 26, 555-560 (1976)
7. GREPE, A.: Cisternography with the non-ionic water-soluble contrast medium metrizamide. A preliminary report. Acta Radiol. (Diagn.) (Stockh.) 16, 146-160 (1975)
8. GREPE, A., WIDEN, L.: Neurotoxic effect of intracranial subarachnoid application of metrizamide and meglumine iocarmate. An experimental investigation in dogs in neurolept analgesia. Acta Radiol. (Suppl.) (Stockh.) 335, 102 (1973)
9. GREPE, A., WIDEN, L.: Effects of cisternal application of metrizamide. An experimental investigation in dogs in N_2O analgesia with and without Halothane. Acta Radiol. (Suppl.) (Stockh.) 335, 119-125 (1973)
10. GONSETTE, R.E.: Metrizamide as contrast medium for myelography and ventriculography. Preliminary clinical experiences. Acta Radiol. (Suppl.) (Stockh.) 335, 346 (1973)
11. GREITZ, T., HINDMARSH, T.: Computer assisted tomography of intracranial CSF circulation using a watersoluble contrast medium. Acta Radiol. (diagn.) (Stockh.) 15, 497-507 (1974)
12. HINDMARSH, T., GREITZ, T.: Computer cisternography in the diagnosis of communicating hydrocephalus. Acta Radiol. (Suppl.) (Stockh.) 346, 91-97 (1975)

13. HINDMARSH, T.: Computer cisternography for evaluation of CSF flow dynamics. Acta Radiol. (Suppl.) (Stockh.) 355, 269-279 (1977)

14. HOUNDSFIELD, G.N.: Computerized transverse axial scanning (tomography). Part I Description of system. Br. J. Radiol. 46, 1016 (1973)

15. JACOBS, L., KINKEL, W.: Computerized axial transverse tomography in normal pressure hydrocephalus. Neurology (Minneap.) 26, 501-507 (1976)

16. JACOBS, L., CONTI, D., KINKEL, W., MANNING, F.J.: Normal pressure hydrocephalus. Relationship of clinical and Radiographic findings to improvement following shunt surgery. J.A.M.A. 235, 510-512 (1976)

17. KATZMAN, R., HUSSEY, F.: A simple constant-infusion manometric test for measurement of CSF absorption: I. Rationale and method. Neurology (Minneap.) 20, 534-544 (1970)

18. ROSENBAUM, A.E., DRAYER, B.P., BANK, W.O., JANETTA, P.J., KENNEDY, W.H.: Computer tomographic cisternography (CTC) using a water-soluble agent (Amipaque). Neuroradiology 12, 48 (1976)

19. ROSENBAUM, A.E., DRAYER, B.P.: CT cisternography with metrizamide. Acta Radiol. (suppl.) (Stockh.) 355, 323 (1977)

20. SACKETT, J.F., STROTHER, C.M.: Computer tomography and subarachnoid metrizamide for evaluation of cerebrospinal fluid flow. Acta Radiol. (Suppl.) (Stockh.) 355, 338-344 (1977)

21. SALVESEN, S.: Suboccipital injection of metrizamide to anaesthetized and unanaesthetized rabbits. Acta Radiol. (Suppl.) (Stockh.) 335, 93 (1973)

22. SALVESEN, S., FREY, K.: Protein binding of metrizamide and the effect on various enzymes. Acta Radiol. (Suppl.) (Stockh.) 335, 247 (1973)

23. SHAH, S., BOWERS, J., ROACH, A., DAVIS, D.O.: CT-study of the intracranial distribution of metrizamide. Neuroradiology 12, 49 (1976)

24. SPRUNG, CH., COLLMANN, H., FUCHS, E.C., SUWITO, S., DUISBERG, R.: Pre- and postoperative evaluation of hydrocephalus using the infusion test. Adv. Neurosurg. 4, 161-167 (1977)

25. STEIN, S.C., LANGFITT, TH.W.: Normal pressure hydrocephalus. Predicting the results of cerebrospinal fluid shunting. J. Neurosurgery 41, 463-470 (1974)

26. TATOR, C.H., FLEMING, J.F.R., SHEPPARD, R.H., TRUNER, V.M.: A radioisotopic test for communicating hydrocephalus. J. Neurosurg. 28, 327-340 (1968)

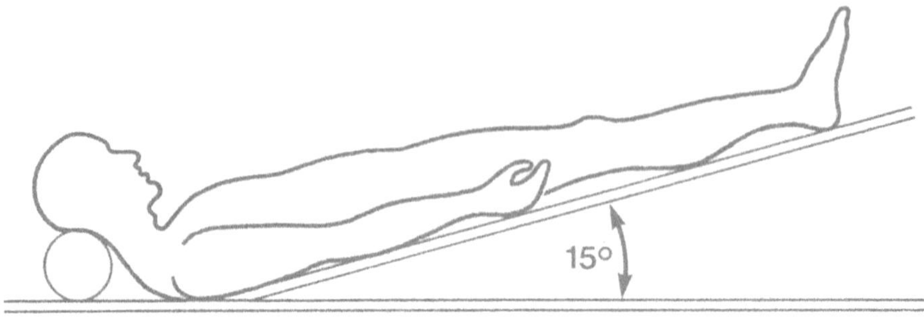

Fig. 1. Position of the patient for 24 h following the lumbar injection of Metrizamide. The neck is slightly flexed and the foot end of the bed raised about 15°. This position is comfortable for the patient and allows collection of the bulk of Metrizamide at the cervicodorsal junction

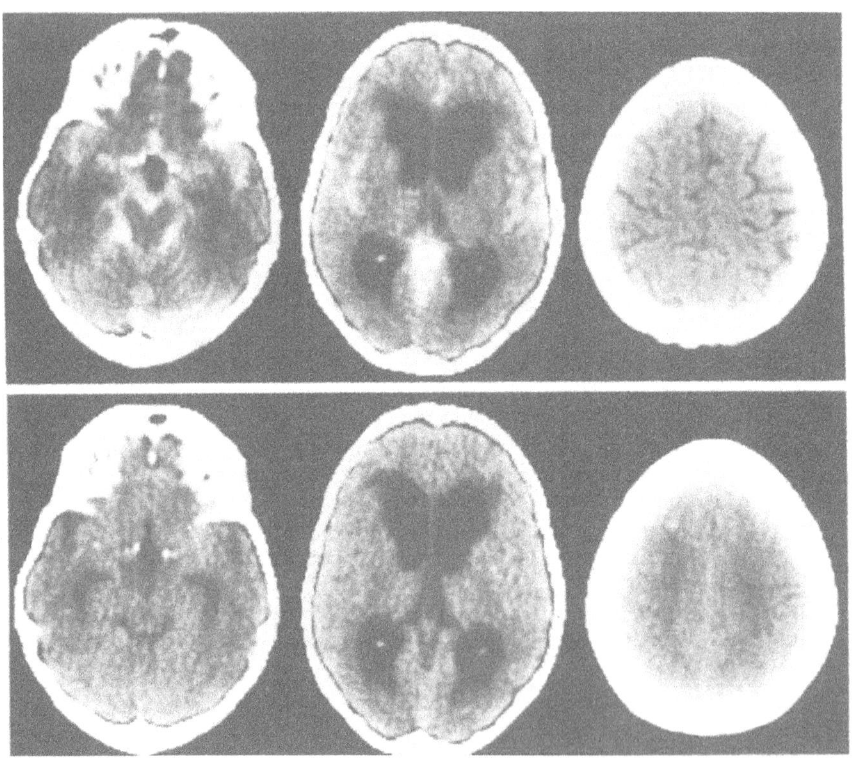

Fig. 2. Normal Metrizamide CT cisternography. *Above:* at 3 h the basal cisterns and the fourth ventricle are filled with contrast medium, which is not the case with supratentorial ventricles. The sylvian fissure is filled with Metrizamide, but the parasagittal region is free of contrast medium. *Below:* at 24 h there is marked decrease in attenuation coefficients of the basal cisterns. The lateral ventricles are still free of Metrizamide, but the parasagittal region shows slightly increased attenuation masking cortical atrophy in this case

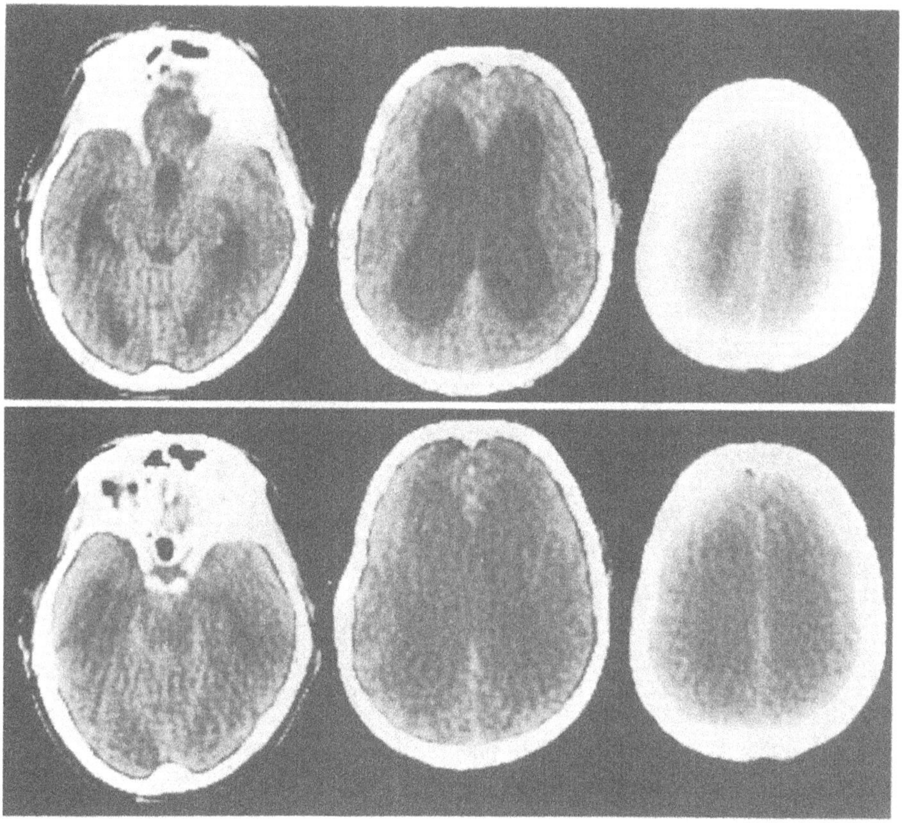

'ig. 3. a Abnormal CSF kinetics in a patient with typical signs and ;ymptoms of NPH. Preliminary CT scan: markedly dilated ventricles and ıormal cortical sulci. *Below:* after 3 h: considerable filling of the ›asal cisterns and fourth ventricle. Brain stem outlined by Metriz-ımide. Slight filling of lateral ventricles, attenuation values below :hat of the surrounding brain. No filling over the convexity

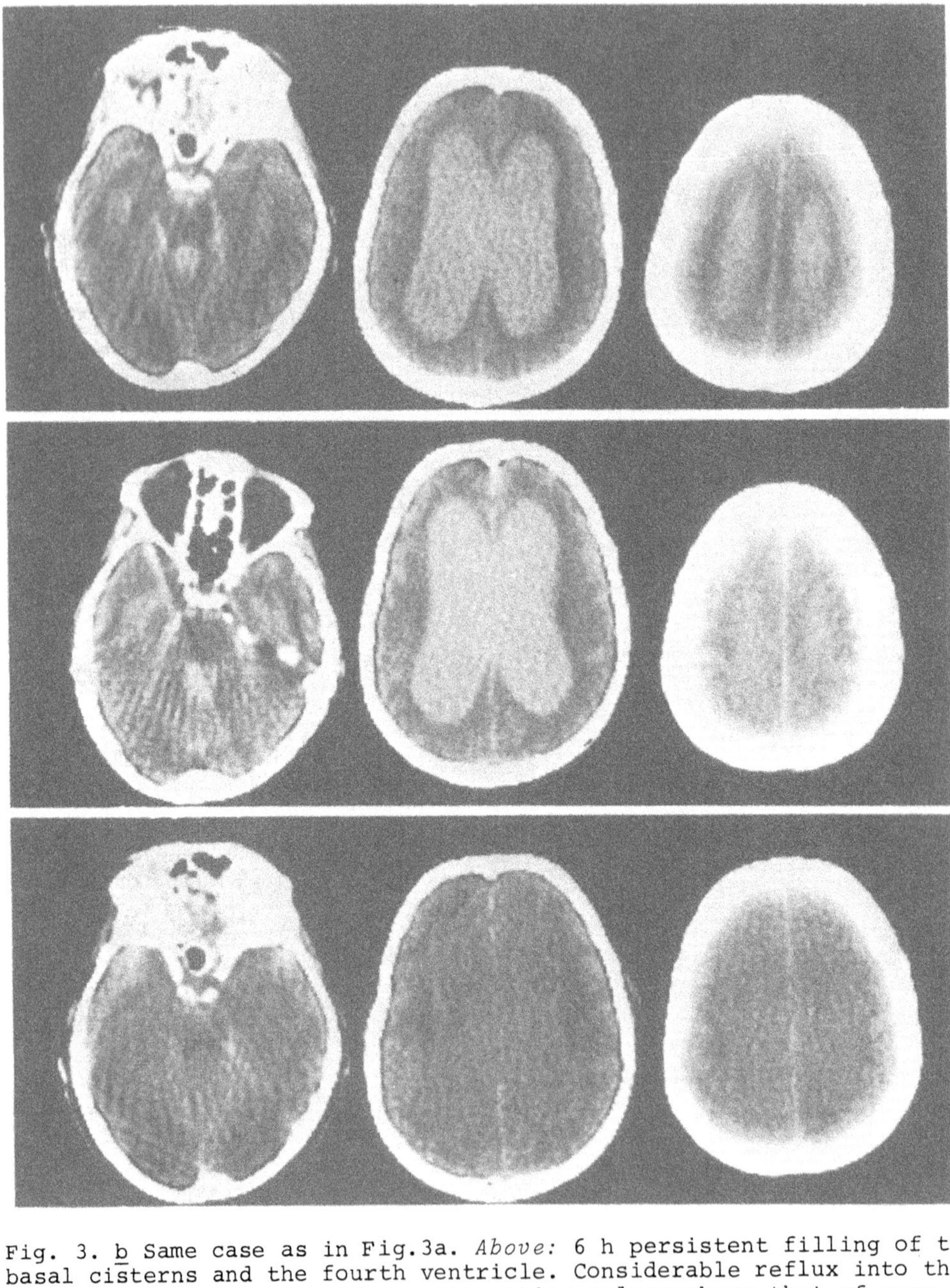

Fig. 3. b Same case as in Fig.3a. *Above:* 6 h persistent filling of the basal cisterns and the fourth ventricle. Considerable reflux into the lateral ventricles, providing attenuation values above that of surrounding brain. Minimal passage of the contrast medium to the subarachnoid space over the convexities. *Middle:* after 24 h: maximal intraventricular CSF attenuation values. Slight "blush" of the parasagittal cortex and over the lateral convexities. Narrow periventricular zone of relatively low attenuation, highlighted between the ventricular Metrizamide and normal cerebral white matter. *Below:* after 48 h: ventricular stasis with decrease pf CSF attenuation to isodense values

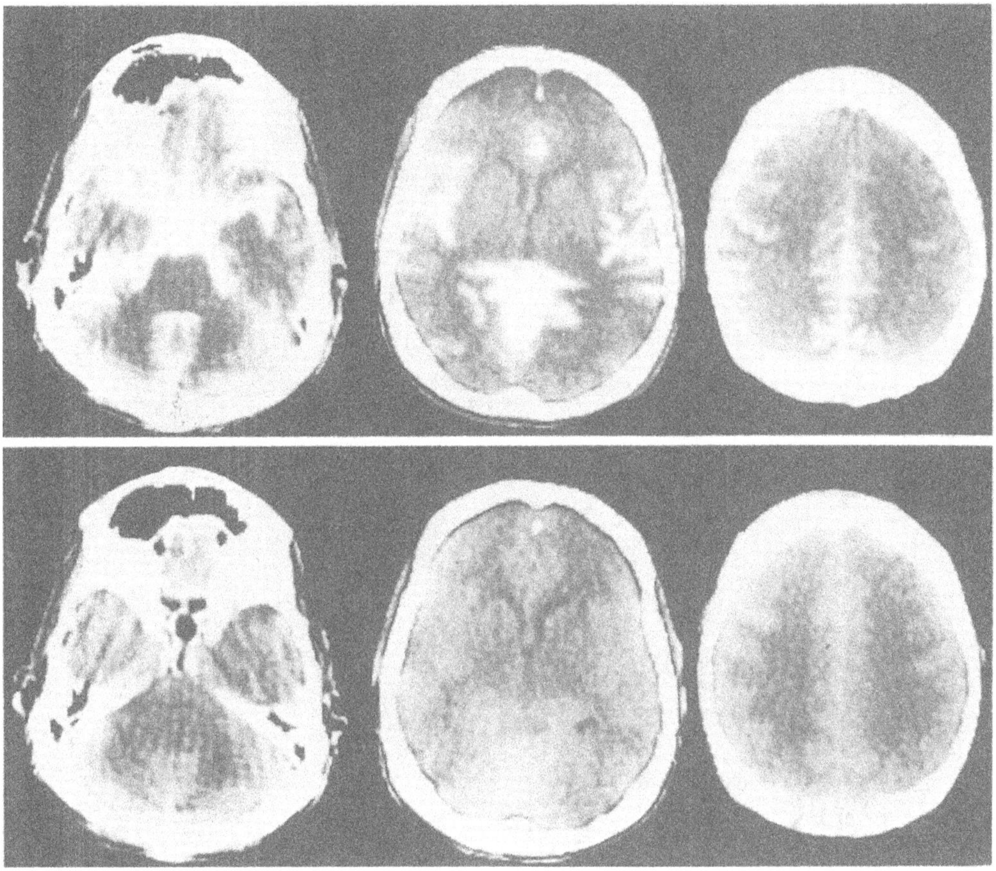

Fig. 4. CT cisternography of a volunteer after routine lumbar myelography with 20 ml of isotonic Metrizamide. No clinical signs of impaired CSF circulation. *Above:* after 6 h: no significant reflux into the lateral ventricles but early appearance of contrast medium in the parasagittal region and on the lateral convexity. *Below:* after 24 h: no reflux in the lateral ventricles, decreased attenuation levels in the region of the basal cisterns and fourth ventricle. Stasis of contrast medium in the parasagittal region and on the lateral convexity, increased "blush" of the parasagittal cortex and over the lateral convexities 20 ml cont. 170 mg/ml = 3.4 gJ

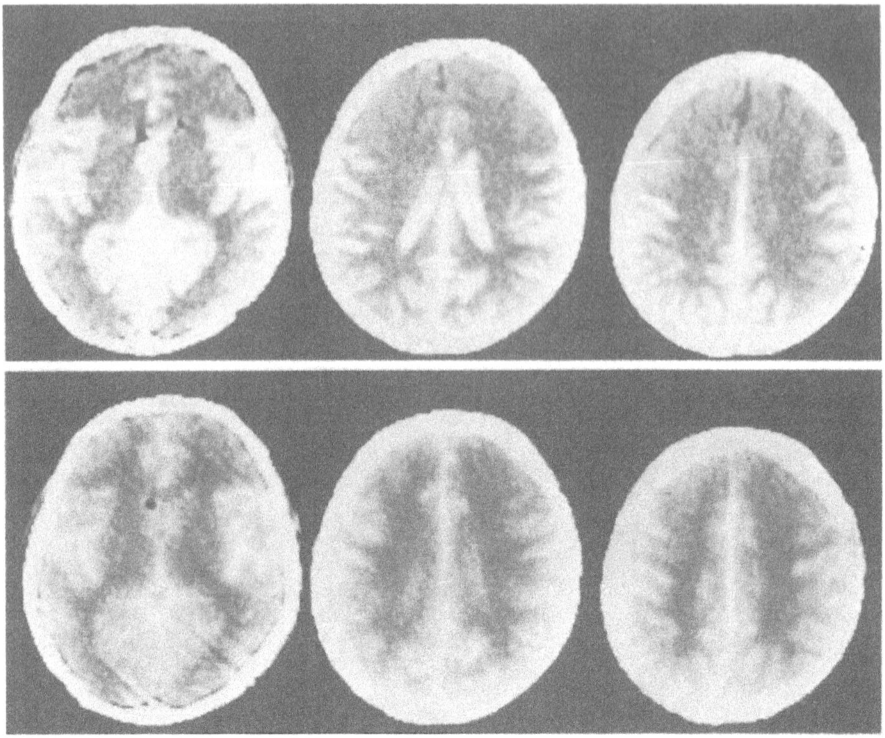

Fig. 5. CT cisternography of another volunteer after routine lumbar myelography with 12 ml of a hypertonic solution of Metrizamide. Preliminary scan showed slight cortical atrophy. *Above:* after 6 h: considerable reflux of contrast medium into the lateral ventricles with increase of CSF attenuation above the level of surrounding brain tissue. *Below:* after 24 h: stasis of contrast medium in the lateral ventricles with decreased attenuation coefficients. 12 ml cont. 230 mg/ml " 2.76 gJ

Identifying Epileptic Foci on Contrast-Enhanced Computer Tomographic (CT) Scans

G. A. OJEMANN, J. OAKLEY, L. MORETTI-OJEMANN, and L. CROMWELL

Introduction

Epileptic foci are commonly identified by changes in scalp electroencephalograms (EEG) and the clinical pattern of the seizure. Recording of spontaneous seizures from scalp or implanted electrodes often aid in this identification. About half of these foci show structural abnormalities on CT scans, such as tumors, focal atrophy, or ventricular dilatation (1). During a seizure, epileptic foci can also be identified by increased metabolism and secondary blood flow changes, using isotopic tracer techniques (2,4). Whether these local metabolic markers are present during interictal periods is controversial (3,6). Our paper is directed at determining whether such interictal local metabolic markers of the epileptic focus might be subtly reflected as CT scan changes with contrast enhancement. Since visual inspection of these scans showed no such changes, numeric analysis of the site of suspected focus and the homologous area of opposite brain on these scans was undertaken.

Materials and Methods

All patients in the University of Washington Comprehensive Epilepsy Center with CT scans were reviewed. From these, several patient groups were selected. Group 1 includes those patients with clearly identifiable foci on scalp EEG, compatible clinical seizures, and normal CT scans (12 patients). Group 2 includes five patients with clearly identifiable epileptic foci but evidence of gross lesions on their CT scan. Group 3 includes seven patients with clinically lateralized seizures but not clearly lateralized EEG foci and group 4 six patients with nonlateralized seizures by EEGs and clinical criteria. Group 1, then, would establish any lateralized CT scan changes related to the location of the focus. Group 2 gives us an indication of the effects of CT scan-demonstrated structural lesions on these changes, and groups 3 and 4 suggest the potential diagnostic usefulness of this technique, if any.

Numeric analysis of the CT scan was obtained by using the region of interest capability of the 1010 EMI CC head scanning unit. The mean CT number was determined for defined radii of homotopic areas of a given tomographic slice for the unenhanced CT scan, and the enhanced CT scan obtained after a bolus injection of 100 cc of diatrizoate meglumine 60% (Hypaque 60). Within this region of interest on each

1 This research was supported by NIH Grant NS 04053 and NIH Contract NO1 NS62341, USPHS/DHEW.

side the mean CT number before enhancement was subtracted from that after and then this change from the right side subtracted from that on the left. The resulting number, after this double subtraction, represents the change after contrast of one side compared to the other, with positive numbers indicating a relative increase in high density CT numbers on the left, negative numbers a relative increase in high density CT numbers on the right. The regions of interest chosen correspond to the epileptic focus on scalp EEG, when this was known (groups 1 and 2), the area suggested by clinical localization if no scalp EEG focus was present (group 3), and superior frontal lobes well away from the ventricles in group 4, patients with generalized seizures. Intrahemispheric specificity was assessed in ten group 1 patients by analyzing additional sites away from the focus.

Results

In this paper, analysis is confined to qualitative differences, that is, which side shows more high-density CT numbers after the double subtraction technique. The magnitude of these differences varies 1% - 41% of the average mean enhanced value.

Control Measures. Data on all patients with measurements in one lobe, frontal, temporal, or parietal occipital, were pooled to see if there were any subtle overall tendencies to right or left numeric CT scan changes in one lobe after enhancement. No statistically significant tendency to lateralization is present in any lobe in these patients.

Group 1. Ten of the 12 cases with clearly lateralized foci and normal CT scans demonstrated relative increases in the change in mean CT density after enhancement on the side of the focus compared to the opposite side. The probability of this finding on chance basis is 1% (sign test (7)). This change is independent of the side of focus (six left, four right). It is present in all four patients who later came to cortical resection with subsequent seizure control. Correct lateralization was present for eight of ten patients with temporal lobe foci and both patients with frontal lobe foci. There is no relation between time of last seizure and lateralization to the side of the focus. Thus, this relatively larger mean CT number after contrast enhancement marks the side of the focus from the homologous area of the opposite side. Intrahemispheric specificity of the CT change to the site of the focus was assessed by obtaining measurements at 16 sites elsewhere in the brain of ten of these patients. Frontal lobe sites showed enhancement on the same side as the focus (in seven of eight), temporal and parietal occipital did not (one of eight). All frontal lobe sites sampled were in patients with temporal foci.

Group 2. The five cases with epileptic foci and gross CT scan abnormalities showed changes only in the direction of the gross CT abnormalities rather than in the direction of the epileptic focus. Thus, the technique does not seem to be usable in the presence of gross CT abnormalities.

Group 3. The seven patients with lateralized clinical seizures but generalized scalp EEG findings showed two with CT scan changes lateralized to the side expected on the clinical findings, five not.

Group 4. Six patients with nonlateralized seizures by both clinical and EEG criteria all showed lateralization to one or the other frontal lobe (four left, two right). This includes one patient with complex partial seizures and bilateral frontal-temporal EEG discharges. Whether this is clinically significant is unknown.

Discussion

A relative increase in mean CT values after contrast enhancement shows a statistically significant association with the side of lateralized temporal and frontal interictal EEG foci. It is not a consequence of some subtle asymmetry in CT values of the hemisphere as no such asymmetry can be shown and the CT change is independent of whether the focus is right or left brain. Within the hemisphere containing the focus, the CT change is not entirely specific to the lobe containing the focus as frontal lobe lateralization to the same side is rather consistently seen in patients with lateralized temporal foci. The technique cannot be used in the presence of a gross CT abnormality, probably because the subtraction techniques are not accurate enough to completely remove the abnormality. Care must be taken to obtain symmetric CT scan cuts with cuts at the same level on enhanced and unenhanced scans if this technique is to be used successfully.

We can only speculate as to what this CT change represents. It is only a relative change. After contrast infusion, mean CT density sometimes decreases on one side, as it did in 28% of our pairs of scans. Thus, it is not always enhancement of the focus but sometimes a relative failure of the opposite side to enhance. Changes in CT density after enhancement have been related to cerebral blood flow and volume (5). Perhaps there is a slightly increased blood flow in the interictal focus as has been reported in some patients using xenon flow techniques (2,6), which accounts for our CT change. However, it may also reflect structural changes in the focus, such as gliosis and blood-brain barrier alterations. Indeed, it may be this nonspecificity that accounts for the greater association of these CT scan changes with interictal foci than is seen with the more specific measures, such as the regional cerebral blood flow.

The major clinical usefulness of the technique would seem to be in those patients where the EEG does not clearly show a focus. These include patients with temporal lobe seizures but bitemporal EEG spiking, without preponderance, and those with clinically focal seizures but no focal EEG changes. These patients show lateralized CT changes in our study that may provide a hint as to the side of focus to be confirmed by further evaluation.

Conclusions

A statistically significant association exists between a relative increase in mean CT value after contrast enhancement in the area of a well-defined EEG interictal focus compared to homologous opposite brain and the side of that focus. This is independent of the side of focus or time of last seizure but cannot be shown if there is a gross abnormality on the CT scan. This technique provides some evidence of lateralization in epileptic patients without clearly lateralized EEG findings.

References

1. GASTAUT, H., GASTAUT, J.L.: Computerized transverse axial tomography in epilepsy. Epilepsia 17, 325-336 (1976)

2. HOUGAARD, K., OIKAWA, T., SUEINSDOTTIR, E., SKINHØJ, E., INGVAR, D.H., LASSEN, N.A.: Regional cerebral blood flow in focal cortical epilepsy. Arch. Neurol. 33, 527-535 (1976)

3. LAVY, S., MELAMED, E., PORTNOY, Z., CARMON, A.: Regional cerebral blood flow in the epileptic brain during the seizure-free interval. INGVAR, D.H., LASSEN, N.A. (eds.), Acta Neurol. Scand. (Suppl. 64) 56, 232-233 (1977)

4. PENFIELD, W., von SANTHA, K., CIPRIANI, A.: Cerebral blood flow during induced epileptiform seizures in animal and man. J. Neurophysiol. 2, 257-267 (1939)

5. PENN, R.D., WALSER, R., KURTZ, D., ACKERMAN, L.: Tumor volume, luxury perfusion, and regional blood volume change in man visualized by subtraction computerized tomography. J.N.S. 44, 449-457 (1976)

6. SAKAI, F., MEYER, J., NARITOMI, H., HSU, M.C.: Regional cerebral blood flow and EEG in patients with epilepsy. Arch. Neurol. 35, 648-657 (1978)

7. SIEGAL, S.: Nonparametric Statistics for the Behavioral Sciences. New York: McGraw Hill 1956

Recognition of Minute (5 mm) Cerebral Gliomas by Advanced Computer Technology

C. H. SHELDEN, G. D. MCCANN, D. JACQUES, and R. KATZ

Introduction

The treatment of primary brain tumors is usually unsuccessful. Great effort has been made to improve the statistics, but results have added only slight prolongation of life and some temporary amelioration of symptoms with essentially no cures. Tumors are found too late and too large. They resist complete removal and do not respond favorably to irradiation, chemotherapy, or immunologic attack (6).

Although it is true that the treatment is ineffective, the fault may lie more with the human tumor model than the methods. A new look might be helpful. We should determine how we can improve the results by finding tumors earlier when their size is expressed in millimeters rather than centimeters. The defense mechanism possibly is being overwhelmed by tumor antigen.

The brain is said to be immunologically privileged (1) in that its response to antigen by antibody and/or T cell is poor. It also is said that the blood-brain barrier prevents the cytolytic elements from reaching the tumor (4). Yet one can hardly imagine that Nature would deprive such a valuable organ as the brain from the protection of its most formidable defense mechanism. Furthermore, it hardly seems likely that the tight junctions of the capillary endothelial cells would prevent lymphocytes from having ready access to the brain since these same cells can easily pass through endothelial cells elsewhere (3). However, it is not certain whether all types of T cells have this capability.

Clinically, a brain tumor must be reduced in volume before any form of adjuvant therapy can hope to be successful. Hence, the smaller a tumor can be found the less tissue that need be removed to reduce the residual cells to an acceptable limit.

It is stated that a glioma of 1 g = 10^9 cells = 1 cm^3 of volume (5). Autograft survival of 10^8 cells is always successful, whereas a graft of 10^4 cells will not survive even though transplanted to a most favorable environment. Considered in terms of exponents, it appears rather simple to reduce the mass or "tumor burden" to 10^4 cells. Yet removal of 99% of a tumor containing 10^9 cells still leaves only 1% of the cells, but this still amounts to 10^7 of 10 million tumor cells. To obtain a residual tumor mass of 10^4 cells (or 10,000 cells), one must remove 99.9% of this remaining 1% of the original tumor mass.

Thus, one can visualize the need for attacking the smallest tumor that can be successfully diagnosed and localized. If additional tissue around the tumor is removed, one could consider it a "complete" gross removal. In spite of such care, there would remain some 10,000 residual cells in the bumor bed. This area would be treated with adjuvant therapy, thus creating an "in-vitro, in-vivo" treatment program that could be visually controlled through an implanted cannula.

Materials and Methods

A microsurgical method must supplant our present open operation with free hand suction removal of a tumor several centimeters in diameter. To meet this challenge, we have developed a method for stereotactic removal of a minute (5mm) intracerebral tumor or hematoma under direct three-dimensional binocular vision.

CT data for preoperative localization is obtained by use of a circular aluminum ring with four pins of varying lengths projecting from the surface (Fig. 1). The ring is fixed to the skull with four screw pins under local anesthesia, similar to the usual bony fixation of the head prior to craniotomy (Fig. 2). An algorithm utilizes pin position and selection for determination of the X, Y, and Z axes.

The instrument (8-9 mm OD) is introduced through a burr hole in the skull and guided stereotactically to the target along through a track previously made by a series of three dilators of increasing diameter. The instrument is passed along the Z axis to the target where expandable blades are opened exposing the tumor. Through a side port microinstruments are introduced under direct vision through an air-filled cavity for removal of the lesion. This method should afford much greater accuracy, less brain trauma, and more complete tumor removal (Fig. 3).

The methodology and technical aspects of handling minute intracerebral lesions has progessively improved. Localization by computer control of the X, Y, and Z axes coordinations, and actual removal of the lesion will not present major problems.

Diagnosis of lesions 5 mm or less is a problem. To my knowledge no gliomas of this size have been recognized on primary routine transmission CT scan. Our numeric experience has been limited to date, but we have seen the scans of a number of patients that were initially and on subsequent review called negative in whom we have been able to verify the lesion by more intense CT investigation.

Our advanced computer efforts have been directed toward accurate determination of the Z axis from data derived from the sets of pins on the skeletally fixed head ring. This simple method would simplify stereotactic procedures. It eliminates the need for coronal or other additional scanning views. It affords coordinates that allow re-entry to the exact site of the planned surgical procedure.

Computer enhancement and enlargement have allowed us to blow up areas with possible tumor. This can be done on the TV screen or on the digital printout for permanent record. Numbers within possible suspect ranges can be separated from those of the surrounding tissue. We have found that assigning a specific color to numbers within a specific range of interest greatly enhances one's ability to distinguish areas.

Three-dimensional reconstruction has also proven of great value. It allows three-dimensional visualization of the posterior configuration of the tumor as well as the surface of the underlying edema (Figs.4-6).

Thus, irregular shape or unsuspected projections of tumor tissue can be determined preoperatively, information that is absolutely essential for accurate stereotactic tumor removal.

Summary and Discussion

This project was begun 3 years ago because the introduction of CT scanning had so enhanced our localizing capacity for minute lesions that it soon would surpass the technical level of our surgical hardware. We now have hardware to cope with the most minute intracerebral lesions; this was as planned, but we hoped that diagnostic methods at this time would include screening and molecular markers to match the hardware. Great progress is being made.

Since it is our goal to find and remove brain tumors before they produce clinical signs, we need a blood-screening test to indicate the presence of a malignant tumor in the brain (8) much like α-fetoprotein or carcinoembryonic antigen in other tissues. If positive, a molecular level test like the emission CT position method would be appropriate (2). Suspicious areas from this method would mandate a detailed local transmission CT study such as we have described. Transmission CT data must be reviewed regarding the unenhanced scan since it seems likely that the events we are discussing occur before the breakdown of the blood-brain barrier, which is necessary for present enhancing views to be positive.

After the tumor is diagnosed, localized, and removed, the 10,000 tumor cells (10^4) must be dealt with by adjuvant direct chemo- or immunotherapies (4,6,7). Though complex, this approach will become better understood as more information is available. If one accepts the probable origin of a glioma from one cell that has changed for some unknown reason from self to non-self, there can be little hope of cure if after a 99% removal over 10,000,000 cells remain. A microstereotactic method is essential. One must start with a very small lesion. After tumor removal, plus immediate adjacent brain tissue, the residuum of cells must be so few in number that local adjuvant therapy can function without the hindrance of great antigen excess. A means of holding the residual cells in limbo, until the adjuvant therapy is effective, must be developed.

References

1. FUDENBERG, H.H., STITES, D.P., CALDWELL, J.L., WELLS, J.V. (eds.): Basic and clinical immunology. Lange 1976
2. GRUBB, R.L.: Emission computed tomography. Neurosurgery 2, 273-280 (1978)
3. HOOD, L.: Personal communication, California Institute of Technology, October 1978
4. MORANTZ, R.A., SHAIN, W., CRAVIOTO, H.: Immune surveillance and tumors of the nervous system. J. Neurosurg. 49, 84-92 (1978)
5. OMMAYA, A.K.: Immunotherapy of gliomas: A review. Adv. Neurol. 15, 337-359 (1976)
6. SHAPIRO, W.R., YOUNG, D.F.: Treatment of malignant glioma. Arch. Neurol. 33, 494-500 (1976)

7. TAKAKURA, K., MIKI, Y., KUBO, O., OGAWA, W., MATSUTANI, M., SANO, K.: Adjuvant immunotherapy for malignant brain tumors. Jap. J. Clin. Oncol. 12, 109-120 (1972)

8. TROUILLAS, P.: Letter: Carcino-fetal antigen in glial tumors. Lancet 11, 552 (1971)

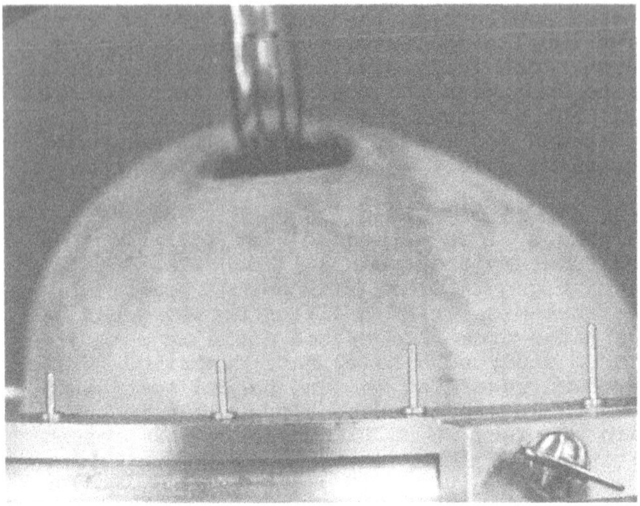

Fig. 1. Circular aluminum ring with vertically projecting pins for calculation of the Z axis

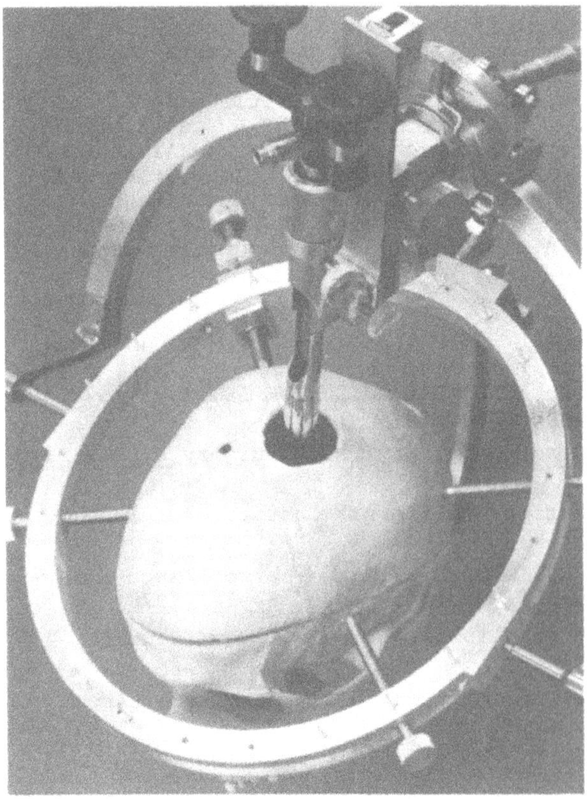

Fig. 2. Circular aluminum ring showing attachment to skull

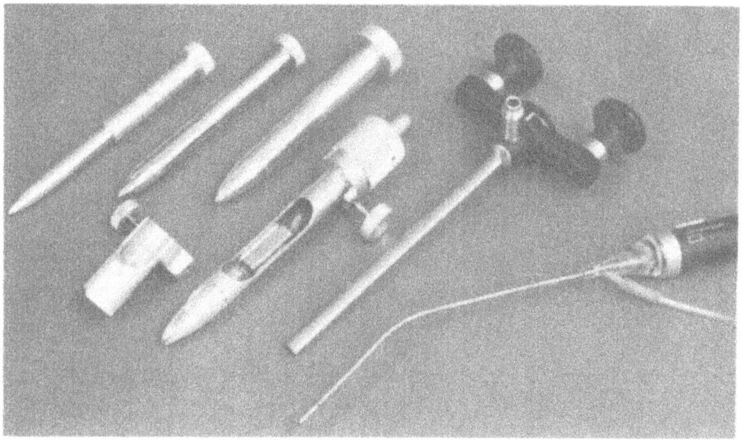

Fig. 3. Tumor scope with associated optics, dilators, and suction-dissector apparatus

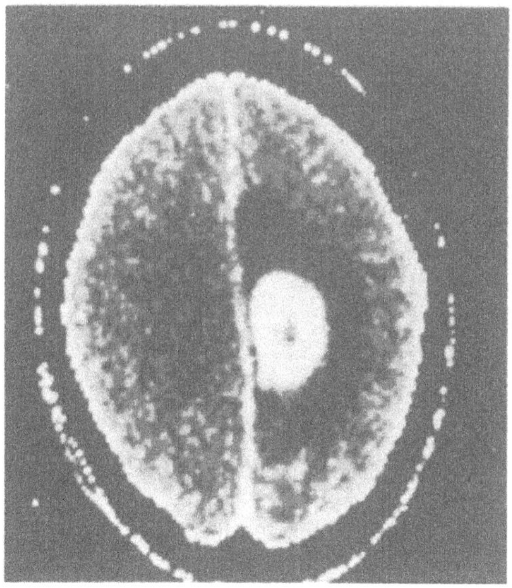

Fig. 4. Routine CT scan of large glioma

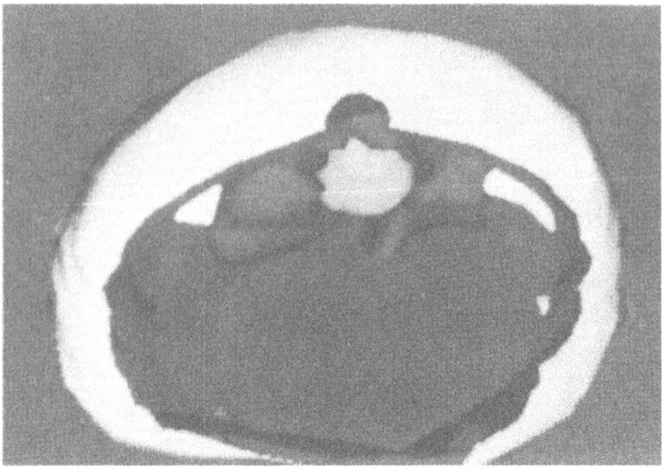

Fig. 5. Three-dimensional computer reconstruction of tumor and edema of lesion in Fig. 4

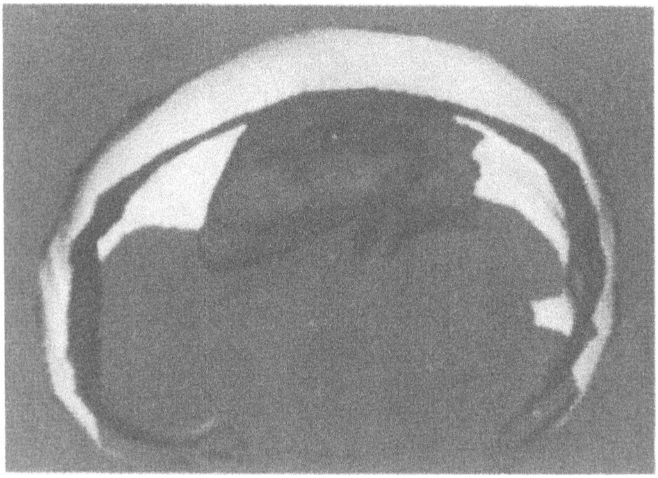

Fig. 6. Tumor "removed" from Fig. 5 revealing surrounding edema

Intraoperative Prophylactic Antibiotic Therapy: a Prospective Study of the Effectiveness, Cost, and Complications

R. C. LLEWELLYN, D. M. JARROTT, and R. P. MERIWETHER

The term "prophylactic" in describing the use of antibiotics to prevent surgical wound infections is well chosen. The mysticism espoused by some groups and the dogmatic, even rigid formulations advised by others to prevent wound infections evokes prescientific notions of family planning. This is compounded in the current surgical literature by the multitude of studies concerning postoperative infection rates with and without antibiotic usage. Approximately 13,000 papers have been published since 1975 concerning this topic. CHODAK and PLAUT have recently reviewed 131 articles dealing with clinical trials and surgical antibiotic prophylaxis but found only 24 adequate in terms of meeting the criteria for appropriately designed prospective double-blind investigations (1).

Guidelines for Peer Review in the use of antibiotics were prepared by the Veterans Administration Ad Hoc Interdisciplinary Advisory Committee on Antimicrobial Usage and published in the Journal of the American Medical Association from March to May 1977. This series of articles was prepared at government expense and described by the authors as "providing a basis for discussion among physicians and to raise the level of knowledge of infectious disease which has been recently reported to be deficient" (4). The first article in the series concerned the use of antibiotics in surgical wound prophylaxis and contained a specific rejoinder to the effect that the material presented was for the guidance of hospital staffs in developing methods of monitoring antimicrobial usage and did not constitute official Veterans Administration policy. Neurosurgical procedures were included parenthetically under "clean operations" after varicose vein stripping, mastectomy, and thyroidectomy and were accorded a 0% indication for prophylaxis. CSF shunts were included elsewhere under the heading of prostetic devices and were accorded a 100% indication for prophylaxis. This means that using intraoperative antibiotics in any neurosurgical procedure other than the insertion of CSF shunts would qualify the chart automatically for peer review by hospitals that had adopted the Veterans Administration guidelines for use by their own infection control antibiotic usage committees (2).

The timing of antimicrobial prophylaxis was also subjected to peer review criteria. Unless the antibiotic was administered 2 - 4 h prior to the surgical procedure and discontinued within 24 - 72 h, an automatic peer review process would be instituted. Thus, the use of intraoperative antibiotics to prevent wound infections following neurosurgical procedures would be subjected to two counts of peer review on the basis of guidelines developed by the Veterans Administration group with the stated suggestion that they "could" be used to construct audits in the context of "Professional Standards Review Organizations". It requires little imagination to envision the potential medical legal exposure and even hospital practice limitations that might follow.

Although scrupulous skin preparation may effectively sterilize the surgical field when the incision is made, the area is rapidly repopulated with bacteria. Any operative procedure that lasts more than 30 min should be considered at least technically as "clean and contaminated". Instrumentation before, during, or after surgery could lead to transient bacteremias with colonization of the postoperative wound. One wonders why postoperative infections are so uncommon considering these factors. Undoubtedly, the tremendous defenses and healing powers of the human body account for the good results so often quoted in surgical series. The term "prophylactic" then cannot refer to the prevention of bacterial contamination of the wound but must imply the prevention of symptomatic infections, particucarly that of wound suppuration and dehiscence (2).

The neurosurgical literature contains several recent references to the use of antibiotics specifically for the prevention of wound complications (6,7,8). Ampicillin, lincomycin, and clindamycin have been reported in studies of postneurosurgical wound infections (7,8). The use of intraoperative garamycin, vancomycin, and streptomycin was first proposed by MALIS at the AANS meeting in 1976. He will soon report 2000 consecutive neurosurgical procedures without infection while using this prophylactic regime (3). His preliminary report was encouraging and was the basis of antibiotic selection for use in this prospective study of cost effectiveness and complications.

From April 1976 to December 1977 an intraoperative prophylactic antibiotic regime was rigidly applied in all patients who did not list specific allergies to the antibiotics used. This prophylactic regime was instituted in a multihospital-based private practice and was compared to a prior 2-year period of time in the same private practice when prophylactic antibiotics were not utilized. In addition, for cross-comparison, the rate of infection experience in our residency-based teaching hospital population was evaluated. In these institutions prophylactic antibiotics are not used. The infection rate in the three series of patients is basically the same, which raises the question of the validity of using prophylactic antibiotics in neurosurgical procedures.

Table 1. Schedule

Garamycin	80 g IM	($ 16.50)
Vancomycin	1 g IVPB	($ 60.50)
Streptomycin	50 mg/1000 ml	($ 8.25)

The antibiotic regime that was utilized is given in Table 1. Shortly after the institution of anesthesia, garamycin in a single 80-mg dose was given IM. An intravenous piggyback infusion of vancomycin was begun and 1 g was administered. Streptomycin was added to the saline irrigating fluid in a dose of 50 mg/liter. While this may seem like a small quantity, the actual concentration of 50 µg/ml is far above the minimal inhibitory concentration required for bacteriocidal activity. The figures given in parentheses are the approximate cost to the patient of these antibiotics. The patient was considered to have a wound infection following surgery if wound drainage or dehiscence occurred and a positive bacterial culture was obtained. Instances of wound swelling or erythemia that were resolved by the patient without the use of postoperative antibiotics were not listed and indeed may reflect missed, but self-limited postoperative "infections". In addition, computer statistics available at one hospital were employed to compare the postoperative fever curve experienced by patients with and without antibiotics.

Table 2. Study results

	No. of cases	Wound infection (%)
Community hospitals		
Without antibiotics	263	1.2
With antibiotics	174	1.1
Training hospitals	1854	0.8

The results of the study are shown in Table 2. In the multihospital-based private practice without antibiotics, 263 cases were performed over a 2-year period with an infection rate of 1.2%. With antibiotics 174 cases were performed with a wound infection rate of 1.1%. There is no statistical difference between the two groups. At the same time, the residency training hospital experience of 1854 cases reported an overall infection rate of 0.8% during which time intraoperative prophylactic antibiotics were not utilized. Two wound infections with staphylococcus were encountered and one gram-negative meningitis occurred following a craniotomy in the nonantibiotic group. During the period in which intraoperative prophylactic antibiotics were employed, there were two wound infections. There was one gram-negative infection with proteus and one infection from which a diphtheroid was cultured (Table 3).

Table 3. Postsurgical infections

	No.	Site	Organism
Without antibiotics	2	Wound	Staphylococcus
	1	CSF	Pseudomonas
With antibiotics	2	Wound	Proteus (1)
			Diphtheroid (1)

Adverse reactions were encountered in a very few cases (Table 4).

Table 4. Adverse effects in 174 cases of "prophylactic" antibiotics usage

Hypotension during vancomycin	2
Skin rash (vancomycin?)	3
Postoperative IV site phlebitis	10

In two instances hypotension occurred during lincomycin administration intraoperatively and was reversed by discontinuance of the infusion. In three additional patients, an erythematous skin rash developed during intravenous administration of vancomycin. This cleared following discontinuation of the antibiotic infusion and the use of antihistaminic agents. Postoperative phlebitis at the intravenous site occurred in ten patients. There were no major complications or signs of toxicity on the ear or kidney with this antibiotic regime. Figure 1 shows the maximum fever experienced by the patients in each group, and it is apparent that the maximum temperature that developed following surgery was not modified by the use of antibiotics. However, when the duration of postoperative fever is examined, it is evident that the defervescence occurs slightly earlier in the group given antibiotics (Fig. 2). The peak defervescence occurred within 3 days in patients receiving the antibiotic regime as compared to 5 - 6 days in the group operated without antibiotic coverage. This is explained on the basis of antibiotics contributing to the overall defense mechanisms and process of wound healing in a "clean but contaminated" wound even if it is not sufficiently significant to be manifested in gross wound infection rates.

Finally, the overall United States wound infection rate in general surgical cases is quoted at 3% - 5% without antibiotics and 1% with antibiotics (5). In a New Orleans survey of all surgical cases performed in the community hospitals constituting the private practice of the senior author, a 2.67% reported infection rate was discovered (Table 5). This is compared to the 1.2% in the series of neurosurgical cases reported here. An exhausting review of the German literature reveals an infection rate approximately equaling that of the United States' series and a 3% figure is presented here as an average. It is concluded that the use of intraoperative antibiotics is a safe and noncostly way of enhancing the patient's wound healing and defervescence following surgery. However, there is no apparent difference in the wound infection rates in 174 cases examined prospectively and given intraoperative antibiotics as compared to a previous group of 263 cases who underwent surgery without prophylactic antibiotic coverage.

Table 5. Wound infection rate

General surgery	%	
United States	2 - 5	Without antibiotics
	1.0	With antibiotics
New Orleans	2.67	All surgical cases
	1.2	Neurosurgical cases
Germany	3.0	Neurosurgical cases

References

1. CHODAK, G.W., PLAUT, M.E.: Use of systemic antibiotics for prophylaxis in surgery. Arch. Surg. 112, 326-334 (1977)
2. GUIDELINES for Peer Review: Veterans Administration Ad Hoc Interdisciplinary Advisory Committee on Antimicrobial Drug Use. 1. Prophylaxis in surgery J.A.M.A. 237, 1001-1008 (1977)
3. MALIS, L.I.: Personal Communication
4. NEW, H.C., HOWREY, S.P.: Testing the physician's knowledge of antibiotic use. N. Engl. J. Med. 293, 1291-1295 (1975)
5. NICHOLS, R.L.: Personal Communication
6. SAVITZ, M.H.: The use of prophylactic antibiotics in neurosurgery. In: Current controversies in neurosurgery. MARLEY, T.P. (ed.), pp. 648-50. Saunders 1976

7. SAVITZ, M.H., MALIS, L.I.: Prophylactic clinidamycin for neurosurgical patients. N.Y. State J. Med. 76, 64-67 (1976)

8. SAVITZ, M.H., MALIS, L.I., MEYERS, B.R.: Prophylactic antibiotics in neurosurgery. Surg. Neurol. 2, 95-100 (1974)

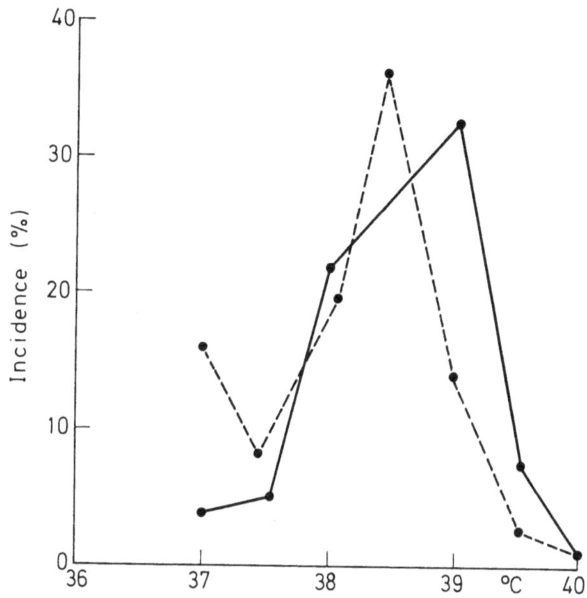

Fig. 1. Maximum temperature after laminectomy. —— without antibiotics (96); --- with antibiotics (96)

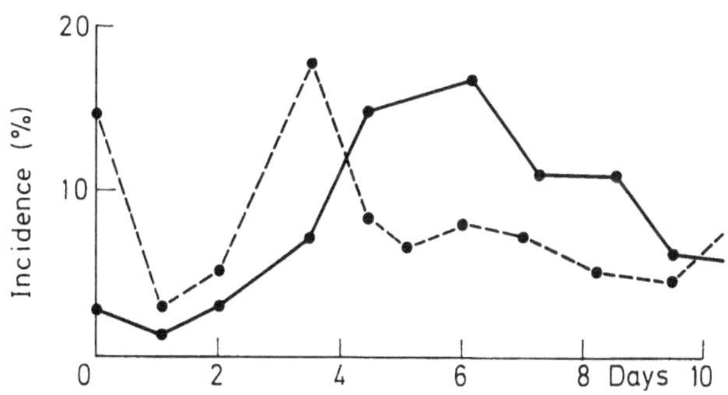

Fig. 2. Duration of postoperative fever. —— without antibiotics, --- with antibiotics

Interferon Productivity of Human Lymphocytes with the Induction of Poly I:C in Cases of Malignant Glioma

K. SANO, N. SHITARA, and K. TAKAKURA

Interferon was originally discovered as a factor or factors that can inhibit virus infection, independently of the immune system, first by NAGANO and KOJIMA (3), then by ISSACS and LINDENMANN (1,2). The latter authors named this factor "interferon".

It was soon found that interferon (IF) belongs to the defense mechanism of the body phylogenetically older than the immune system and that all cells are supposed to have the ability to produce this substance. It has also been shown that IF has not only an antiviral effect but also an anticancer effect by preventing nucleic acid aberrations as related to carcinogenesis or viral infection inside the victim cells. This paper deals with studies on IF productivity of human lymphocytes with the induction of poly I:C (polyriboinosinic acid · polyribocytidylic acid) in glioma cases and will discuss a possible therapeutic application of this sustance.

Method

The mononuclear cells of enriched lymphocytes were harvested with Ficoll-isopaque gradient, and the cells ($1 \cdot 10^6$/ml) were cultured in serum-free RPMI 1640 containing 5 μg/ml of poly I:C (Yamasa Lot No. 9) and 20 μg/ml of DEAE-dextran, for 1 h at 37° C. After washing out polyI·C, the cells were refed into the RPMI medium containing 10% calf serum for 23 h. The value (I.U.) of IF produced by the above cells 24 h after the initial 1 h exposure to poly I:C was measured by the 50% plaque reduction technique.

Results

The value of IF produced by lymphocytes with the induction of poly I:C in 11 patients with gliomas was 177 ± 162 (mean ± SD) I.U./ml, whereas that in 11 patients without neoplasms was 425 ± 299 I.U./ml (Fig. 1). Thus, IF productivity of lymphocytes in glioma cases was significantly lower ($P < 0.05$) than that in nontumor patients.

Among glioma cases, the IF productivity of lymphocytes was definitely low ($P < 0.001$) in glioblastoma cases (the value being 27.5 ± 5.59 I.U./ml) as compared with that in rather benign glioma (astrocytoma grade I, II, oligodendroglioma) cases (the value being 358 ± 177.8 I.I./ml) as seen in Fig. 2. One-third of these glioblastoma cases showed still positive purified protein derivative (PPD) and one-fifth of benign glioma cases showed negative PPD.

Animal Experiments

Experiment I. Similar results were obtained in rats implanted with C6 glioma (N-nitrosomethylurea induced cell line) and in rats harboring no tumor. The former rats receiving an intramuscular injection of 10 mg/kg poly I:C showed a plasma value (per milliliter) of 1790 ± 340 I.U., while the rats with no tumor receiving the same injection showed a plasma value of 4360 ± 609 I.U. ($P < 0.01$) as shown in Fig. 3. The IF induction with lower concentration of poly I:C (2.5 mg/kg) did not show a significant difference in this value.

Injection of poly I:C (2.5 mg/kg), however, produced more than 100 I.U./ml plasma value of IF in both groups of rats. This value is effective for preventing tumor growth as will be shown later. The experiment suggests the clinical use of poly I:C injection in human brain tumor cases.

Experiment II. Plasma levels of IF in rats receiving an intravenous injection of homogeneous spleen cells ($8 \cdot 10^7$/250 g) that were treated with 5 μg/ml of poly I:C in the same medium as described in human cases were 170 - 175 I.U./ml (at 4 h after injection). Plasma levels of IF in control rats (without polyI·C) showed 0 I.U.

Cytostatic Effect of Human Interferon

A cultured human melanoma cell line (Seki II) was exposed to 100-1000 I.U./ml of IF induced from human lymphocytes. As shown in Fig. 4, a remarkable cytostatic effect of IF was observed with these concentrations. Probably, an IF concentration of more than 100 I.U. will be effective as a cytostatic agent.

Cell cycle phase analysis of these melanoma cells using the pulse cytophotometer revealed that the S-phase cells were accumulated when exposed to IF and that this accumulation was parallel to the concentration of IF and the exposure time.

Discussion

From the above data, it can be stated that patients harboring malignant glioma showed a very low value of IF productivity of lymphocytes with the induction of poly I:C. Similar result was found in experiment I in rats. This fact may suggest that the low IF productivity of glioblastoma cases is not due to administered chemotherapeutic agents but rather that the nonspecific defense mechanism of those cases is weakened, nearly independently of the condition of their immune mechanism. Injection of poly I:C, even in lower concentrations (2.5 mg/kg), however, was shown to produce a plasma level of IF that is effective in preventing tumor growth. This may suggest the clinical application of polyI·C in human brain tumors.

Experiment II suggests the possibility that the transfusion of human lymphocytes treated with poly I:C may be used for the treatment of patients with malignant brain neoplasms. The cytostatic effect of human IF (at more than 100 I.U./ml) was confirmed by the last experiment on cultured melanoma cells. The mechanism of the cytostatic effect of IF has not been clearly elucidated yet. It is propounded, however, that IF acts by preventing nucleic acid aberrations related to carcinogenesis inside the victim cells. From the data of the pulse cytophotometer, it may be presumed that IF may block the S phase of the tumor cell cycle or of the aberrant cell cycle inside the tumor cells.

Conclusion

1) The IF productivity of lymphocytes induced with poly I:C was significantly lower in cases of glioblastoma than in benign glioma cases and nontumor cases.
2) Rats implanted with C6 glioma showed significantly lower plasma levels of IF when injected with 10 mg/kg of poly I:C as compared with the control rats. The injection of poly I:C, however, produced more than 100 I.U./ml plasma value of IF even with a lower concentration (2.5 mg/kg), both in the control rats and in rats with a C6 glioma.
3) The injection of homogeneous spleen cells ($8 \cdot 10^7$/250 g) treated with 5 µg/ml of poly I:C was able to produce a significant plasma level of IF in rats.
4) The cytostatic effect of human IF at a concentration of more than 100 I.U./ml was confirmed on human melanoma cell line (Seki II).
5) Cell cycle phase analysis of these melanoma cells using pulse cytophotometer revealed the accumulation of S-phase cells. This may suggest that IF may block the S phase of the tumor cell cycle.

References

1. ISSACS, A., LINDENMANN, J.: Virus inference. I. The interferon. II. Some properties of interferon. Proc. Roy. Soc. Ser. B. 147-267 (1957)
2. ISSACS, A., LINDENMANN, J.: Virus interference. The interferon. II. Some properties of interferon. Proc. Roy. Soc. Ser. B. 268-273 (1957)
3. NAGANO, Y., KOJIMA, Y.: Pouvoir immunisant du virus vaccinal inactivé par des rayons ultraviolets. Compt. Rend. Soc. Biol. 148, 1700-1702 (1954)

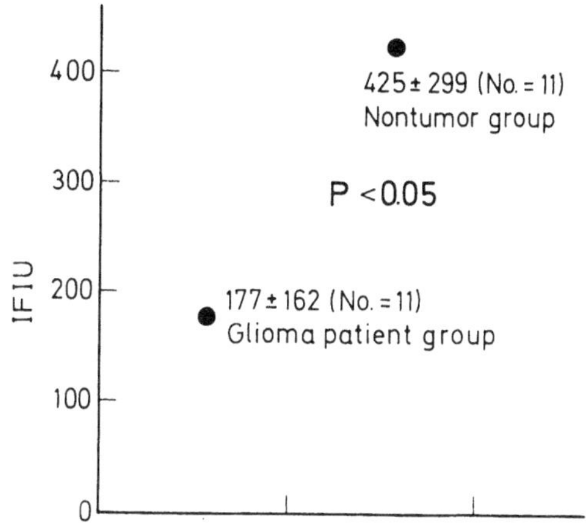

Fig. 1. Interferon productivity of human lymphocytes with poly I:C

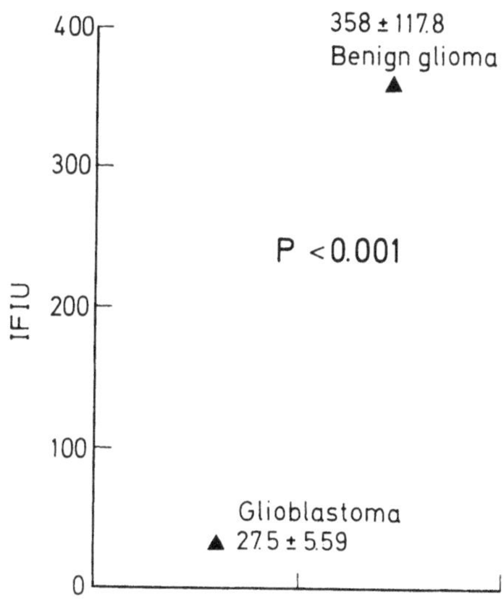

Fig. 2. Interferon productivity of human lymphocytes with poly I:C

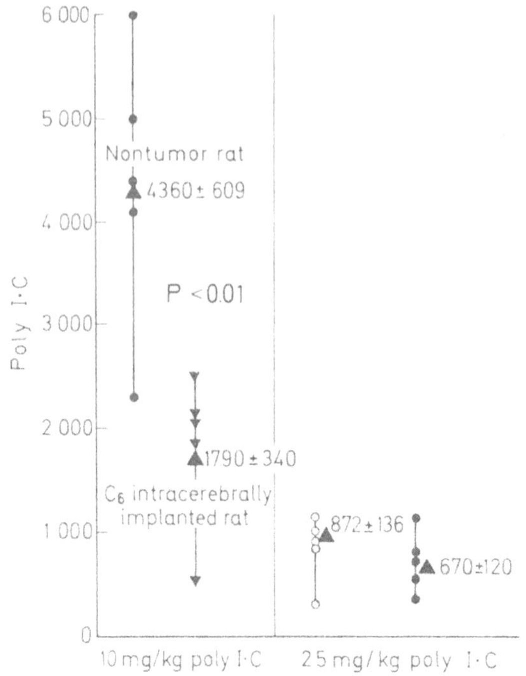

Fig. 3. Plasma levels of interferon in nontumor rats and in rats with tumor induced by polyI·C

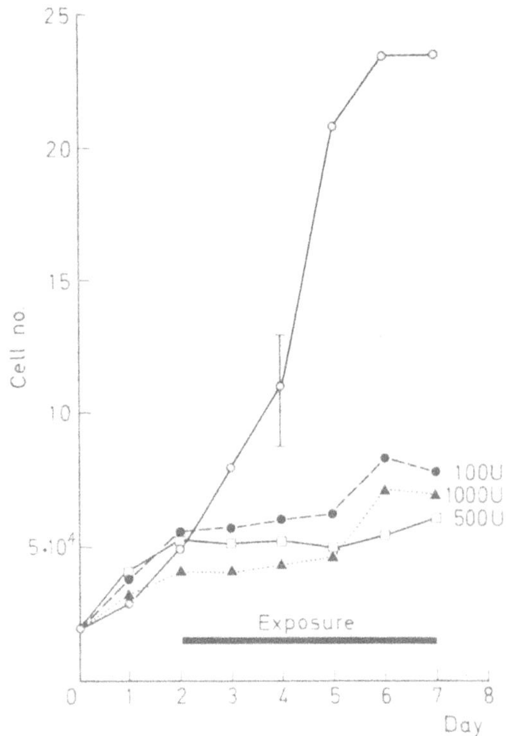

Fig. 4. Cytostatic effect of interferon

How to Handle Brain Tumor Classifications

O. STOCHDORPH

Classification of brain tumors has manifold purposes. It brings a body of observations into a manageable order, it facilitates comparison between observations from different observers, and it may provide clues for prognostic evaluation.

There are very many possible bases for classification, e.g., age and sex of the patient or even his initials, site, clinical behavior, macroscopy, and histology. The fundamental principle evolved from histology is classification according to histogenesis, i.e., identification of the tissue of origin. One should not equate histogenesis with cytogenesis in the sense of defining a presumed cell of origin for a given tumor cell population. It is true, of course, that "omnis cellula e cellula eiusdem generis nascitur".

However, this is not equivalent with "e cellula eiusdem speciei".

Certainly, with an experimental tumor, we may kill an experimental animal by inoculation of a single tumor cell, e.g., by diluting a Yoshida sarcoma in its ascitic form to a degree where a minute quantity of injected fluid contains only a single tumor cell. Most primary tumors, however, and this is especially true for brain tumors, are derived not from a single cell, but from a number of cells distributed over fields of origin. Furthermore, we have to take into consideration the scope of possible differentiation of growing cells into several directions. If, for example, we find within an osteogenic sarcoma osteoid, chondroid, myxoid, and fibrous areas, we call such a tumor an osteochondromyxofibrosarcoma. However, nobody presumes in such a case that an osteoblast and a chondroblast and a myxoid cell and a fibroblast have conspired and united to build up a tumor. We are quite certain that within the proliferating osteogenic matrix there is differentiation along several lines. In a similar way, brain tumor tissue containing astrocytic, oligodendrocytic, and in-between cell types has not evolved out of one astrocyte, one oligodendrocyte, etc. but is the result of proliferation and concomitant differentiation of cells of stem cell quality. In brain tissue, the glial stem cell is probably of an oligodendrocytic aspect.

In brain tumor histology, the number of possible patterns is nearly infinite. This is why any classification has its shortcomings. However, there are a few typical pitfalls. Any organ tissue is a composite structure made up of parenchymal and stromal elements. Meninges, for example, are such an organ tissue. One should not call each and every tumor arising within the meningeal tissue a menigioma. There are among the meningeal tumors quite a number of tumors derived from tissue structures also found elsewhere, e.g., hemangiopericytomas, and calling these tumors meningiomas would amount to trading histogenesis for mere topography.

With any classification problem, we meet the opposing factions of "lumpers" and "splitters".

Brain tumors are no exception in this respect. Both sides have their strong and their weak points. In one regard, the lumpers are at an advantage. There are, apart from the ependyma as the lining of the ventricular cavities, only two glial cell types commonly known and taken for granted, viz., the astrocyte and the oligodendrocyte. The specialized neuroanatomist is familiar with glial cell types that have not yet gained access to the brain tumor classifications in use. The tanycyte (from the Greek root *tany* for "slender"), for example, is found in the circumventricular organs and bears a striking resemblance to the so-called pilod astrocyte, which is said to build up the pilocytic astrocytome of the cerebellum, etc. However, this cell is not well enough known to be admitted to brain tumor nomenclature.

The splitters, on the other hand, have a very strong hand in the older literatur. BAILEY and CUSHING (2) have split up the central group of glial tumors into four apparently separate entities (Table 1). In 1949, histologic grading as introduced by BRODERS (3) was adapted to brain tumors by KERNOHAN et al. (5) (Table 2). What was said earlier about intermutability of type among proliferating glial cells is an argument against any strict separation of this type. HENSCHEN (4) has pointed out that "splitting" of tumor patterns according to the prevailing type of differentiation has its undenied value with tumors of low-grade malignancy. Higher grades of any pattern, however, merge into the so-called glioblastoma multiforme pattern (Table 3).

Table 1. Patterns of brain tumor classification (I) (2)

Fibrillary Astrocytoma protoplasmic	Oligodendro- glioma pleomorphic	Ependymoma
Glioblastoma Multiforme		

Table 2. Patterns of brain tumor classification (II) (5)

Astro- cytoma	Oligo- dendro- glioma	Ependymoma
I II III IV	I II III IV	I II III IV

Table 3. Patterns of brain tumor classification (III) (4)

Astrocytoma	Oligodendro- glioma	Ependymoma
Glioblastoma		

One should avoid what may be called cross-contamination of nomenclature. If we come to recognize certain brain tumor patterns in computerized tomography, we should not use the term grade 2 or a similar term borrowed from histology.

Another deplorable contamination has been introduced by ZÜLCH (6) into the forthcoming WHO brain tumor classification. He uses the term "grade" for a comparison of the prognostic value of different tumor types. As has been the experience with other tumor categories, grading is a very useful tool for subdividing such tumors as, for example, with astrocytes as predominant type of differentiation, according to a lower or higher degree of dedifferentiation. The term becomes devoid of meaning when applied for example to medulloblastomas, which do not show, from case to case, any appreciable difference in dedifferentiation. We cannot call a medulloblastoma a grade 4 tumor since there is no such thing as a grade 1 medulloblastoma.

In general, we should abstain from too rigid subclassifications based upon an "either-or" principle. The basic type of the brain tissue's own tumors is a glioma. ACKERMAN and ROSAI (1) point out that in some brain tumors of presumably astrocytic lineage "the dedifferentiation is so great that an astrocytic origin cannot be established". They draw the following conclusion (Table 4):

Table 4. Patterns of brain tumor classification (IV) (1)

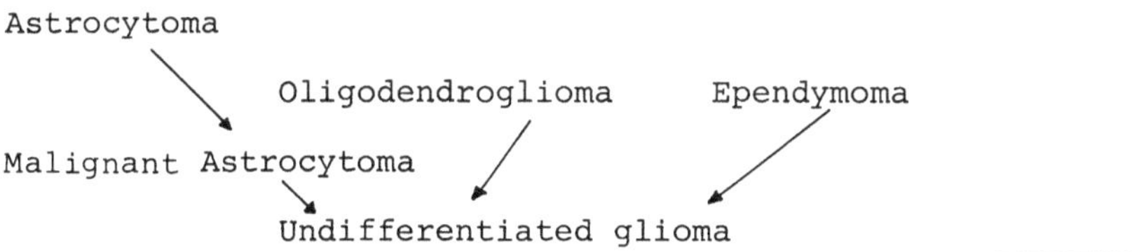

The designation of glioblastoma multiforme has traditionally been given to this variety. This term is unsatisfactory for several reasons. First, it implies an origin from (or at least a relationship with) the embryonal glioblast which probably does not exist. All the available evidence seems to indicate that this tumor is instead the result of progressive dedifferentiation in a neoplasm that originated in an adult cell. Second, it conveys the impression of a specific tumor type when it simply represents the undifferentiated form of all types of gliomas. Admittedly, the large majority of tumors called glioblastoma multiforme are of astrocytic origin, as demonstrated by special stains, tissue culture, and electron microscopy, but oligodendrogliomas and ependymomas may result in an identical microscopic appearance. Therefore it seems more logical to simply call these tumors undifferentiated gliomas.

No terminology - and therefore no classification either - is entirely free of preconceived notions. A basic hazard of any attempt to introduce a standardized classification without suitable consideration of all pertinent aspects is canonization and therefore petrification of obsolete, for example, embryogenetic concepts. At the present time, "lumping" seems more appropriate in brain tumor classification than "splitting".

References

1. ACKERMAN, L.V., ROSAI, J.: Surgical pathology, 5th ed. pp. 1248-1249. St. Louis: Mosby 1974
2. BAILEY, P., CUSHING, H.: A classification of tumors of the glioma group on a histogenetic basis with a correlated study of prognosis. Philadelphia: Lippincott 1926
3. BRODERS, A.C.: Carcinoma: grading and practical application. Arch. Pathol. 2, 376-380 (1926)
4. HENSCHEN, F.: Tumoren des Zentralnervensystems und seiner Hüllen. In: Handbuch spezieller pathologischer Anatomie, Vol. XIII/3, pp. 413-1040. Berlin, Göttingen, Heidelberg: Springer 1955
5. KERNOHAN, J.W., MABON, R.F., SVIEN, H.J., ADSON, A.W.: A simplified classification of the gliomas. Proc. Staff Meet. Mayo Clin. 24, 71-75 (1949)
6. ZÜLCH, K.J.: Atlas of the histology of brain tumors. Berlin, Heidelberg, New York: Springer 1971

Subject Index

Advances in Neurosurgery

Volume 6

Treatment of Hydrocephalus Computer Tomography

Editors: R. Wüllenweber, H. Wenker, M. Brock, M. Klinger

1978. 111 figures, 86 tables. XXXI, 230 pages
ISBN 3-540-09031-2
Distribution rights for Japan:
Nankodo Co. Ltd., Tokyo

Contents: Treatment of Hydrocephalus. – Computer Tomography. – Free Topics. – Subject Index.

Volume 6 of **Advances in Neurosurgery** is devoted to two important topics in neurosurgery today. The first part of the book looks at hydrocephalus. The papers focus on research results and early and late sequelae of therapy. Methods of treatment play a lesser role. Collective reports from several clinics and a comparison of the results achieved by Dutch and British neurosurgeons make this an unusually comprehensive treatment of the subject.

The second part studies the importance of computerized tomography to neurosurgical diagnosis. Again detailed comparative reports are the basis for this section. Sources of error to be looked for in using this technique are discussed at length.

The third section of this volume offers papers on numerous clinical and experimental topics of current interest from the entire field of neurosurgery.

Springer-Verlag
Berlin
Heidelberg
New York

www.ingramcontent.com/pod-product-compliance
Lightning Source LLC
Chambersburg PA
CBHW061154240926
51846CB00006B/1012
* 9 7 8 3 6 4 2 6 7 4 5 7 0 *